INJECTION!

by Carol Givner
Editor: Gary S. Goldman, Ph.D.

A fictional account based on a
Researcher's 8-year experience on a project funded by the
Centers for Disease Control and Prevention (CDC)

P.O. Box 847
Pearblossom CA 93553

Library of Congress Control Number: 2006931730

ISBN-10: 0-9788383-0-0 (paperback)
ISBN-13: 978-0-9788383-0-0

Printed in the U.S.A. by Medical Veritas International Inc.
Phone: 1-800-309-3569
Website: http://www.injectionbook.com/

Disclaimer

Acknowledgement

Gary S. Goldman, Ph.D. wishes to express thanks to Paul H. Connett, Ph.D., Boyd E. Haley, Ph.D., Harold E. Buttram, M.D., Mark R. Geier, M.D., David A. Geier, Teri Small, Marc Girard, M.D., and Pearblossom Private School, Inc. for granting permission to re-publish and include their authoritative material in the appendices of this book. A special thanks to F. Edward Yazbak, M.D. for his technical assistance with the narrative.

Also, a gracious thank you to the courageous parents, scientists, and researchers who have actively sought reforms in vaccine safety, who have carefully documented adverse vaccine reactions, who have published data demonstrating deleterious results despite (1) attempts at censorship, or (2) being targeted to be discredited through use of political maneuvers that are tied to power and profit motives rather than interests of public health

Prologue

While this book is written in a fictional setting, the core of the material has a scientific basis. *INJECTION!* presents a potentially unique and often candid look at aspects of the pharmaceutical and medical industries with the goal of revealing major disease trends that are already endangering the health of millions of unwary people. The text investigates how certain medical interventions affect the population at large. More specifically, the narrative addresses issues pertaining to birthing, specific vaccines, adverse vaccine reactions, fluoridated water and more.

The fictitious town of Sycamore Springs, while somewhat rural, is not unlike most urban U.S. cities—including the city in which you, the reader, reside. The water supply is fluoridated (see Appendix I. Fifty Reasons to Oppose Fluoridation) and public health officials strive to achieve their goal of administering all vaccines to all children in a timely fashion according to the childhood immunization schedule. The town physicians all believe that the Universal Varicella (Chickenpox) Vaccination Program is completely safe and will lead to better health of not only children, but all individuals in the community.

The fictional account that you are reading is based on a researcher's true-life experience. In 1994/1995, the Centers for Disease Control and Prevention (CDC) initially funded a Varicella Active Surveillance Project (VASP) to study chickenpox and the effects that the chickenpox vaccine had on each of three U.S. communities: Antelope Valley, California; West Philadelphia, Pennsylvania; and Travis County, Texas. The VASP gathered reports of chickenpox cases from sources such as public and private elementary, middle, and high schools, daycares, private physicians, health maintenance organization's (HMOs) offices, hospitals, and other locations so that important trends could be discerned following licensure of the Varivax® vaccine (manufactured by Merck & Co., Inc.) by the U.S. Food and Drug Administration (FDA) on March 17, 1995. Gary S. Goldman, Ph.D., serving as the sole Research Analyst on one of these projects, initially reported dramatic declines in chickenpox cases and other findings associated with increasing administration of the chickenpox vaccine during the first five years following licensure. These data and positive results were welcome and included in manuscripts prepared by the CDC and the local health department for publication in peer-reviewed medical journals. Goldman was listed as a co-author and was encouraged to contribute additional findings that could lead to publication. In 2000, he discovered a preliminary deleterious trend. When Goldman reported this deleterious effect and submitted draft manuscripts for review, these were treated much differently. At first, he stood alone with his preliminary findings. Later, additional studies would corroborate his hypotheses, translating into increased pain and suffering among millions of individuals throughout the United States.

Seeking to independently publish his research findings in a peer-reviewed medical journal, Goldman first made inquiry at the VASP as to whether the project co-principal investigators as well as those at the CDC desired co-authorship credit. Some months later, after having received no response from his colleagues, Goldman received a letter from the county legal department ordering him to "cease and desist from publishing in a medical journal." Goldman first tried reasoning with the health department attorneys, suggesting that the experienced medical journal editors and assigned peer-reviewers decide whether or not the submitted studies were scientifically sound and sufficiently robust to warrant publication. One attorney replied, "You don't understand, Goldman… they [co-principal investigators of VASP] do not want the studies published." Goldman had his attorney intervene and the issue seemed to be resolved. Goldman's attorney had reasoned, in part, that since the research was funded by the CDC, all results should be available to citizens via the Freedom of Information Act. Three of Goldman's manuscripts were subsequently accepted and published on 18 consecutive pages in the peer-reviewed journal *Vaccine*. This would not be the last time attempts would be made to suppress Goldman's research and manuscripts.

In Sycamore Springs, as in other cities, many children will fail to be properly diagnosed. Instead, they will demonstrate behavioral difficulties and some will be labeled as troublemakers. This leads to discipline problems in schools, reducing the time that teachers have available to teach. Schools must expand their "opportunity" and other special education classes, leaving few funds to support standard educational programs.

Leading officials from the Centers for Disease Control and Prevention (CDC) have stated in their presentations that the varicella vaccine has maintained a protective effect for 20 years in Japan. "Reliable" sources have also cited several studies that show there have been no *statistically* significant increase in shingles incidence in the years following licensure of the varicella vaccine.

As the story unfolds, you will learn how chickenpox and shingles are related and the important role played by annual epidemics or outbreaks of chickenpox in the community. Using studies with flawed methods and improper statistical techniques, public health authorities produce what appears to be supportive documentation for the Universal Varicella Vaccination Program. This keeps confidence high among physicians and patients to encourage the maintenance of high vaccination rates.

If you had been the researcher and had recognized that several key assumptions underlying the Universal Varicella Vaccination Program were invalid, and that eliminating chickenpox would cause an epidemic of a far worse disease, would you have stopped it? Would you have allowed the program to continue, knowing that to ameliorate the deleterious effects experienced by adults, a second vaccine would be needed (along with subsequent booster doses) to offset the effects caused by the first vaccine? Would you have allowed the delicate balance of childhood disease and the natural protection it afforded to be disrupted in the first place, possibly never able to return to the balance that existed in "mother nature" prior to the initiation of the chickenpox vaccination campaign? Or would you have sat back, enjoyed your paycheck, and done nothing to the experimental program that was already in full swing, just watching the epidemic of suffering and death it would bring to the generation of adults who never received the chickenpox vaccine?

Gary S. Goldman, Ph.D. resigned after nearly 8-years on the Varicella Active Surveillance Project (VASP) in October of 2002 on ethical grounds because as he stated,

"Whenever research data and information concerning potential adverse effects associated with a vaccine used in human populations are suppressed and/or misrepresented by health authorities, not only is this most disturbing, this goes against all accepted scientific norms. It also dangerously compromises scientists' professional ethics."

INJECTION! presents information that some have tried to suppress and that others would like to cover up. By 2018, you, the reader may likely be affected even though you did not expressly consent. Unknowingly you became a participant in a vaccine experiment for which the long-term consequences were dismissed in exchange for short term profits. Oh, you think, "No one has vaccinated me recently, so this scenario is not plausible and is simply an attempt to create undue fear." To that, the researcher, along with other experts corroborating his hypothesis, would respond: "Paradoxically, over the next 50 years, millions of adults in the U.S. population that did not receive the varicella vaccination will be most affected by the administration of varicella (chickenpox) vaccine to virtually all healthy children starting in 1995."

Without the publication of this book, by the time 2018 rolls around, you might have thought to yourself or outright expressed to others: "Why are so many of us becoming ill? Why are we experiencing such excruciating pain?" You might have blamed the adversities on stress, on poor eating, or perhaps on unhealthy lifestyles. These factors certainly play a contributing role. But, you would never in your right mind have suspected that the majority of suffering and in some cases the fatal outcomes were at the instigation of "health" initiatives by authorities and institutions you had trusted implicitly.

Rising healthcare costs, and numerous other implications, are not unique to Sycamore Springs. They will likely affect all U.S. communities. The problem started when objective research was ignored by the healthcare authorities in office in 2001.

By 2018, many individuals and families will be stressed in order to afford medical insurance coverage. Healthcare premiums will have to rise considerably to compensate for the increases in average annual medical costs. The book's fictional character, Dr. Leviticus, will have seen numerous epidemiological reports corroborating or substantiating the preliminary data reported by "Craig" the researcher documenting the increased incidence of shingles during the early stages of the universal varicella vaccination program.

It is entirely possible that in the real life scenario, these reports will be downplayed to the public, but the HMOs and hospitals will quickly notice the overflow of shingles patients and their related medical expenses. Certainly both the physicians and pharmaceutical firms will be in a quandary as to how to proceed. When the true source of the increasing disease burden is uncovered by the public, the possibility of a class action lawsuit will be real. In all probability, health officials and politicians will recommend laws preventing individuals from seeking compensation for the increased risks of shingles due to implementation of the universal varicella vaccination program. Also, the divorce rate will climb as the stress of raising vaccine-injured children burdens households both emotionally and financially.

Might Dr. Leviticus, with his hero complex, reap the consequences of committing an injustice by injecting the measured 0.5 ml (milliliter) liquid containing live varicella virus into his patients? The Bible book bearing his name, Leviticus 19:35-36, warns, "YOU must not commit injustice in judging, in measuring, in weighing or in measuring liquids."

The motivation in writing this book is neither to gain prestige nor profit. Rather, the researcher felt a moral obligation to warn his family, friends, community, and the world at large that we all must take a more active role in decisions relating to our health and that of our children. It is a call that ordinary citizens should not give carte blanche support and put misguided trust in healthcare authorities and their suggestions, which may be mandated by the state. It also is intended to sound an alert to healthcare and political officials of the consequences of the vaccination policies and programs they have intentionally or unwittingly set in motion and the responsibility they ultimately bear for increased suffering and death. Lastly, it is also a call for research reform: to have independent investigators corroborate research data and results, immune from the influence of sponsoring agencies and health departments with their vaccine profit motives, and other conflicts of interests that ultimately stem from pharmaceutical enrichment.

INJECTION! does not promote anti-vaccine views. Just because a child is unvaccinated, however, does not mean that the child is unprotected—he or she still has their natural immunity. This book's narrative, supported by published peer-reviewed research and literature provided in the book's appendices, contains practical, cautionary, and balanced admonition that each new vaccine should be thoroughly tested as to its safety. The appendices (see Table of Appendices on the following page), authored by leading scientists, researchers, and medical doctors, highlight relevant information supporting the medical issues discussed and will help you to be more fully informed on important health topics.

Whether or not the possible future that *INJECTION!* presents becomes reality will largely depend on what you as the reader learn and do based on your informed conscience.

A brief "Primer" on Chickenpox and Shingles

Here are brief sketches of chickenpox and shingles, because understanding the close linkages between these two will be critical to your grasp of the vital issues this book deals with.

Varicella (chickenpox) and herpes zoster (shingles) both derive from the varicella-zoster virus (VZV). Varicella is typically a benign disease characterized by a rash that appears in crops, progressing from macules to papules, vesicles, pustules, and eventually to crusted lesions—all of which may be present during the peak of the clinical phase. Lesions are often concentrated on the trunk, scalp and face and symptoms resolve in 7-10 days. Chickenpox is highly contagious and occurs most often among 3- to 8-year-old children. It's transmitted through the respiratory system when a person who's susceptible to the disease comes in close proximity to an infected person who coughs, sneezes, or even breathes. The average incubation period is14 days, however a chickenpox case can occur between the 10th and 21st day after exposure. Varicella is most contagious one to two days prior to rash onset, so quite often a person does not know precisely who transmitted the infection to whom. Ordinarily, the only treatment for uncomplicated chickenpox in healthy children is application of "anti-itch" lotions that help keep children from scratching the rash too avidly. (Scratching can introduce a bacterial infection, causing physicians to prescribe antibiotics.) Occasionally, in more severe cases, doctors prescribe antiviral drugs such as acyclovir (Zovirax®) or famciclovir (Famvir®).

Following primary infection with varicella, the VZV goes dormant in the body's cranial nerve and dorsal-root ganglia. When VZV immunity declines below a certain threshold level, the virus can reactivate in the secondary infection, shingles. Individuals have a 20% chance of developing shingles during their lifetime. Unlike chickenpox, the shingles rash is often confined to distribution along one or several adjacent dermatomes on one side of the body. A dermatome is an area of the skin supplied by sensory fibers from a specific spinal nerve. An illustration of the various dermatomes is provided on page x. Post-herpetic neuralgia (PHN), or persistent pain following the shingles rash, occurs in 20% of patients.

A person who has never had chickenpox cannot have shingles. However, a person who has never had chickenpox can become infected with chickenpox by exposure to a person with either chickenpox or shingles.

Based on five years of data collected prior to licensure of the chickenpox vaccine in 1995, there was a mean of 4 million cases, 11,000 hospitalizations, and approximately 100 deaths (50 children/50 adults) attributed to chickenpox annually. Approximately 1 million cases of shingles occur annually, representing about 75% of medical costs due to VZV. Thus, morbidity and mortality due to shingles far exceeds that due to varicella. Although shingles can occur at any age in individuals with a previous history of varicella or in those who have received the varicella vaccine, the majority of shingles cases occur among adults aged 50 years and older.

Those at highest risk for complications of chickenpox and shingles include the elderly, patients with compromised immune systems (e.g., AIDS, and leukemia) or serious illness (e.g., Hodgkin's disease, bone marrow transplants), and pregnant women. Chickenpox in newborns is a life-threatening condition. Although chickenpox can still be very dangerous in older infants, most are protected by antibodies in breast milk from mothers who have had chickenpox. Children under age one who develop chickenpox are at higher risk for childhood shingles.

The varicella-zoster virus belongs to a group of herpes viruses that are similar in shape and size and reproduce within the structure of a cell. The eight herpes viruses include Herpes Simplex virus (HSV-1—causes cold sores involving the lip and cankor sores in the mouth; HSV-2—is sexually transmitted and causes genital herpes), Varicella-Zoster virus (VZV) which causes chickenpox and shingles and is found among 95% of adults, Cytomegalovirus (CMV) which infects 50% of children with no symptoms, Epstein-Barre virus (EBV) which causes infectious mononucleosis, Human Herpesvirus type 6 (HHV-6) which causes roseola (a skin rash with associated fever), Human Herpesvirus type 7 (HHV-7) which infects all children by age 3 years and persists lifelong, and Human Herpesvirus type 8 (HHV-8), also known as Kaposi's sarcoma herpes virus (KSHV), which is found in the saliva of many AIDS patients. The last three herpes viruses were discovered only recently in the 1980s.

Sometimes shingles is difficult to diagnose, because even without a visible rash present, a person with shingles can experience pain so severe, it's at first mistaken for gallstones or kidney stones, appendicitis, pleurisy, or even heart attack, depending on which nerve(s) it affects. Often, even before shingles erupts with its classic rash (usually on only one side of the body), a sufferer's skin is painfully sensitive to clothing or to touch.

Here are some additional complications that may arise from shingles.

Postherpetic Neuralgia (PHN)

Postherpetic neuralgia, or PHN, has been defined as persistent pain in the area of the rash after the rash has healed. PHN develops in as many as 60% to 70% of patients with shingles older than age 60 and is the most common complication of herpes zoster. PHN may also occur after an interval of no pain and may last for months and sometimes years. The pain from PHN can be debilitating and if it persists for years, it may lead to physical, occupational, and social disability, along with distress and depression. PHN has been described as a constant burning, aching, boring, or tearing sensation; or as shooting or stabbing pain. Allodynia occurs in approximately 90% of patients with PHN and is triggered by clothes touching the skin or other light stimuli such as a slight breeze.

Postherpetic Itch (PHI)

A particularly interesting case of shingles arose in a 39-year-old woman who experienced what is now referred to as postherpetic itch, or PHI. Instead of experiencing pain following the rash, known as postherpetic neuralgia (PHN), the woman developed severe itch on her forehead where a shingles rash had appeared. The itch persisted and within one year, she had scratched through her skull to her brain. She was treated for herniation of the brain and an intra-cranial infection, subsequently followed by skin grafts placed over her brain. Her intractable scratching damaged these grafts and only through use of hand restraints and a helmet was she prevented from further self-injury. It has been suggested that shingles particularly on the head or neck, in rare cases, causes chronic focal itch due to neural damage with loss of protective pain sensation. This condition is often resistant to treatments and can be disabling.[1]

Ramsay Hunt Syndrome

This syndrome is associated with shingles on the face, scalp, or neck in combination with facial palsy. There is often involvement of shingles on the external ear, or *herpes zoster oticus*, or the soft or hard palate, around the mouth. Complications such as hearing loss (ranging from partial to total) and vertigo (dizziness ranging in duration from days to weeks) are common due to involvement of the eighth cranial nerve. Other symptoms may include severe ear pain, ringing in the ear, loss of taste, nausea and vomiting. While these symptoms, including facial paralysis, usually resolve without problems, in some cases, the facial paralysis may be permanent.

Bell's Palsy

Bell's palsy is diagnosed when shingles causes paralysis to usually one side of the face. Individuals with Bell's Palsy at first believe they have suffered a stroke, however, the fact that only muscle weakness on one side of the face has occurred without loss of mental function confirms the Bell's Palsy diagnosis. Initially, Bell's Palsy and Ramsay Hunt Syndrome may be indistinguishable.

Meningitis and Encephalitis

Inflammation of the membrane around the brain, or meningitis, and inflammation in the brain itself, or encephalitis, are rare complications in individuals with shingles. The encephalitis is generally mild and resolves in a short period. In rare cases, particularly in patients with impaired immune systems, it can be severe and even life-threatening. Both meningitis and encephalitis due to the varicella zoster-virus (VZV) have been shown to occur even when a shingles rash is not present.

Eye Involvement

Shingles with involvement of the eyes is called *herpes zoster ophthalmicus*. It occurs when the virus affects the ophthalmic division of the trigeminal nerve. This condition is difficult to treat and in 65% of cases can threaten vision if it spreads to the cornea of the eye, or *herpes zoster keratitis*, a potential cause of blindness if not recognized and treated promptly (within 72 hours of rash onset). Patients with eye involvement should seek examination by an

[1] Oaklander AL, Cohen SP, Raju SV. Intractable postherpetic itch and cutaneous deafferentation after facial shingles. Pain 2002 Mar;96(1-2):9-12.

ophthalmologist, especially when shingles involve the tip, side or base of the nose (Hutchinson's sign).[2]

Shingles can also cause a devastating infection in the retina, or *imminent acute retinal necrosis (ARN) syndrome*. Interestingly, this complication can develop weeks or months following the resolution of a shingles rash that occurs anywhere on the body, not just the face.

A condition uveitis, or inflammation and scaring of the iris, can last from several weeks to years and is often associated with elevated intraocular pressure.

In rare cases, shingles affecting the third cranial nerve causes ophthalmoplegia, a partial or in some cases, a complete paralysis of the muscles controlling the eyes and eyelids.[3]

Jaw Involvement

Shingles affecting the maxillary and mandibular divisions of the trigeminal nerve can cause *osteonecrosis* and spontaneous tooth exfoliation.[4]

Leg, Bladder, and Bowel Involvement

Lumbosacral zoster can be accompanied by leg weakness as well as bladder and bowel dysfunction. In rare cases, herpes zoster infects the urinary tract and causes difficulty in urination and bladder retention. This condition is usually temporary but may require a catheter to eliminate urine in some patients who have prolonged difficulty in urinating.[5]

Disseminated Herpes Zoster

As with disseminated chickenpox, disseminated herpes zoster, which spreads to other organs, can be serious to life-threatening, particularly if it affects the lungs. While this condition is very rare in those with healthy immune systems, patients with compromised immune systems are at greatest danger, with risk ranging from 5-25%.

Stevens-Johnson Syndrome (SJS)

In very rare cases, shingles has been associated with *Stevens-Johnson syndrome*, an extensive and severe systemic disorder in which widespread blisters cover mucous membranes and large areas of the body.

Congenital Varicella Syndrome (CVS)

Pregnant women who contract varicella or herpes zoster in the first or second trimester of pregnancy can pass on varicella to the developing fetus. In a low percentage (0.4% before

---

[2] Shaikh S, Ta CN. Evaluation and management of herpes zoster ophthalmicus. American Family Physician, 2002 Nov. 1; 66(9):1723-1730.

[3] Shin HM, Lew H, Yun YS. A case of complete ophthalmoplegia in herpes zoster ophthalmicus. Korean J Ophthalmol. 2005 Dec; 19(4):302-304.

[4] Pallai KG, Nayar K, Rawal YB. Spontaneous tooth exfoliation, maxillary osteomyelitis and facial scarring following trigeminal herpes zoster infection. Prim Dent Care. 2006 Jul;13(3):114-116.

[5] Ginsberg PC, Harkaway RC, Elisco AJ 3rd, Rosenthal BD. Rare presentation of acute urinary retention secondary to herpes zoster. J Am Osteopath Assoc. 1988 Sep; 98(9):508-509.

13 weeks gestation; 2.0% between 13-20 weeks gestation) of births to mothers with VZV infection, this results in limb deformities and infant death.[6,7]

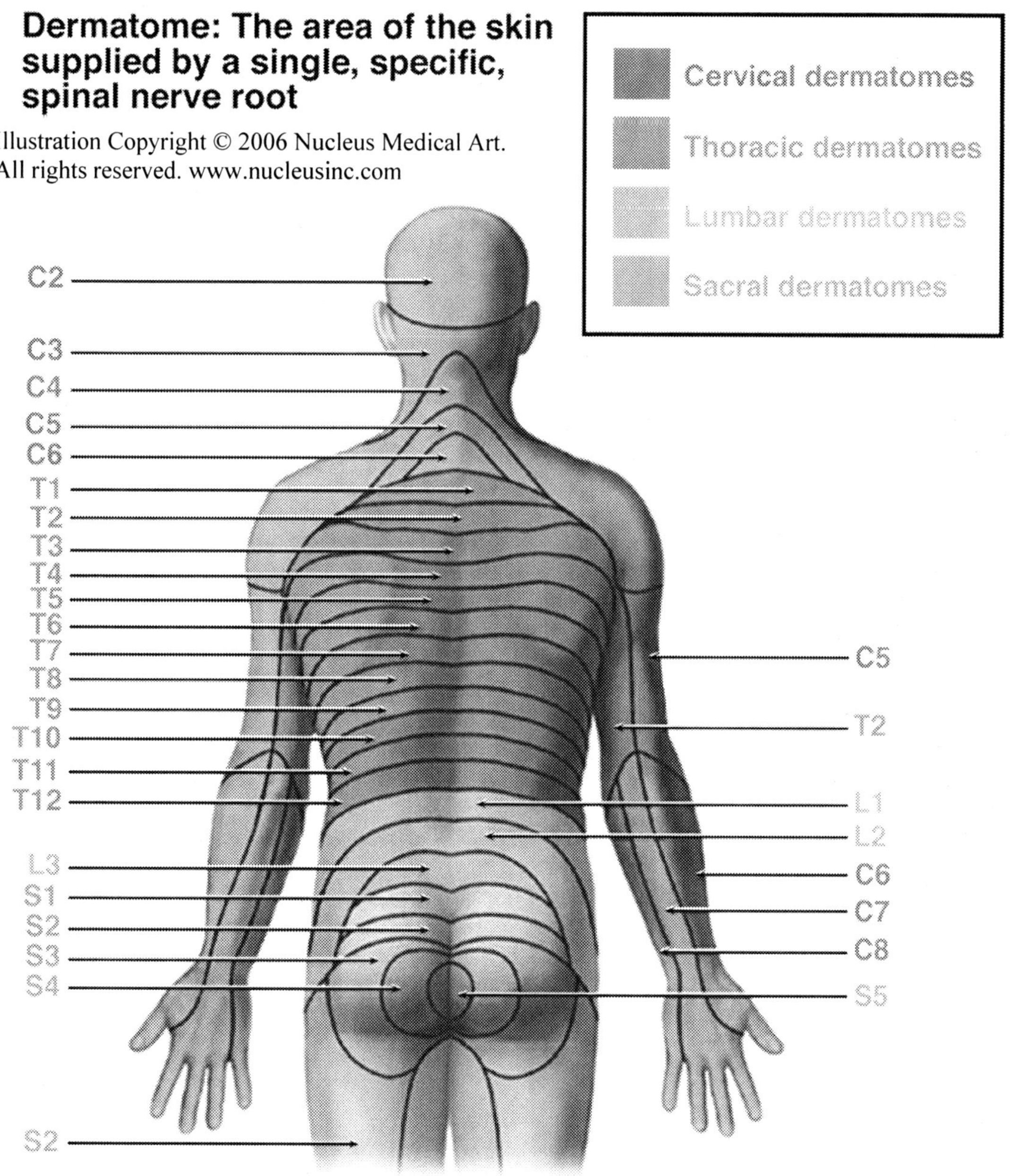

[6] Meyberg-Solomayer GC, Fehm T, Muller-Hansen I, Enders G, Poets C, Wallwiener D, Solomayer EF. Prenatal ultrasound diagnosis, follow-up, and outcome of congenital varicella syndrome. Fetal Diagn Ther. 2006;21(3):296-301.

[7] Enders G, Miller E, Cradock-Watson J, Bolley I, Ridehalgh M. Consequences of varicella and herpes zoster in pregnancy: prospective study of 1739 cases. Lancet. 1994 Jun 18;343(8912):1548-1551.

Table of Appendices

But man, proud man,
Dressed in a little brief authority,
...Plays such fantastic tricks before high heaven
As make the angels weep.
-William Shakespeare, poet and dramatist (1564-1616)

Chapter 1

Sycamore Springs, California
2018

"Lies, lies, lies."

Damon Leviticus threw the offending report against the open file cabinet. The weight of the bound volume rattled the window and dislodged a spider from the complacency of its afternoon web. A bowl of paper clips and a picture of a teenage boy fell off the neat desk and clattered to the floor.

Millie jumped and hit her knee on the corner of the desk. She winced. *Why did people end up getting hurt around Dr. Leviticus? Whatever he did caused pain. Did he have to be so melodramatic? So hyperbolic?* She'd known him all her life, and he still scared her. His raspy voice was thick with sarcasm even during the few times he was not talking about himself. His eyes sat emotionless in their sockets, watching everything, but seeing nothing. With thick eyebrows pulled together in the middle of his thin face, he looked like the miserly contradiction she knew him to be, cheap with his actions but extravagant with his promises.

"I will not tolerate these stories you have been inventing to discredit me, Millie, even if my son has made you his wife through the holiest bonds of matrimony. You are an ever present thorn in my side."

Talk about a loving father-in-law.

"Damon, you know these stories are not my invention. They are based on studies and research done by my own father. He can back up every word in them with hard facts and documented evidence of observable data. His work has been published in prestigious journals and quoted in countless articles."

He reached her with two long strides and stared her down. "You can bring me all the articles you want, you can manipulate them to fit your own agenda, but you will never change my mind. I know your father has a doctorate degree in computer science, but he is not qualified to draw these conclusions. I know you're going to defend him and his degrees, but he is still not a *medical* doctor." He shook his fist at the report he'd thrown to the floor.

She bit the inside of her mouth to keep from flinching. No amount of desensitization through countless Thanksgiving dinners had made even the slightest dent in the anxiety she felt whenever she looked at the man her son called Grandfather. He'd never evolved into a true human. The years away from Sycamore Springs had only furthered his resolve to remain obstinate. Shouldn't he have changed after all the havoc he'd brought to the town through his own egotistical agenda?

"You can rant all you want, Doctor, but the truth is evident, and once my father's latest article is published in a peer-reviewed U.S. medical journal and available on the National Library of Medicine's search engine, www.Pubmed.gov, you will have an entire country questioning what you did in Sycamore Springs two decades ago. You're going to be held accountable for your actions, and you're going to pay with your reputation." Millie's voice shook with anger. She'd warned Brandon that she was going to go through with the investigation to vindicate her father's work, and she wasn't going to be intimidated, no matter how ugly her father-in-law got. Some people had lost their lives, others had lost their minds. Damon could have been a part of the solution and helped stop it all, but instead he was part of the problem. He'd plowed ahead like the stubborn, egotistical man he was, certain of his opinions even in the light of irrefutable proof to the contrary.[8]

Her father's preliminary studies and manuscripts written in 2000 and 2001 had been disregarded and dismissed by the majority of those responsible for insuring public health, even though she believed with every fiber of her being that he was correct. People who had put their trust in the myth of public confidence, had their lives sacrificed by the very professions and organizations that were sworn to protect them.

I will not back down. I will not give in. I am right. Millie repeated the mantra she had learned alongside her childhood reading. No one was going to make her go against her logic and reason. Facts were facts. People were growing sicker and many had died, and Damon had been the cause. He had lined up the entire town and shot them full of a future of pain and suffering. He'd shortened their lives and doomed them to illness and disease.

"You should have listened to both sides of the issues. Yours wasn't the only opinion on the issue of vaccinations. They've been linked to autism for a long time. Vaccines have caused unnecessary deaths since the first one was developed. My father looks at all the facts, not only the ones that would give him a profit. He has no bias. People come to him because they know he will tell them all the facts, instead of selectively picking and choosing the ones they ought to know."

"Your revered father is a troublemaker," Damon ground out, his eyes slits of hate. "If all of his research reaches the public, do you know how many people will be hurt? Do you know how many good citizens will listen to him and in doing so jeopardize their health? It isn't a good idea to give the general population a choice. Most people are not qualified to make any decisions whatsoever, let alone those dealing with their health. Lay people are common people. They have no medical training. They don't know how to conduct studies and gather research. They certainly don't know how to interpret what they see. It takes years of training to. . . ."

"Cover up the truth?" Millie interrupted. "To manipulate the data? To misquote? To out and out lie for profit?"

"Enough," he thundered, his voice shaking her insides with anger. "Doctors and drug companies don't lie. We have watchdog agencies that keep us on our toes, not that we need it. We're squeaky clean."

Millie was certain of the validity of her father's conclusions—conclusions corroborated by a few others conducting careful research. *She reflected for a moment on a quote she once read, "When great changes occur in history, when great principles are*

---

[8] See Appendix VIII. A Summary of Scientific Literature Supporting the Exogenous Boosting Hypothesis

involved, as a rule the majority are wrong."[9] She felt the bile of fury rising in her throat. "How can you say that? Deceit and cover-ups are reported every day."

He slammed one of his fists into his other hand, open and waiting for the rehearsed gesture she'd seen him use more times than she could believe. "By whom? By hack reporters like you. You never even went to college. You know nothing about life. You allowed yourself to be impregnated by my son and trapped a wealthy kid into marriage. Well, I hope you're satisfied. You've turned a star football player into a doormat, following you around, hanging on your every word as if he loves you."

Tears stung her eyes. "He does love me. You're the one who's alone. Your wife ran from you in the middle of the night. When she wants to see her grandson, she stays with us, not with you." She bent down and carefully picked up the picture from the floor. "Mark loves her, but he's afraid of you."

"You turned him against me, Millie. I will not forgive you for that."

She wanted to laugh, but the tension in her body was too tight to allow it. "We've taught him from the day he was born to stay away from you and people like you. We want him to have a long and healthy life." Millie had previously done research that revealed doctors were the third leading cause of death in the U.S. with an estimated 225,000 iatrogenic deaths annually; *iatrogenic* meaning the deaths were induced by a physician or caused by the U.S. healthcare system.[10]

"He'll never be healthy, because you won't consent to letting me give him the necessary vaccines and take care of him."

She shook her head vehemently, loosening the modest bun at the nape of her neck, driving her glasses farther down her nose. "You are an evil man. You've made us all sick. Not only those who took your defective and flawed immunization, but now virtually all the adults in Sycamore are at greater risk of developing (a) chronic autoimmune disorders[11] and (b) shingles[12] which can be a source of excruciating pain. Heaven only knows what else your misuse of your power and forced respect has done to us. We trusted you, Damon, and you betrayed us."

He advanced, causing her to back up, seeking safety, leaving her desk the only fortress between them. "You are a pre-menopausal woman suffering from delusions of self-importance. You have a meaningless journalism job, and you think it gives you the right to pry into people's lives and to invade their privacy. If you print one word of this in your small-minded paper, I'll sue you for libel. You have no real evidence. You can never destroy me. I am invincible, because I have the power of the medical and pharmaceutical

---

[9] Quoted from Eugene V. Debs (1955-1926).

[10] Starfield B (of the Johns Hopkins School of Hygiene and Public Health). Is U.S. health really the best in the world? Journal of the American Medical Association (JAMA) 2000 Jul. 26;284(4):483-485. Of the 225,000 deaths, 12,000 were due to unnecessary surgery; 7,000 due to medication errors in hospitals; 20,000 due to other hospital error; 80,000 due to infections contracted in hospitals; and 106,000 due to prescribed pharmaceutical drugs.

[11] See Appendix XII. Vaccination and Autoimmunity: Reassessing Evidence.

[12] See Appendix VIII. A Summary of Scientific Literature Supporting the Exogenous Boosting Hypothesis.

establishment behind me. They will back me no matter what you print. You'll run out of money giving it to lawyers for their outrageous legal fees before you can make a dent in my bank account." His face was red, and his eyes bulged out of his face with intense emotion.

"For heaven's sake, calm down, Damon. Try to see my father's point of view for once in your life."

He stood his ground silently for a change, watching her every move, his chest heaving, his breath coming in short, agitated gasps.

Millie wished she had one of the new offices in the building with the built-in alarm button under the desk to summon building security. The security team would know how to deal with a temper tantrum. She didn't think Damon would harm the mother of his grandson, but she didn't think he'd do a lot of things.

But he had.

And now there was cause for much suffering and anguish.

##

"Mark, where are you going?" Brandon followed the carbon copy of himself into the living room of the home he loved. He was truly blessed. He had a wife who loved him as much as he loved her. He had a son who had every good characteristic he had hoped to find in himself, but rarely did. He had a career with a built-in future, coaching the high school football team where he had made eight winning touchdowns in the championship season of his dreams.

"Got a date with Hallie, Dad, why?" Mark turned back to him with a touch of impatience in his blue eyes. They were kind eyes, and Brandon knew they looked at the world with loving kindness.

"Just worried. You need some time off," Brandon said, taking the football that had made the last winning touchdown in senior year out of its moorings on the pedestal on the mantle. "I thought you might like to try out a few of the old plays, throw a few passes." His voice dwindled to nothing as he watched the disinterest on his only child's face. He doted on Mark. He would have made a pact with the devil to insure his son's safety. Did his son look tired? Did he need an herbal elixir to pep him up? He hadn't been feeling well himself lately, and he wondered if the family had picked up a virus as the children of Sycamore returned to school in the autumn, and unintentionally contaminated each other with their various germs and illnesses.

Maybe he should talk to Millie about him. She always had the best ideas. Too bad she spent so much time in her office instead of home loving him. He worshipped her. Millie was his soul mate, even if he had made every mistake known to courtship rituals before they were married. Looking back now, he knew he had behaved like a lovesick schoolboy because he was a lovesick school-boy. He had fallen in love with Millie when they ran through Sycamore in the early years. The city was new and fresh. The people were hopeful and generous. What had gone wrong with the vision of the future they all had? So much had changed, and not for the better.

If it hadn't been for Millie, he would have ended up alone as he'd gotten older. She'd saved him from a life with his father. She hadn't done it with force or insults. She had helped him with her intelligence and commitment to the common good, as she called it.

"I'm fine. You worry too much. It's making you old. You look really tired today. I'll be home late. Hallie and I are going to a boondocker. Don't wait up."

Brandon felt a familiar tug. The boondocks. His old playground. Mark wouldn't be standing in front of him right now if it wouldn't have been for his impulsive behavior with Millie on a star-filled night many years ago when they were all young.

"I'm going to wait up. I want to be sure you get home safely." He always waited up, no matter how late. Millie did, too. She pretended to be reading, but she had the clock in front of her on the nightstand when she brought her work to bed.

Mark shrugged. "That's what I get for having grandfathers who have doctorate degrees. No one lets me have any fun. I want to give every girl in town a chance to get to know me before I go to college." He flexed his muscles and stared at his own face in the glass of the front door. "You wouldn't want any of them to miss the experience of me, now would you?"

Brandon laughed. They were so much alike. He was a great kid, just like his mother.

Mark started for the door and paused. "You gotta talk to Mom. She's giving me grief about the health requirements for college applications, you know the immunizations and the chest x-rays. She said to forget any college that won't take a philosophical or religious exemption as a reason to opt out of the meningococcal vaccine given to college freshmen who are going to live in dormitories. I don't want to cross that many universities off my list. Will you talk to her? I know she believes what she believes, and most of the time I agree with her. Actually, all of the time I agree with her, but when she interferes with my chances for getting ahead in the world, I think she should back off. I'm an adult, soon, and I can do whatever I want anyway, but I don't want to get her mad at me if I go against her beliefs. She always backs them up with facts and figures, charts, graphs, study after study.[13] I feel like an idiot if I don't agree, but sometimes I just gotta. You know what I mean?"

Great. Another battlefield revisited. "I'll talk to her, but I'm warning you, I don't disagree with her as much as I used to. Over the years she's been right on most occasions. I remember when we went to enroll you in elementary school. The Public Health Department

---

[13] The FDA News, dated September 30, 2005 warns, "The FDA and CDC are alerting consumers and health care providers to five reports of Guillain Barre Syndrome—GBS—following administration of Meningococcal Conjugate Vaccine A, C, Y, and W135, trade name Menactra, manufactured by Sanofi Pasteur." CDC next reports in *Update: Guillain-Barre syndrome among recipients of Menactra meningococcal conjugate vaccine—United States, October 2005-February 2006*, MMWR Morb Mortal Wkly Rep. 2006 Apr 7;55:364-6, "During the 4 months since, three additional confirmed cases of GBS have been reported." Authors Scott II RD, Meltzer MI, Erickson LJ, De Wals P, and Rosenstein NE reported, "The net cost per death averted ranged from $7 million to $20 million" in Vaccinating first-year college students living in dormitories for Meningococcal disease: an economic analysis, published in Am. J. Prev. Med., 2002 Aug., 23:98-105.

and school nurse knew that in California (as well as in most states) a parent can claim a philosophical or religious exemption and not have their child vaccinated—just by signing the reverse of the Immunization Card. However, the Public Health Department and school nurse were not obligated to inform parents of this exemption option. You either had to know your rights or your rights were waived. Fortunately, because your mom exercised her rights, you have always been healthier than most of your vaccinated classmates. It's scary. She often discuses medical interventions with Craig first. I know her father's right most all the time too, but sometimes I wonder how they know what they know."

"Just smart I guess. I gotta go."

Brandon caught the door before it closed completely and watched Mark jump into the expensive convertible he'd bought for him over Millie's objections. With a great deal of apprehension, he watched his son screech out of the driveway on his way to meet his girl of the hour.

Brandon blinked the irritation out of his eyes. Must be from the smoke that the tires created on the concrete. He covered his eyes, the light overwhelming him again. Blame it on the smog from Los Angeles creeping over the hills and into the valley of Sycamore Springs.

He closed the door and made his way to the sink in the downstairs guest bathroom. With his eyes shut, he found the faucets and turned the water on full blast, dipping his head closer so he could splash his face with water, hoping to clear the sting and unfamiliar gritty feeling. His fingers brushed against a strange sore on the tip of his nose. It had developed almost overnight, and it produced a sensation like nothing he had ever felt.

He turned off the tap and dried his face with the ends of his shirt. His eyes felt too irritated for him to open them. He moved cautiously down the hallway back to the living room and inched toward the sofa in the memorized room. Fortunately, they hardly ever rearranged the furniture.

Gratefully he sank down into the depths of the couch. The stinging sensation made him wince. A little nap. That's what he needed, and he'd be fine. He thought about his beautiful wife and quarterback son and smiled through the discomfort. He relaxed in the afternoon sun, listening to the sounds in the neighborhood—kids playing and yelling, cars stopping and starting near the traffic light on the corner, a distant radio, a nearby conversation.

Life never changed in Sycamore Springs. Some people were born while other people died. Some got sick, others got well. It was a roll of the cosmic dice, some said, but he wasn't one of them. Luck had nothing to do with it. Intelligence and individual responsibility made the difference between life and death, sickness and health. Things went wrong all the time. What bothered him, though, was that he knew the perpetrator of the most evil offenses committed in town. It wasn't a stranger or a someone he could easily dismiss.

It was his father.

Chapter 2

Sycamore Springs, California
17 years earlier: 2001

"Lies, lies, lies."

Damon Leviticus slammed the thicket of papers onto Barbara's desk, ignoring the scattering that fell into her lap. "I will not tolerate deceit and greed in my town."

He was Dr. Demon tonight, she thought, wishing she could find a destination that didn't start with the words growing town and end with the surety of boring. "Why do you call Sycamore Springs your town? It isn't yours to control. Most of the people don't know you personally. They only know about you. It isn't the same thing. There are over thirty thousand people here. We have a statue of Benjamin Franklin in the center of the city on West Main Street. The talent show over at the high school is our cultural activity, and this little city's idea of a big time sporting event is our own son making yet another winning touch down, chalking up another victory for dear old Sycamore High."

She bit back a yawn. Why bother explaining normalcy to a man like Damon. He had his own ideas, and he never deviated from them. When he was right, he let everybody know it, and when he was wrong, he ignored it. As a result, he was as interesting as a mailing label, thin and frequently illegible, but he, to himself, was always certain where he was going.

Damon, with no indication he had heard a word Barbara said, sank into the sofa that cost two tonsillectomies and a hernia. "Veritas,[14] my dear wife. Veritas."

Another evening at home. Just what she always wanted. Certainly she could think of somewhere to go. Maybe Lisa wasn't taking a class, maybe Aileen wasn't entertaining anybody, maybe even Brandon would go for ice cream with her. She could go alone, just as she usually did, but tonight she needed company. Sometimes the emotional isolation got to her. Sometimes the crowd was too much to bear alone.

Nothing much to buy in Sycamore. No expensive clothes, no tasteful decorating items. Even the basics had to come from the drugstore instead of an upscale department store, especially on late nights like this when the Shop-For-Less was closed.

Unfortunately, Tippy's Ice Cream Freeze would be populated with Brandon's friends. He wouldn't like his mother standing in line for a Rainbow Cone on a blistering Saturday night along with his girlfriend, Millie, a candidate for Ivy League anonymity.

Damon gestured to the sheaf of paper. "Take a look at that, and then tell me I don't have any rights here. I delivered nearly every kid within the city limits for the last two decades. These people are my responsibility."

"Why don't you let them take care of themselves? They seem to do a good job of it when you're away."

---

[14] Veritas is a Latin word meaning "truth". On occasion, instead of calling his wife by her real name, Dr. Damon Leviticus will affectionately use the term "Veritas".

He ignored her. She could have been a lamp or a pillow. Unless she challenged him, he stormed by her comments.

"These good citizens are helpless without me. They trust me to make their health decisions for them. Remember Sam Perkins?"

Who didn't. An obnoxious little man with lechery on his mind and inadequate bus fare in his unwashed pockets.

"His wife needed an operation, and he didn't know what to do, so I made the decision for him," Damon continued, searching for his glasses on the lamp table.

"Sarah Perkins died on the table," Barbara reminded him unsteadily, remembering her friend and the fear on her face when they wheeled her toward the operating room. She hadn't wanted the surgery. It was elective by most standards. She didn't need it.

She had been pressured into it by Damon raising his voice at her, "Are you sure you want to take that chance with your life?"

Sarah's life had never been in danger. She could have gone comfortably into old age with a little encouragement instead of a heavy dose of mind-boggling fear that led to her death.

"But she needed the surgery. That's what the protocol says." His voice was firm and resolute. And blind.

"She could have lived for years. There were other ways to approach the problem."

Damon whipped his glasses off and flung them to the floor. "I don't want to hear anymore from you about other ways. There are no alternatives to good medicine."

Barbara recognized the curdle of resentment where her stomach met her common sense. Being a doctor's wife had its advantages, even in a small town where the most coveted commodity was preferential treatment at the post office. She could speak up, or she could remember how long the lines could be in Los Angeles, where the most prized privilege was anonymity.

Sycamore Springs had been a drive-through collection of diners and tall grass where she and Damon had settled in the housing boom after his return to California from Vietnam. Alone, on their down-filled mattress in the silence of neglect before Brandon's birth, he filled her mind with tirades of disappointment instead of filling her body with love.

He'd told her that every man he'd healed in the defoliated jungles had been a hero except him. Patching up the shock and mutilation had not been rewarding, he'd said more times than was necessary, as they lay together into the darkness of their top-of-the-line model home, after the housing developers had taken down the flags for the night, but before the bulldozers returned at dawn to carve yet another promise of prosperity out of the virgin hills.

No, his new doctor status had been abused, in his opinion. No glory for him. Only endless hours and tedium. What kind of a life would that be for him, just another medical flunky in the aftermath of endless training. He hungered for something he deemed intrinsic to his service to humanity.

Beyond the money, beyond the prestige, he wanted fame. He craved recognition, and by all that he held holy, he was going to have it.

She'd heard it all before, and she was weary of it. Brandon had just turned eighteen. He was her prize, her reward. She'd never thought much of being Damon's wife, but she was indeed Brandon's mother, and that made her walk with pride down West Main Street, right into the post office.

"Have you read it yet?" He peered into her thoughts, his eyes demanding slits of suspicion. He didn't trust anyone, because, as he told it, no one was trustworthy, one hundred percent certainty rate. She thought that was short-sighted for a man of science to misuse statistics.

Nothing is ever one hundred percent, dear, she'd tell him as he ranted nightly about the people he had to instruct about good health practices.

He didn't hear her, but it gave her something to do.

"I tried to read it, but you interrupted me too many times to finish."

He shoved his thin fingers through the papers and pulled out the cover page. "It's a study, a statistical analysis of immunizations in this country."

She read a few words on the paper he held in front of her face and nodded. Something about chickenpox. Damon had been exposed to this virus often due to the very nature of his profession.

Her thoughts sought a refuge. Maybe she could meet Aileen at the new strip mall on the Burgess off-ramp. She'd heard they had an antique store run by a couple of no-taste attorney's wives. Clearly a tax write-off for them, but maybe she could find something interesting to brighten the fireplace in the living room, anything to elevate track-home tacky.

Damon pushed his glasses closer to his eyes. "Let's see what we have here," he muttered in the same tone of voice he used for his patients.

An arrogance permeated the library, and Barbara looked away toward the pictures on the desk. She and Damon on their wedding day, Brandon when he won his first game for the Junior Varsity Football Team, and Brandon with Millie, the girl he loved.

Barbara squirmed in her chair. Millie. That girl was going to bring destruction to the House of Leviticus, of that she was quite sure. From the child's uninteresting features to her enviable intellect, Millie was hardly the daughter-in-law of her dreams. Good thing she and her son were so young, just turning 18, or they would have been married already. College would cause a major rift in their relationship. She'd see to that.

"…and that's the gist of my speech. What do you think?" Damon looked up, waiting for her typical praise.

What had he been saying? It didn't matter. Whatever opinion he had expressed, and it was always an opinion of his own, she was expected to worship each syllable he uttered.

"I agree with you completely, Doctor."

He smiled smugly, stroking his chin, looking for the beard that had never been on his face in the first place. How did he see himself? As some bearded savior with a desire to rescue humanity by destroying it first, placing its fate in his hands, and riding to the fore with a bottle of pills and a hypodermic?

She should have married Lindsey Fellows. He was a self-educated man, proud of his family and his career. Fitness Trainer wasn't a real job, according to Damon, but she knew that Lindsey was in far better shape then her husband, who had never led a healthy lifestyle and relied on medications to put the bloom of middle age in his cheeks.

"Where's Brandon?" Damon asked abruptly. "I'd like him to hear my speech."

So it had been a speech.

"He's with Millie."

Damon's face clouded with cumulonimbus warning. "I have plans for him. I want him by my side."

##

"This town is uninspiring and boring."

Brandon crumpled the Smoothola cup into a cardboard mess and shoved it to the floor of his car on the plush mat. He turned the CD player to low and tilted his seat back. The look on his face reminded Millie of the many days she had watched him at practice when he was trying to out-play the team's plays and fix the flaws he saw in the original strategy.

Millie sighed. Two burgers and a drink of something chemical and vile upset the usual belligerent manner he had lately and turned him into the iconoclast she loved. He was interested in the world around him, politically and environmentally. Together they had helped Sycamore Springs recycle their aluminum cans. They had rescued feral cats, begun a sanctuary for wild birds, and taught reading to people who didn't have any skills in that area.

Brandon was obviously different from many of the other boys at school. He was a football hero and a good student at the same time. He had many relationships with willing females, but he treated them all with respect. He was close to his parents, but saw them as they really were, not as heroes, but as people. He tried to have the best of all possible worlds.

"No one here has any sense," he continued, impatiently punching the buttons on the CD player on the dash. "These people are lemmings, following any toad-made-king by public decree of indifference right over the cliff of conformity to their doom."

"Anyone in particular?"

"Doesn't matter. They're all the same. Each one knows it all. My father's the worst one, but you already know that."

"You're traditional, Brandon."

"I am not. I'm progressive."

"Same thing."

He snorted. "How can they be the same thing? One is stuck in the past, and the other is committed to the future."

"That's minor. That's not why they're the same. They share a common factor."

"Which is?"

"They're labels. If you can label something, then it's already known. You're looking for an unknown, like in scientific research. You have controls for everything except for one variable."

"It's always science with you."

"That's all I understand."

Brandon watched nothing in particular out the window. "I understand you. You're traditional in your clothes and in your scientific method, but you're progressive in wanting to investigate the truth and bring it to light. If you weren't in pursuit of the truth all the time, you'd be more comfortable with your traditional roots."

Millie sighed. "You're beginning to sound like your father, mixing up the past and future, the irritation of the truth with the complacency of tradition. You'd fit right into an old guard school in the East. You should talk to your father. He wants you to go to a good school. Then we can be together all the time."

Brandon shook his head. "He'd never go for it. He thinks state universities are just as good. He's one of those people who wants the best for himself, and to make sure he's the best, he has to make everyone else as small as possible."

What a contrast to her own father, who wanted to elevate everyone to their highest level of achievement with praise and encouragement. "Damon went back East, didn't he?"

"Of course. He's a sainted doctor. Where else would he go but to some pompous private college covered with poison ivy?"

Millie took his hand as he switched the music to the radio. "Why does he make you so angry? Why can't you just walk away and live your own life? If he influences everything you do, how will you ever be your own person?"

He scowled at her. "Because my own Father never tells me what he thinks."

Millie laughed out loud and took his hand. "He always tells you what's on his mind, but only what he wants you to know. He believes he's educated, and what he's been taught is gospel. He talks all the time. Some of what he says may have value, but most of it is his interpretation of the facts. He's also been taught how to be selective in what he reveals. He wants to be a hero, the champion of health for an entire town. That's got to go to his head."

Brandon pulled away from her. "Don't laugh. I hate it when people laugh at me. You know that. What bothers me is that he doesn't think for himself. He honestly believes he does, but he only reads what his peers tell him, churns the information he's gleaned around in his narrow mind, and then spits it out to his advantage. Do you know what scares me? That one day it's going to be me or Mom or even you or people we love, and he won't put us first. He'll put himself first, and his reputation above all."

"You sound like him when you talk like that," she said quietly, knowing he wouldn't like that either. "Do you know why? Because it isn't logical. He's not the only saint in town. We can call up any number of people for their opinion at a moment's notice. You're not trapped. You are free to do whatever you please whenever you want."

He grabbed at her fingers, in a contradictory move pushing her away. "I'm not like him, and I'm never going to be like him. He's got something mixed up in his mind. He confuses the people he should love with the people he wants to impress."

"And he doesn't impress you?"

"How can he, when he lost the ability to fool me years ago."

Millie adjusted the height on the seats of the unnecessarily luxurious car of Brandon's non-materialistic dreams and eased into the depths of the leather buckets. Most of the citizens of Sycamore believed every word Brandon's father uttered, no matter the intention. From her own vantage point, she believed Damon was a complex man.

And she didn't like him.

"He has nice taste in cars," she murmured, aware she couldn't push Brandon too far. He had a temper, but he had to keep it to himself in front of his father. Unwillingly, he had learned limits. He didn't do what he wanted. He couldn't. He wanted his father to love him, but his father only used him.

"You know I didn't want this. I wanted him to give up his self-appointed post of school doctor instead. Coming in every week, embarrassing me, giving those ridiculous lectures on safe sex, as if anyone in Sycamore High is still a virgin."

"I would be, had we not secretly married as soon as we both turned 18."

"Our strong moral character and chaste conduct prior to marriage is what will keep us faithful in marriage," he added at the same moment, absently grazing her tummy with a gesture of acknowledgment. "While we are still living under our parent's roof, it is not the time to start a family now, but when we both graduate and confront our parents about our marriage, this situation will change."

"Brandon, I still remember our wedding day, when we visited the County Clerk's office together to get our marriage license. You told me most people get married believing a myth: that marriage is a beautiful box full of all the things they have longed for—companionship, intimacy, and friendship. The truth is, that marriage, at the start, is an empty box. You must put something in, before you can take anything out. There is no love in marriage. Love is in people. And people put love in marriage. There is no romance in marriage. You have to infuse it into your marriage."

"Yes, and we agreed that a couple must learn the art and form the habit of giving, loving, serving, praising—keeping the box full. If you take out more than you put in, the box will be empty."

If she didn't love him, she would have stopped trying to get his attention from the early days when he ignored her during class and resented her ability to answer more questions from the teachers than he could.

"I am yours, Brandon. Remember, when you gave me your pep rally tag and proposed to me." She cared about him.

"Yeah," he whispered out the window, however he'd had enough mental exercise, and it had never made him any healthier. He felt the best in a huddle listening to the coach, who had more common sense than his own father.

Every pill shoved down his throat, every injection stabbed into his body since his birth had reinforced his desire to live a life free of medical interference. And that's why he was attracted to Millie.

She questioned every system from local government to medicine. Just because someone had a degree or an office, didn't mean they had a brain, she'd told him frequently, and he agreed. She was smart, and he half-resented, half-respected her for that. She followed her own scientific method based on observation and relentless research.

Yes, she'd reach her goal of investigative reporter, no matter what obstacles came her way.

But when they each went their separate ways to their parents' house, the nights were long and lonely for them in Sycamore Springs, especially now when the summer was over and autumn's sunlight took on a waning hue. They both had to complete high school during a season when increased crime and higher rates of communicable illnesses occurred in the shorter, colder days. When would be the right time to tell their parents their secret? When would they be able to live together in their own house and start a family?

Chapter 3

"Please, welcome to the podium, Sycamore Springs' recipient of the Key to the City Award for the eighth year in a row, Dr. Damon Leviticus."

A spotlight moved from the center of the stage to where Damon sat with Barbara at a long table covered with white linen and sterling silver.

"They love me," Damon said under his breath to his wife and moved to the center of the dais. Applause filled the Spartacus Club, and in appreciation he gave his admirers a toothy smile and a wave. He stood beaming as the applause continued, doing nothing to stop the din of appreciation she heard and resented.

Like a shark, she thought, politely clapping, uncomfortable after a mediocre dinner. For the money they had to pay to be there, the dinner could have been more than unrecognizable chicken, peas, and soggy potatoes.

Finally, Damon held his hands up in a show of supposed modesty and stepped back like a shy little boy. He shook his head from side to side and shrugged in helpless submission as the applause went on and on.

What an act. I wonder what's for dessert.

"My dear friends," he began, and the sound system squawked feedback in protest. "I stand before you today as your mentor and as your friend as well as your doctor. I have had the privilege and the honor of delivering your children, treating you and them when all of you are sick, and doing my best to ameliorate sickness and suffering—trying to keep all of you in the best of health. I stress preventive medicine, and I expect to see you all in my office on Monday for your checkups," he quipped.

Polite laughter filled the hall. Barbara wondered how many people in Sycamore really believed in preventive medicine. From what she had seen, the medical profession perpetrated illness and disease. How many times had the good citizens walked into the doctors' or dentists' offices in perfect health, and come out crippled, maimed, coughing, with broken teeth and broken lives? More times than not.

Damon continued. "I have in my possession documented evidence that medical science has triumphed once again, this time against a feared disease that has been one of the scourges of mankind. These are not frivolous facts, my fellow citizens of Sycamore and esteemed members of the Spartacus Club. In fact, these are dreaded numbers, frightening in their power, unavoidable in their implications."

He paused for effect, gathering his flock. Barbara watched the faces at the front tables. Helen Porter and her third husband Lyon. Michelle and Travis Beaumont. Lisa and Paul Christiann. Almost all loyal friends and supporters of her husband.

She didn't think Lisa particularly liked Damon, even though they were in the same profession in many ways. Lisa was a well-liked school nurse, who knew every child by name. She and Damon frequently discussed trends in the health of the kids in the community, especially if any epidemics hit the school system. Lisa was honest and careful. She put the kids' confidentiality above Damon's insistence on knowing everything that went on in her office, as if he were her superior.

Damon leaned forward over the podium, raising his voice for emphasis. "Do you hear me, Sycamore Springs? We are in trouble. We are in the middle of a plague upon the House of Sycamore, and the name of the pestilence is varicella, or as you call it, chickenpox. It leaves some children scarred for life with disfiguring pits on their innocent faces and unsuspecting bodies. It ravages their inner organs and varicella pneumonia can result in death. Most importantly, parents often lose out on income from missed work when taking care of their children with chickenpox."

No stopping him now. The Preacher of Panic had hit his stride. Barbara looked for the remnants of the dinner roll on her plate. Not much else had been palatable, and her stomach growled noticeably.

"Every year four million unprotected people in the United States are stricken with varicella and there are approximately 11,000 hospitalizations due to this disease. An unconscionable fifty children and fifty adults, or a total of one hundred precious lives are lost. The annual cost savings due to vaccinating against varicella totals $380 million.[15] Of this total, $80 million is due to medical costs and $300 million is due to societal costs in the form of lost wages from parent's missed work."

Each time he mentioned the official name for chickenpox, he divided it into syllables and enunciated each one – VAR-I-CEL-LA – as if he were instructing a group of idiots. With the exception of for Barbara, no one else in the audience had bothered to do the math to compute the true death rate associated with varicella. The 50 deaths, out of 4 million per year that varicella causes in children, is quite low.[16] In perspective, a person has a greater chance of dying by being struck by lightning in the U.S. (mean of 90 cases annually in the U.S.)[17] than of a child's dying from contracting varicella.

He went on. "Once again, the great and glorious profession of medicine has risen to the challenge and formulated an immunization that will eradicate the disease by sensitizing the immune system to a weakened or attenuated strain of the live virus. We and our children will be free of the pock marks of this disease that occurs in annual epidemics."

Applause thundered through the arena, and Barbara felt obligated to join the din. Not that it mattered. People got sick. People got well. It was *how* they are healed that disturbed her. Left to their own devises, allowed to mend according to their immune systems and the ecological balance of nature, she figured most people did pretty well. But once the marketeers and profiteers plundered the database of recovery, well, then the problems fed on

---

[15] Lieu TA, Cochi SL, Black SB, Halloran ME, Shinefield HR, Holmes SJ, *et al.* Cost-effectiveness of a routine varicella vaccination program for U.S. children. JAMA 1994 Feb 2; 271(5):375-381.

[16] Seward JF, Orenstein WA. Commentary: The case for universal varicella immunization. Pediatr. Infect. Dis. J. 2006;25:45-46.

[17] Curran EB, Holle RL. Lightning fatalities, injuries, and damage reports in the United States from 1959-1994. U.S. Department of Commerce, National Oceanic & Atmospheric Association (NOAA) Technical Memorandum, 1997; NWS SR-193. Available online at http://www.nssl.noaa.gov/papers/techmemos/NWS-SR-193/techmemo-sr193.html

each other. Would this be another one of those chains of unstoppable events, beginning with a shot in the dark, and then leading the unsuspecting victims of the very drugs that were touted to help them into an endless prison of side effects?

She had seen it all before, and she didn't like it any better as she got older. Who was running the show anyway? Who mandated the shots and pills that made their way into the mainstream under the guise of good medicine?

Years before, when Brandon was born, Damon had taken charge from the second he had personally decided a c-section was better than the natural childbirth she had spent her entire pregnancy learning. No real reason, he told her as she begged him to let her have her baby her way. Just a gut feeling. Didn't she want a perfect baby? Did she want to risk the possibility of a low-oxygen problem? Besides, with a c-section, he would personally lift the baby right out of her, no risk to the baby at all, and statistics proved that generally, it was safer for the mother and less legal liability for the physician that way, too.

She'd been hysterical.

She'd been ignored.

Damon had delivered Brandon while she was unconscious, because her husband had told her he didn't want her to be afraid, he didn't want her to have any discomfort whatsoever.

She wasn't sure she had ever forgiven him for that.

Or the hysterectomy he had performed at the same time to spare her any female problems in the future.

And any more children.

"Yes, my dear friends," he droned on, "with the new chickenpox inoculation, no one in Sycamore Springs will ever suffer the ravages of the disease again. Do you know why? Because I have personally arranged for every man, woman, and child who has not had a previous history of chickenpox to receive a free vaccination. One month from today, starting at eight o'clock in the morning, the street in front of my office will be closed, and tables will be set up. My nurse and I will personally administer the injection to each of you as a front line of defense against the plague of chickenpox. No more marked little faces, no more chances for the complications of encephalitis and varicella pneumonia. We are going to be a model for the entire country, yes, the entire world. History will be made here, and we will be on every news channel, in every newspaper. We are the Sycamore Springs Injection Day model, and we are confident that we will prevail."

He'd done it again, just the way he had in the past. Everyone from Helen to Travis was on their feet. Paul Christiann was making whooping sounds the way he did at the football game. Porter was the first to rush the stage and pump Damon's arm up and down in congratulations.

But Barbara stayed seated. Her husband didn't need her anyway. He had his fans.

She put the last bite of the stale roll back on her plate and patted the empty space in her abdomen where her dreams had once been.

##

"Come in, Millie, dear."

Barbara led her into the ornate foyer. The home she created as a doctor's wife was far from the refuge she envisioned. It was cold and foreboding. The furniture was complicated and confusing, surrounded by somber colors and old objects owned by many people. Nothing was new or innovative. Nothing brought warmth or happiness. The only emotions were control and the accumulation of wealth in the oversized rooms.

She closed the door behind Millie, cutting off the fresh air of Sycamore, leaving them both in the gloom of the house. The younger woman Brandon loved smiled at Barbara. Millie seemed genuine, a little on the cautious side, but Barbara assumed that was because someday Millie would probably be her mother-in-law, an uncomfortable position for any girl.

She liked the child, but she didn't want Brandon to end his plans for college by becoming a father too early in his career. Not that she thought Millie would trick Brandon into fatherhood, and not that she thought her son was careless. Just motherly worry and precaution. Better to prevent a problem, than have to deal with one later. She knew that Damon had taken care of the father-son talks when Brandon reached puberty, because he said that was the best time – studies showed – to take care of such matters. She, of course, had discussed it with her son much earlier than that, guided by his natural curiosity and questions.

"Thank you, Mrs. Leviticus."

Always so polite, constantly correct, that was the best way to describe Millie—the love of her son's life. Barbara had seen the pictures Brandon had of her in his pajama drawer. Had they been intimate together? She didn't think so. Millie was too shrewd for that. Even at her young age, she knew she had Brandon for life, so why marry him early and take on more financial and emotional responsibilities?

"I heard Dr. Leviticus gave an impressive speech at the Club last night."

Barbara led her into the kitchen. "Would you like a bran muffin? Yes, his little talk brought him a standing ovation. He talked about preventing the yearly epidemics of chickenpox and the varicella vaccination he wants everyone in Sycamore Springs to have."

"You must have been very proud." She took the muffin and nibbled.

Millie was smart, no doubt about that. Barbara was aware of her father's research. Craig Manchester was an internationally respected scientist. He was unbiased and maintained a truly scientific objectivity despite pressure and criticism. She admired his adamant stand on the issues of the day – nutrition as a first line of defense against disease and truly informed consent when it came to considering any medical interventions..

Damon hated him. They were on the opposite sides of every debate, which meant an argument to her husband every time he saw Craig.

Millie took another dainty bite out of the muffin. How did she do that without grimacing? Now that oat bran was medically sanctioned as heart healthy, Damon put it on everything. In just the prior years before this, when Millie had advocated fiber in a good diet, he had ridiculed her, and said it was part of a left-wing, radical, socialist plot to pollute the food supply.

She didn't think Millie cared much about what she ate. She was thin and fit.

And young.

And she had Brandon.

"I suppose I'm proud of my husband. He blusters and postures, but . . . ."

"Deep down you know he's right?" Millie supposedly finished her thought, mumbling through another bite of tasteless dough.

Had she said that with contempt? Millie always sided with Craig. Had she said it to humor her, placate Barbara? Millie didn't like doing that; she hated being manipulated, even if it went under the guise of good etiquette.

Did Millie really believe Damon was evil and Craig was good, with no shades of gray? How innocent were the young to divide the world into right and wrong, good and evil. No shades of intention or malice of forethought, no qualifications of a difficult life or a childhood burdened with hardship.

Pride and shame, how close they were on the spinning wheel of daily living, turning and blending until no one could tell them apart. Society frequently found a way to justify wrongdoing such that sins were acceptable—"bad" being called "good".

Barbara knew where her loyalties stood. She was ashamed of Damon Leviticus, the man who slept far away from her in their lonely bed. He put his professional life above his family, and she resented it. How many times had he forced medication on her and Brandon just because he had samples in his pocket? Sometimes she worried what he could do if he had free rein in a gullible society. Would he knock them out with his rhetoric and remove their future from their unconscious bodies as he had done to her?

"I know he thinks he's right," she answered, moving the muffins closer to Millie. "How is your family? I didn't see them at the Club last night." Her parents were inseparable, never away from each other unless it was unavoidable. Craig was not tyrannical. He exercised his headship in a loving way, earning the respect of his wife Faith. How different a marriage like that must be.

"They're out of town celebrating their anniversary. It's so romantic. Dad bought Mom a necklace, and then he surprised her with a trip."

Her eyes glowed with respect, and Barbara felt a gnawing in back of her rib cage. Talking to Millie upset her. Their families led parallel yet unfamiliar lives. Craig and Faith loved their only child, Millie, with undisguised fervor. They were the fairy tale family that could put counseling out of business. They shared, they supported, they encouraged each other. Craig had a doctorate degree, too, but he had worked his way through the university to attain a Ph.D. in computer science combined with a B.S. degree in engineering. He devoted his life to his family whenever he wasn't on a computer implementing algorithms[18] for the common good.

Craig and Faith saw more of each other in one week than she and Damon had in the last ten years. Millie had discussions with her father; Brandon had confrontations with his.

"Mrs. Leviticus, can I ask you something about Brandon?"

---

[18] An algorithm is a step-by-step procedure for solving a problem implemented in either a computer language such as PASCAL or a rapid application development environment such as DELPHI.

Great, a heart-to-heart with yet another woman she didn't like. "Of course, dear."

"Brandon and I are getting sort of, you know, closer, and he's mentioned several times that something happened between him and his father that led him not to trust Dr. Leviticus."

Barbara hoped the silence in the ultra-modern, sterile kitchen would be the answer Millie wanted.

"I don't mean to pry, but you know I want to be a reporter, not one who just puts together a story from the Associated Press, but one who investigates and researches the who, what, when, why, and how of the piece to be sure the reporting is unbiased and fair with no political or corporate backing or funding to sway the actual story." She stopped for a breath.

Barbara sighed. Millie was going to make trouble for them all. She questioned, and wasn't that a futile and useless thing to do. The Damons of the world got their way, by virtue of the authority vested in them by the institutes of higher learning and the power of Daddy's money. What chance did even a well-to-do kid from even an above-average, prosperous city like Sycamore have? So she'd uncover something. Big deal. Then she'd have to get it on the air, get it to the people. Did she think that would be easy? They'd come out of the woodwork trying to stop her.

"What type of investigating and reporting would you like to do?" Barbara asked, attempting to steer the conversation into more neutral territory for the sake of brevity. She had plans to meet Aileen and have their nails done. Nothing could be more innocuous than that. The afternoon should move pleasantly forward with neat cuticles.

"Medical journalism, of course." Millie blinked, obviously disbelieving anything else could exist.

"Of course." Millie's cuticles could use some attention. The rest of her needed a little more care, too. What was Faith thinking of, letting her daughter leave the house dressed like a librarian? At least her clothes were pressed and clean, but most of the kids in Sycamore wore tattered jeans and t-shirts with lewd or musical slogans on them. Didn't she feel left out?

"How about something for yourself instead? What do you plan to major in when you go to college?"

Millie felt the familiar signals of impending indigestion. It happened every time she spoke with the woman who unknowingly was already her mother-in-law. She and Barbara had nothing in common except Brandon. Barbara dressed like a typical doctor's wife in designer suits that emphasized how elderly they really were, or were about to become one day. The fabrics of these clothes were as artificial as the color of their hair. The best laboratory-made plastic clothes and hair dye that money could buy, all topped with trendy labels for the geriatric set. Barbara was tall with a well-disguised, unfit body. She had her share of wrinkles and jowls, and tried to offset them with a halo of short blond hair, teased into a static helmet.

Fortunately, Millie's own mother neither dressed nor acted that way.

Millie knew Barbara thought she was some kind of dorky kid with no sense of glamour, but she always was quite sure that Brandon's obviously jealous mother was wrong about her.

Barbara knew all about glamour.

No, all that time Barbara spent putting on makeup and stylish outfits wasn't for Millie. Millie had a brain, and she intended to use it, small town upbringing or not. People had the opportunity to make choices every step of the way in their lives. Good and evil were not necessarily mandates from a genetic predisposition or environmental influences.

Millie had chosen to remain chaste until she married Brandon. She had chosen to answer every question in school, no matter the ridicule she received from her uneducated peers. She had chosen to speak out against lies, deceit, and injustice, and to live by all that she believed to be true and right in the world.

Chapter 4

"Did you ever have chickenpox?"

Paul looked up from the classic car parked in his driveway, a rag covered with hand-wax poised over the white surface. "Sure, I did. Every kid gets chickenpox. I had it for two weeks. My whole family did, at least the kids. It's a good disease, too."

Damon made a note on the clipboard he was carrying. "There's no such thing as a good disease. If there were, I'd be out of a job." Lisa's husband wasn't the brightest guy in the city. He often wondered why she married him, probably because opposites attract, although he had never seen a psychological study that could prove that beyond a shadow of a doubt. That's what mattered in medical as well as behavioral studies – proof, documented evidence that could be quoted with confidence. Why, he built his entire philosophy on related information supplied to him by drug company research on how best to treat illness and disease.

"Pox are good, and here's why." Paul swiped at the mirrored surface and dug the heel of his hand into the cloth. "You can stay out of school longer, because the nurse has to okay that the pox marks have completely crusted over and are no longer contagious. That's good for at least 10 days, maybe the whole two weeks. The worse the case, the longer the vacation from Mr. Wilkes' boring chemistry lectures. Did you know I've heard recent rumors that he changed his identify before moving to California because that guy was convicted of molesting students? He's always keeping the girls after school." He grinned and licked his lips.

Damon ignored his asides. Paul was the kid he always wanted to be, if he hadn't wanted to be a doctor so badly, the one with the noisy motorcycle and the bevy of the biggest collection of women in town following him into the boondocks for evening exercises. Too bad he didn't look like Paul, big and beefy, or he'd have had all those women and wild nights, too, instead of his respectable marriage. Of course, he'd never force anyone to do anything they didn't want to do in the first place. He wasn't that kind of man, and Paul wasn't either. However, Lisa's husband looked the part of a bad boy.

"That's no reason to let a disease run rampant, when we have the means to stop it." Ah, yes, how Damon loved invoking the collective "we". No matter, he didn't look like an advertisement for a work-out infomercial. He had intelligence, and that's what made the world spin on its financial axis. That's how and where he bested Paul. He could think, and he did. Paul bypassed thinking and went straight for physical demonstration. That was why Paul's wife had to work to contribute to their upscale lifestyle and membership in the Spartacus Club and why *his* wife did not have to bring in a dime. She was free to have her nails done at any time of the day. He was proud of that.

Damon believed that Barbara was just as smart as Lisa, but neither of them were as intelligent as he was. He'd never tell either of them that, but he knew it was true. He could control both women if he occasionally allowed them to believe he valued their opinions.

"Listen," Paul said leaning over the car, "why waste your time on a disease that doesn't kill people. Why not find out how to stop that AIDS thing going around." He resumed polishing, scraping a nonexistent spec from the hood with his fingernail.

"Paul," Damon said patiently trying to keep the condescending quality out of his voice, "AIDS doesn't go around like the flu. You have to be careful what you say when it comes to medicine. People might get caught up in a wave of misinformation and alter their entire lives built on a falsehood, either intentional or unintentional. Just because you read something unfounded in the paper or hear something on the news doesn't mean it is valid. We wouldn't want people to lose their lives because of an unproven theory, now would we? We would want to be sure we have unbiased data, and that those data are corroborated by studies conducted in other studies and populations. Then it takes experience to derive conclusions that demonstrate balance and reasonableness. At this point, we know that AIDS is caused by unprotected sex and shared needles."

"Chickenpox is different," Damon continued. "It's spread by the respiratory system of an infected child who sneezes, coughs or breathes, usually one to two days before the rash has even broken out, in close proximity to someone susceptible." Hadn't Paul paid the smallest amount of attention in school? He had to have taken at least two science classes to graduate.

"Yeah, right. Someone sneezes pox and scabs into the air, and they stick to someone's arm." He polished with fervor, obviously wounded that Damon was either kidding him or ridiculing him for his lack of knowledge.

How uneducated were some people, Damon thought. No wonder they needed him and trusted him. The whole city, maybe the entire world, would be lost without him.

People like Lisa, the School Nurse, were his helpers. They knew a little bit about a few things, and they did an adequate job. However, they had to confer with doctors on the big questions. School nurses knew about skinned knees and elbows, perhaps a sprained ankle and other emergency care. But when an epidemic struck, like the chickenpox epidemic we had a few years earlier, he, Dr. L, as he was affectionately known by some, had to go through the painstaking educational process of telling Lisa how to observe children returning to school. A cursory examination wasn't enough. She had to ask parents pertinent questions: What was the highest temperature at the peak of the illness? What medications were given? Were there any complications and pre-existing medical conditions? Then she had to chart everything and keep permanent records. She hadn't liked that, and she'd let him know it.

He remembered she'd constantly reminded him that the schools themselves didn't require her to go through such a complicated procedure. He'd told her that he was of a higher authority than the school system. He was a medical professional who was also a representative of the local county public health department.

She infuriated him by stating that she was part of the medical profession as well, and her research and data collecting methods, which she willingly did at Craig's request, were more extensive than the ones Damon suggested. When Damon angrily asked her why she felt that way, she had replied because she and Craig consider all possibilities—cases where the vaccine appeared to provide protection as well as cases involving vaccine failure. This yielded a more balanced and circumspect view. Also, she insisted that she and Craig had no scalpel to grind, no biases or ties to the pharmaceutical firms, thus their research truly placed the health interests of the students above pharmaceutical profits.

"Where's your wife, Paul?" Damon asked, looking around the carport into the kitchen window. "School's out for the day."

"Yeah, but she's still there. First day back after Labor Day. She had to check all the immunizations for the new students, and all the boosters for the returning students. You know the routine."

Damon knew. He set it up. Sycamore Springs had one of the best school health programs in the county, courtesy of the long hours he put in. "I'll go over and see how things are doing. It's a little late in the day even for a school nurse. I thought she'd be home by now, and I have a world-changing idea that I know she'll appreciate."

Paul looked up from his endless polishing. "Yeah? Free antidepressants for all the parents?" He howled with laughter.

Damon sighed. He would have given his left femur to have been like Paul.

##

"Busy, Nurse Lisa?"

"Damon, am I glad to see you."

She heard him chuckle. He always thought it was personal, but it never was. She wasn't fond of Dr. L, but she had to see him professionally and socially. Sometimes she'd purposely avoid him if she saw him first in town before he saw her. He was depressing, always making her work for him specifically, instead of letting her do her job or have free time away from her work.

"How did the first day of scraped knees and bloody noses go, Nurse Lisa?"

She hated when he called her that. Years ago she had paid off her college student loans which meant she could now support her family. If she had waited for Paul to provide monetary support, they would have starved. She worked hard at her profession, and she felt he degraded it when he gave her a pet name.

"The usual number of patients, Doctor. Wayne Porter skinned his elbow in a fight, and Dexter Lowell chased two girls with his motorcycle, teasing that he was in love with them and wanted to take them riding. One of them fell, and he drove off. She isn't badly hurt, but she'll need stitches."

Damon commented, "Boys will be boys. That's why sutures and bandages were invented. I'm sure she'll turn up at my office later. Who's Dexter Lowell?"

"Aileen's son from her first marriage. He's come to Sycamore Springs to live with her at least temporarily, because he was expelled from school in Los Angeles."

Damon's face took on his most self-righteous expression. "What first marriage? Was that ever legal?"

Lisa pulled two chairs over to one of the cots in her office and gestured to Damon to sit down. "Don't judge so harshly, Dr. L. You may not know the whole story."

"I see what's in front of me, and that's enough." He sat down and crossed his arms over his belly. With a look of disdain, he peered over at the clipboard in her hands. "What's that? School business?"

"Not exactly. It's more in your territory."

He held out his hand for the information, but she ignored him. "Damon, something doesn't make sense here."

"Let me see that."

"They're only my notes. I've been at this school for a long time, and the first day is always the hardest. Not to mention that later in the week, I'll go around and ask the teachers if there were any health concerns expressed by the parents during the parent-teacher conferences. Also, as you know, one of my responsibilities is to follow up with those parents indicating any medical problems or issues that have surfaced during the summer—anything that may have some bearing on their children's behavior, performance, and general well-being." The first day had been exhausting.

"Now I bet you can appreciate the excellent training I have given you. It's because of my complete involvement in the school health program that you are so well trained. You and I carefully constructed the evaluation program in the Sycamore School district. We watch for the signals of poor health that parents often miss. Things like mental alertness, lethargy, behavior abnormalities. Any symptom that would say without words that something's wrong with our kids."

"Yes, and...." No use. He wasn't really listening. They weren't his kids anymore than they were hers. They were individuals with their own families. He wasn't supposed to make their health decisions in a dictatorial fashion.

"And other things, too, Lisa, like needle marks on the arms of older students trying to hide them with weekend tattoos, teenage pregnancy, or requests for condoms, and...."

"Damon," Lisa interrupted and grabbed his arm to make him stop. "You know I don't want to interfere in their personal lives, especially when they get to high school. Parents have to take responsibility through education and awareness. The school nurse can't do everything. I really care about all the students, and when they're so young in my kindergarten through third grade sector, then I don't mind being extra eyes and ears. Now that I'm also the nurse for the high school because of budget cutbacks, I'm getting a clearer picture of some problems we might not have thought about."

"Like what?" he broke in at the first opportunity.

"Like the mandatory immunization program and the lack of follow-up."

"What do you mean the lack of follow-up? We track these kids from their first Hepatitis B (Hep B) and Diphtheria, Tetanus, acellular Pertusis (DTaP) vaccines, *Haemophilus influenzae* type b (Hib) to the varicella vaccine, Measles, Mumps, Rubella (MMR) vaccine, inactivated poliovirus vaccine (IPV), and Pneumococcal conjugate vaccine (PCV), and Hepatitis and Meningococcal vaccines colleges often suggest."

"I know, but the Report has some disturbing inconsistencies this year."

"That's the SHOT Report that I developed," Damon said with obvious pride in his voice.

"The letters in SHOT stand for Sycamore's Health On Top."

Lisa cringed. He was so unaware of how amateurish his marketing campaign for immunizations sounded. He even had Pep tags he gave out at the game with SHOT and his name on the reverse side of cardboard hexagons that said "Go Sycamore Saints".

"Right, well, this year Sycamore's health isn't going to be exactly on top, if what I suspect is true."

Leviticus stood up straight as a ramrod, personally wounded it seemed by her comment. "My town has always been the leader in community health," he said evenly. "And I have every reason to believe that it will remain a trend setter in the welfare of body and mind of every citizen within the city limits."

Pretty rhetoric, she thought, absently flipping the pages of her notes. *Wait until he hears what I've got to say.*

Chapter 5

"Just one night, Millie."

"Brandon, stop it."

"Just one. I'm going to be drafted tomorrow. I'm going to enlist in the Peace Corps. I'm going to enter a monastery."

She laughed. "Am I supposed to pick one lie to justify sleeping with you?"

"They're not lies. They're possibilities." He grinned and cupped his hands over her shoulders, pinning her to his locker, and taking the second kiss of the afternoon from her lips.

She pushed him away, laughing. "Stop it. Possibilities are a lot different than probabilities."

He popped another breath mint into his mouth. "Here, these are wintergreen. You're supposed to feel a spark of electricity if you chew one. Maybe that'll turn you on."

The hall was deserted, and if it would have been anyone besides Brandon she might have worried for her personal safety.

"Look, Millie, it's a possibility that I love you, and it's a probability that it's true. It's a possibility that you've given me a physical problem I can't walk away from," he said, "and it's a probability you're the only one who can put me out of my misery before I'm drafted into the Peace Corps or on my way to the monastery."

She slid past him. "I don't like when you talk like that. I'm not a prude, but that doesn't make me naïve. Five percent of girls under the age of 20-years-old in this town become pregnant before they graduate high school. About 80% of these pregnancies were unintended and I don't want that to happen to me."

He caught her in his arms, leaned close. A wave of his dark hair fell in a seductive pattern over his forehead. He had gray eyes that haunted her with the hurt she knew he suffered at the hands of Leviticus. All she ever wanted to do was protect him, to ease the pain she knew he carried in his heart, but she had to curb his baser instincts when he wanted her to give up part of herself.

She wanted to laugh. He was so shallow, so sex-oriented. So normal. How did repressed parents like his ever raise a typical football playing, virgin-chasing kid?

Worse, why did she love him?

He wasn't like her at all. She was all mind, and he was all body. If they ever revealed their marriage to their parents and got their own place, how would they ever live together?

It didn't matter. She was satisfied being his wife, but not really desiring to start a family until later, when she had her college degree. How would she keep him away from her?

How would she stay away from him?

##

"Stop talking in puzzles, Lisa. What are you so secretive about? Let me see the clipboard."

"Just a minute, Damon. You can't read my notes. Let me pull them together for you. Did you know that Lindsey Fellows had shingles over the summer? He was filming a pilot in the Arizona desert, and I think the excessive heat lowered his immunity and caused him to break out in a terrible case of shingles."

Damon snorted. "Lindsey Fellows. Wait until Barbara hears about this. 'Lindsey is so fit, she's always saying,'" he said in a high-pitched voice, mimicking his wife. "'Lindsey this, Lindsey that.' I guess his immune system isn't as strong as he thought."

Damon's jealousy level rose higher than his ability to control it. He hated Lindsey, because he knew that Barbara would have preferred a life with him instead of the path she had chosen. He was convinced she thought about Lindsey more often then she thought about him. However, he consoled himself with the thought that he had structured their lives so that Barbara would be his wife and that was all there was to it. Lindsey had had shingles? Well, then. He probably hadn't taken care of himself properly. It was always the patient's fault if something went wrong with the medical blueprints of their lives. If they didn't follow through on their doctor's advice, they would not get the good outcome they expected.

Lisa shook her head. "You know that is not the entire story. Everyone who has had chickenpox is a candidate for the rest of their lives for having the latent virus reactivate as shingles. The virus hibernates or stays dormant along nerve endings, and if conditions are right, due to waning immunity or possibly stress, the virus can reactivate as shingles, often characterized by excruciating pain and leaving scars. In 20% of adults having shingles, a residual pain called post-herpetic neuralgia (PHN) can occur after the rash has disappeared."

Damon's face clouded. "Don't be telling me my business, Nurse Lisa. I know very well how shingles occurs, and that's why I came to see you today. Not because some fitness trainer got shingles, but because no other kid in the world is ever going to get chickenpox. There's a vaccine now, and we're going to promote it. If Lindsey never had chickenpox, he never would have gotten shingles, right?"

"Possibly." She wouldn't give him more than that. She knew the fact that Varivax® was an attenuated or weakened live-virus vaccine. This allowed for the possibility that vaccinees could reactivate with shingles—just as those having a history of the natural wild-type chickenpox could do so. However, preliminary data suggested that the risk of shingles among vaccinees was lower than those having a history of natural chickenpox. She had Craig's research, and that's what mattered, because Craig looked objectively at all health issues. He never made hasty conclusions on the basis of superficial or surface findings; he took great pains to try to understand the biological mechanisms involved that explained the observed trends in the data.

"Don't show your ignorance, my dear. Varicella is the primary disease caused by the varicella-zoster virus (VZV). After a period of latency, usually when an adult is 50 or 60 years old, the secondary disease, herpes-zoster,[19] occurs. Herpes-zoster is suppressed so long as the body boosts itself by the internal mechanism known as asymptomatic endogenous reactivation. In simple language, when the body's immunities decline below a certain

[19] Hepers zoster is commonly known as shingles.

threshold, the immune system senses this low level and automatically and internally boosts itself back up to a protective level. Since there are no discernable symptoms that this boost has occurred, this reactivation is referred to a being asymptomatic."

"What if that's not all that's involved? What if there is another *outside* boosting mechanism that occurs each time an adult is exposed to a child with chickenpox. What if such an exogenous or outside exposure plays a significant role in boosting immunity to help suppress the reactivation of shingles?"

Damon jumped to his feet. "Are you questioning me?" he thundered.

Lisa felt a spark of anger start in her shoes and shoot up her spine. "Yes, doctor," she said quietly, in contrast to him, hoping he'd be calm if she kept her composure. She had information that could seriously impact the health of the town that trusted her. If she lost her temper, more people would be hurt. The citizens relied on people like her and Craig, even Millie, to investigate and speak the truth.

"You have no right," he said, ready to burst. "I can have your job."

Damon was not an attractive man, but when he became angry, he crossed the line into disturbingly ugly.

"No, Damon, you can't. I'm an employee of the District. You'd have to bring evidence that I haven't done my job properly, and you don't have that evidence. I, however, have observations that question the reasonableness of your interventions."

Pure fire shot from Damon's eyes, and Lisa wondered if she'd gone too far. She had never defied him openly before, but this time she had overwhelming evidence that he was wrong.

"I'll deal with you later," he said tensely, turned, and walked out.

##

"I hear you've got a house guest." Barbara hugged Aileen outside Nails For All.

The strip mall was crowded with small-town women who spent their spare time getting a manicure and pedicure instead of exercising or watching what they ate. As a result, they were well groomed but in poor health. Barbara could spend hours watching them back and forth in between beauty salons and take-out food. Somehow, it never made sense. She'd once mentioned it to Aileen and had been rewarded with a shrill laugh and some advice. Aileen had told her, "Never comment on another woman's appearance or personal habits. She won't change, and she'll probably say more to you about your inadequacies than you could ever devise about hers."

Yet, other women appeared to be happy with their lives. They grew up, got married, and seemed to thrive. What filled her life with despair? Being married to a despot? Brandon was the only shining light in her existence.

"Until Dexter can find his own apartment, for now he's staying with me. His father has a new girlfriend. They don't want him around. His father never wanted him in the first place."

Barbara opened the sliding door, and the cleansing power of artificially cold air hit her summer skin. Another change of seasons, yet nothing changed in Sycamore. The atmosphere outside always seemed parched to her. People were distant, never friendly. She assumed it was because she was the wife of a man who brought disguised hurt to the community. On the surface what Damon said seemed like a good idea, but once people peeled away the layers, they found that his advice always benefited him financially, but rarely, probably accidentally, did it have any good effect on them.

"Good and bad news, I suppose," Barbara surmised, flopping into a comfy chair in the waiting area after signing them both in. They'd have to wait, but she was glad about that. Nothing much to do in town. She was too intelligent to match the slow living pace, and too impatient to try.

"No, it's good and good. I've got Dexter, and some nameless slut has Mr. Deadbeat Dad." She laughed and made herself comfortable. Aileen had the knack of being at ease in any situation. She could triumph no matter what was going on around her.

"Why did the court ever give the father custody in your case?" That had always puzzled her. Aileen was an honest, careful woman. There was nothing bad about her – no drinking, no drugs, no problems, except one.

"Because I have more problems than the father." Aileen admitted taking the seat next to Barbara. "I like men. The Dad likes women, but he'll stay with them long enough to get tired of their cooking."

Aileen was restless, and that made her look undependable. Nothing was further from the truth. Barbara could rely on her for anything, day or night.

Yet, so many years of knowing each other, and Aileen had never told her the name of Dexter's father. Barbara had the feeling it wasn't that Aileen was being evasive. She simply didn't care. As long as Dexter was healthy, what difference did it make who the father was? As far as Barbara was concerned, it was okay that Aileen had left the man nameless.

"When was the last time you and Damon were intimate with each other?" Aileen had once asked.

When faced with that question, Barbara had changed the subject. She'd long forgotten. Damon was not a loving man. He was selfish, conceited, and hardly romantic. He didn't understand how there could possibly be more happiness in giving than there is in receiving.

"I guess you and Dexter's father weren't meant to be together."

Aileen shook her head. "I don't think that at all. Anybody can stay together. No reason to give them an award. Men stay for the same reasons they got married in the first place – sex, cooking, a younger version of Mom, and public opinion. No man wants to be the object of ridicule by his peers. They want approval, and what better way to attain it than to have tangible representations of their social status, like an advanced degree or a complacent wife. What person, husband or wife, wants a spouse who points out his shortcomings? Men, especially, leave immediately if they can't be heroes to their wives, but what if their friends and colleagues are watching? Then they stay, telling themselves that what goes on in their own lives is private, and they're content with that, as long as they can hold their heads high in the community."

She was right about that. Barbara could recount numerous occasions where Damon would have walked out on her, but she knew he couldn't have done that. He had a reputation to uphold, along with a strict set of public values. He wanted to be a hero to his patients. He probably knew that she no longer respected him, and he may have even drawn the conclusion that she never had, but to him it didn't matter. He had taken a young woman in matrimony and turned her into the prototype of a doctor's wife. That was all that was important to him.

Barbara was jolted out of her thoughts by a puzzled look on Aileen's face. Aileen's eyes made a nondescript color by a bold shade of contact lenses, stared directly at Barbara, which was unusual in their conversations. Most of the time, Aileen's attention wandered around the room, checking out the nosey details that gave her a daily dose of gossip. Frozen, unmoving in ever detail, she looked like a mannequin with her dyed red hair in a dated bouffant, welded in place by hairspray.

She cleared her throat in an attention-getting move. "I saw Damon leaving Lisa's office when I picked up Dexter after his mishap. Aren't you worried he might be fooling around?"

Barbara gasped. What an unexpected thing for Aileen to say. She knew that her friend boasted a never-ending series of men in her collection. Perhaps she could spot a fellow philanderer? How humiliating that would be for her. "What makes you say that?"

"Well," Aileen began and unwrapped a generic mint from the bowl of stale customer treats at the edge of the Salon's reception counter, "Maybe Lisa gets lonely."

She did. Barbara knew that, because she and Lisa showed up at every community event and enrichment class in town every night of the week.

Lisa was the last to leave these activities. Did that mean she was cheating on her husband, getting even with him for his own philandering ways?

"Even if she did get lonely, it wouldn't mean she was with a man other than her husband. Surely, she could find something else to occupy her time. She's got her work to keep her company. She really loves the school children, like they'd be an extension of her own family. She spends more hours concerned about their health and well being than any other nurse, from the school district or not, in town. Remember last year during the chickenpox epidemic when too many parents just couldn't afford to take time off from work to stay home with their young children? Lisa asked for and was granted time off from the district to care for the children of these families at her home in a sort of make-shift infirmary. She and her children had already had the chickenpox the previous year. That's dedication for you."

"I know. I remember that. She was written up in the paper for her efforts. But what about her personal life? She can't be a nurse twenty-four hours a day, can she?"

Barbara shrugged. "I'm not so sure she can't. Damon is a doctor twenty-four hours a day. Some people become their professions, as in a marriage, for better or worse." In Lisa's case it was for the better, but in Damon's case it was indisputably for the worse.

Aileen looked at the clock, bored with any conversation that was not about her. So Lisa was dedicated—big deal. So she was intelligent—even less of a deal. What difference did it make in the long run if Lisa helped a family with chickenpox? It didn't matter, and she'd like to tell Barbara why, but she didn't think her friend had evolved to a great enough degree in her dealings with the world to understand the truth.

Evil always won.

Lisa could set up cots to cover her entire home. She could spoon-feed each child chicken soup until it came out of their ears, but it wouldn't change the facts. If evil people were the reason and the intention from the beginning, then what possible chance did good people have to change what had been set into motion? Didn't wise Solomon write, "That which is made crooked cannot be made straight, and that which is wanting cannot possibly be counted."[20]

Everyone in town thought Aileen was all body and no brains, but Aileen knew differently. She'd learned to hide her intelligence to get what she wanted from the establishment, the powers in power. What good could she do? None. So, why try?

Aileen was aware of Craig's studies, and if she were any judge of character and men, and she knew she was the best judge in Sycamore Springs because of and also despite her experience with men, Craig was dedicated to his profession. He was honest and had nothing to gain personally from his work. From the gossip, she'd heard that he'd observed some shocking trends in the medical community concerning vaccinations, and she'd bet her alimony that he was correct.

But what could she do about it? Nothing. Darned if she tried, and darned if she didn't. She had taken Dexter for his mandated inoculations before she learned that she could have legally complied by filing a religious or philosophical exemption. In California, that meant simply signing a statement on the reverse side of the child's immunization record. While both the school and medical authorities knew this exemption existed, they were not under any obligation to inform the parents of this legal provision. No one had the right to tell her she had to pump her son full of dangerous biological substances in vaccines, all of which carried some undisclosed adverse health risk. No one could be totally certain of any given vaccine's safety and she did not for a minute trust the FDA report stating "there has never been a 'hot lot' or a contaminated batch of vaccines in the United States." Dexter seemed healthy, and she was grateful, but very sad for the families whose sons or daughters had died or experienced late-onset autism or other neurological developmental problems because of the positive propaganda that the shots were completely safe and the diseases they protected against were more of a risk than the vaccines themselves.

It depended on whose bull was being gored, she assumed. If children were fortunate enough to avoid vaccines with Thimerosal—such as the flu vaccine, Hep B, as well as other vaccines utilizing this mercury "preservative", then she still doubted the risk was worth it; but

[20] Ecclesiastes 1:15

at least these children had a reduced risk of experiencing adverse reactions or experiencing a dysregulation of their immune systems attributed to the Thimerosal.[21]

She shuddered thinking about the other possibilities. What if the vaccinated child had been given a Thimerosal-containing shot such that the child suffered a needless death or experienced a severe adverse reaction leading to a tragic life just to add funds to the medical community?

She knew the truth, that doctors, schools, regulatory agencies, watch-dog agencies, and everyone involved, from the onset of the production of the vaccine to its stab into the flesh of trusting people, got a kick-back, a portion of the money in some way, usually out and out cash or funding stemming from the Federally-funded Vaccines for Children (VFC) program that provided reimbursement to physicians who administered each and every vaccine specified in the childhood immunization schedule to qualified children. If one parent refused to let their infant, toddler, or child be a victim, then everyone involved had less money in their pockets. What a racket. The tragedy was that lives were lost everyday, beautiful and promising lives of people who had every right to live, because of the vicious deceit and outright lies concerning safety studies indoctrinated into the medical profession and sometimes flagrantly manipulated by the pharmaceutical companies themselves.

Aileen felt her heart beating too hard in her chest. Why was she getting so worked up? Hadn't she promised herself long ago she wasn't going to get involved anymore? She already knew too much concerning the corruption and greed in the medical field. Aileen's sharp mind could recall a flood of examples. One case that especially stood out was how Dr. Andrew Mosholder of the FDA had discovered a link between use of some antidepressant drugs and child suicides. The FDA management disagreed with his findings presented in a February 2004 meeting and they cancelled Dr. Mosholder's presentation to the advisory committee. Dr. Mosholder's findings were suppressed by the FDA, but were proven correct months later. Aileen also recalled that the findings of another FDA scientist, Dr. David Graham, were stonewalled following his discovery of an increased risk of heart attacks and strokes in patients taking Vioxx®. Aileen reflected on the courage of these two individuals from the FDA who reminded her of Craig Manchester. She thought of the guts it must take for honest scientists to go against their supervisors, possibly undermining their careers. It would take many more individuals with their courage to achieve any improvement in public health. In the meantime, she felt discouraged and downhearted knowing these individuals would be treated with disrespect because they were guilty of being committed to telling the truth. She had firsthand experience of Solomon's words, "... so that he that increases knowledge increases pain."[22]

Let people think she was mindless. It was better than the truth.

---

[21] Mutkus L, Aschner JL, Syversen T, Shanker G, Sonnewald U, Ashner M. Department of Physiology and Pharmacology, Wake Forest University School of Medicine, Winston-Salem, NC 27157-1083. In vitro uptake of glutamate in GLAST- and GLT-1-transfected mutant CHO-K1 cells is inhibited by the ethylmercury-containing preservative Thimerosal. Biol Trace Elem Res. 2005 Summer;105(1-3):71-86.

[22] Ecclesiastes 1:18

She had been a doctor's wife.

Dexter's father had been a prominent physician working with the pharmaceutical companies. She knew the insider treachery he perpetrated. That's why she left him. That's why the courts gave her doctor ex-husband custody, because he had the supposed prestige of his seriously flawed profession shine as a blinding light in the judge's eyes.

He was a flawed doctor, a flawed husband, a flawed father, and a flawed man.

Aileen sat back and took a few breaths, hoping to calm down. She still felt helpless in the face of the life-taking and hideous misuse of power that the medical, pharmaceutical, and legal professions got away with. Someone had to stop them. Only occasional bursts of public outcry had a chance, if they resulted in people simply not going along with the deceitful scams. Only an informed public boycott of deceitful practices could bring about their eradication and ultimately improve pharmaceutical drug and vaccine safety. Aileen subscribed to the futuristic thinking espoused by the inventor Thomas Edison, "The doctor of the future will give no medicine, but will interest his patients in the care of the human frame, in diet, and in the cause and prevention of disease."

She sighed. She had to remember she was getting her nails done with the unenlightened wife of yet another selfish man. She better think in smaller words so she doesn't give herself away. Someday she and Barbara might be able to meet on more common ground, but at the moment, the only thing they had in common was the ultimate manicuring experience at Sycamore Springs' finest, and only, nail salon.

Chapter 6

"I'm glad you're home, Brandon. I want to talk to you."

"Dad, I'm busy." Brandon paused on the stairs and looked toward the landing. "Millie's waiting. We're going to do our homework together, and we want to get an early start."

Damon shook his head and stood his ground, as usual. "You can't fool me. No one does homework on the first day back from summer vacation. You must have something else planned, and whatever it is, it can wait. I have something to tell you."

Caught. He'd be in for at least an hour of haranguing and argument. No use trying to slip out the door. "I guess I have a few minutes, if it can't wait."

"It can't. I've always had all the time in the world for you," Damon said self-righteously, wounded.

Where did he get an idea like that? Brandon knew he couldn't remember a single instance when he'd had his father's undivided attention. Too bad he didn't get in and out of the house without being seen. He knew his father would only remember his own side of the conversation, and not a word of whatever he himself had to say.

"What is it, Dad?" His father was dressed in his Saturday clothes, a combination of golf course and studied day-off attire. His slacks and collared shirt belonged on the links, but his Eastern school loafers set him apart as an uncoordinated misfit in his attempt at a social life, his need to fit in with the common herd.

"Sit, Brandon, and listen. I have a new project for Sycamore, and I know you'll be interested in it."

Why? I've never been interested in anything you've done before.

"It's innovative, yet tried and true. It's new to the city, but not to the medical community. You'll be impressed, I know it."

Damon opened the window shades and let a blast of late summer sun into the stale room.

Why does this house smell like a doctor's office, full of chemicals and depression? Brandon thought, trying to decrease his lung capacity.

"What's your project?" he asked, knowing he couldn't rush Dr. L. His father had his own agenda, no matter who was inconvenienced. He thought his career made him knowledgeable, when it only made him undesirable except to his own kind.

Damon paused and looked through Brandon.

I'm over here, Dad, he wanted to say.

"Son," he began with a word as a father he didn't understand. He just as well could have called him stranger.

"Son," he repeated. "This is my idea."

Brandon wanted to bolt. "Which is?"

"I'm going to save Sycamore Springs from its annual epidemics, and when we have significantly reduced morbidity and mortality of disease in this town, I'm going to save the world."

"From?"

"Chickenpox."

Great, more interference by man. More assault on the balance of immunity naturally occurring in the present community. He paid just enough attention in Old Man Wilkes' class to learn enough about science to stay out of its way. He didn't get a good feeling about this.

"That's great, Dad. I gotta go."

"Not yet. Don't you want to know how I'm going to do it? How you're going to play a major role?"

"No." How many months had he been of age? How many more years was he going to be used a pawn for his father's excessive, worthless heroism?

Damon's face clouded up, and his eyes turned to familiar slits of anger. His breathing became erratic, and Brandon could hear his breath rattle in his lungs. "How dare you defy me. I've given you everything you've ever wanted."

Brandon felt the bile rising into his throat as his stomach constricted with unspoken anger. He had been reaching a level of high anxiety faster as he got older. Yet, each time, he had to tamp it all down, make it fit into the tiny storage compartment his pride had become. What had his father done to him, and why was he even more unable to control his feelings?

If he could be honest with his mother, he might ask her, but, as is, he only had his own thoughts as his guide. He hated his father, but it wasn't yet the right time to do anything about it. When he had a son one day, he would be the best dad in the world. He'd never yell, he'd never administer harsh punishment in anger. He'd encourage and love.

"You certainly have not, Dad," Brandon muttered, wondering if he could make it to the door before his father could stop him, wondering if he could get to the safety of Millie's arms before he exploded with the pressure building in his throat. He had never openly defied his father. What would happen if he did?

The rattle again. "What did you say? Are you talking under your breath so I can't hear you? You know how I have to know everything that goes on, because you and your mother are too weak to think or act for yourselves."

Brandon's heart rate doubled in the space of a few seconds. His anxiety was out of control. He had to get out. He felt impending doom, and it had his father's name all over it.

To shake himself back under control, he swore softly.

Damon closed the distance between them in an instant, grabbed him by his shoulder blades, and shook him. "How dare you curse in front of me, you whelp."

Brandon jumped to his feet, his legs shaking and his arms weak. "I've heard you curse when you don't think anyone hears you."

"You dare to defy me, your father?"

"I've heard you defy anyone too vulnerable to leave your office under their own power. You've never been a father to me. The only time I hear from you is when you want to bully me, to use me for one of your community experiments. Other times, you hide in your office like the coward you are. If your sick patients could fight back, they'd have you six feet under by now instead of them. I won't be part of any more of your projects. Because of you, I've had enough needles, medications, and x-rays to make me sick for the rest of my life."

He shot past him, intent on the front door, but Damon was faster and tackled him roughly by tugging furiously on his arms and pulling him down. "Where are you going, young man? To your little mousey girlfriend?" he said venomously.

Brandon shoved his father's hands off him. "Wrong, Dad. You don't know the first thing about my relationship with Millie? You're completely wrong. Shows you how much you know."

"You're an irresponsible idiot," Damon shouted.

"You think so? Well, just watch me, now. It's time for someone in this house to set the standard for 'good father', and I can see that person is going to be me."

"You dare to…."

Brandon yanked open the door and slammed it back against the foyer wall. He heard the crystal shudder in the breakfront, a fitting pretense for the phoniness that went on in the entire house.

"Good night, Doctor."

Chapter 7

"Great night for crickets," Millie said snuggling down in the front seat. The air was clear, and she could hear their sweet song in the evening breezes.

The park was empty except for them. Where was everybody? She'd heard vague rumors of a boondocker, and she assumed the entire high school had left the city limits in search of privacy.

Nothing could be more secluded than the farthest parking space by the thicket of trees. No one could see them, and no one could hear them. They'd parked there many times and listened to music or talked about nothing at all. Brandon would steal a kiss, she'd pretend he'd gone too far, he'd kiss her again, and she'd put a stop to it. That was about it. Would tonight be different?

Brandon played with a strand of her hair that he'd pulled loose from her usual bun and arranged it around her shoulders for a change. He thought he had never seen her more beautiful. Her eyes sparkled. She was young and fresh, clean and new. She didn't have the smell of intolerance and the sound of ignorance. Her soft skin felt like velvet under his fingertips. Here was the one woman he wanted by his side for the rest of his life.

Why was he attracted to her beyond the physical? Easy. She was the opposite of his parents. She questioned, she didn't accept. Damon embraced his profession with absolute faith, and Barbara stayed in a marriage, which was loveless to even the most casual onlooker, with complete resignation.

But Millie. What fire, what passion she had for the truth.

She'd never lie to him. She'd always fight for him.

And she'd love him until the day he died, just as she had stated in the wedding vows on the day they were married..

"Great night for a lot of things," he whispered, watching her pulse flutter under the pale skin of her neck. He pressed his lips to her ear. "I have a theory," he whispered, inhaling the scent of the jasmine cologne she wore.

"Does it have to do with football?" she asked, kidding, but he heard the catch in her breath. He could get to her, as innocent as she was, he could make her lose her train of thought on that repressed locomotive of academics she allowed in her on-the-track intelligent mind.

"Kind of. It has to do with touchdowns."

She giggled. "In the end zone?"

Got him. Okay, so she maybe wasn't as naïve as he thought. All the better.

Millie heard her own quiet laughter ring though the car and fill the empty park with life. Sycamore Springs had many lover's lanes, mostly out in the boondocks on the way to Los Angeles, except for a few choice local places in City Park under a grove of trees that the city kept watered even in the heat, courtesy of Dr. L and his Park Project. That man had more projects going than the rest of the citizens put together. Most people thought that he was a great humanitarian and a fine citizen because of them, but she had her own opinions of him.

As far as she was concerned, he was an excessive blow-hard who never saw the forest of despair of others for the well-watered trees he perpetuated for himself.

"Brandon, this isn't a good idea. You know I want to wait. It's getting late, and it's time we started back to my house."

"You know what they say about time. It's relative."

She squirmed, wanting to push him away, wanting to pull him closer. "That's not exactly the Theory of Relativity."

"Sure it is. I'm no Einstein, but I bet he developed his ideas sitting in the moonlight with a beautiful woman."

She shook her head. "Of course he didn't. Einstein's work had to do with physics."

"Exactly, physical stuff, just like I said. His level of passion was directly proportional to the time he spent next to his girl friend."

"You're wrong," she managed to say, adroitly avoiding a perfectly placed kiss.

"Discredit me. Prove me wrong, that the longer I sit here is inversely proportional to the amount of love I feel for you."

He was such a contradiction—a jock on the football field, a leech in the park, and a hurt and lonely man desperately trying to keep from being like his father. His intelligence frequently surfaced when he tried to hide it the most, in a joke or a political statement.

She better reply in kind. He had a look in his troubled eyes she hadn't seen before.

He needed her.

In more ways than the physical.

"You know what Einstein said?" she asked.

"Tell me," he answered softly, watching her mouth, waiting for the love he knew she had for him.

"After he read a book of essays written in the 1930s by physicists in Germany who wanted to debunk his Theory of Relativity," she said, "Were my theory wrong, it would have taken but one person to show it."

Brandon muttered something under his breath and moved away.

"What's the matter? Do you disagree with Einstein's remark?"

"Stop it, Millie. Why do you always sound like a professor? Couldn't you be a woman first and a journalist, or a teacher, or whatever it is you want to be, later, for once in your life? I don't want to make love to a news anchor. I want to make love to a real flesh and blood woman. For the first time since I met you in the second grade, would you please let me take the lead?" His eyes blazed fire, his chest moved up and down with the emotion he tried to contain.

Stung, Millie pulled the rest of the way out of his arms and huddled by the door. "Sorry, I thought you knew how much getting to the truth means to me. I have lots of quotes that inspire me to do what I want with my life. I didn't know that bothered you." She had to keep calm to recognize him when he was upset. Only his father could alter his sense of reality to such a degree.

"You're so smart, Millie, the only person in town smarter than I am. Am I the one you want to discredit? Are you going to prove me wrong?

"In this car, tonight?"

"No, in this town, tomorrow and next month and next year."

"What are you talking about, Brandon? I thought you were trying to have sex with me, the way
you do every time we're alone."

"You're wrong, tonight. I wanted something more."

She blinked.

"Millie, I wanted you to tell me that you love me, and that we have a future together, and that we're going to make Sycamore Springs take note of a beautiful reporter and football player who is just as important off the field as on, no matter what the reputation of his father."

Brandon's words echoed in her ears. So that's what it was about again. His pride. What had his father done to him this time?

"Was Dr. Leviticus home when we stopped at your house."

"Yeah."

"Did you talk to him?"

"Yeah."

Oh, no. One word answers. She hated it when his father stole his resolve. Thank heavens her parents never did that to her.

"Whatever he said, he isn't right, you know," she said softly.

"I know that. But he thinks he is, so he is."

She snorted. "That's ridiculous. That would make every lunatic on the face of the earth right."

"They are." Brandon continued, "That's what's wrong with the system, and that's why you'll never be able to stop it, no matter how many noble women and men you quote."

"You're saying that the person spouting off decides if he's right or wrong? Not the community? Not the collective good?"

He was going to lose his temper with her, and that was something he didn't want to do. "What is this 'collective good' you're always talking about? Good isn't collective. Evil is. Evil runs in packs, because evil is a coward. Good is solitary and lonely and hides in the beaten hearts of do-gooders like you. When are you going to admit you don't have a chance against them. They've been evil longer than you've been good. They have a methodology you couldn't begin to understand. They have a jargon all their own, and funding all their own, and rules all their own. You don't have the table stakes, sweetheart."

Poor man, even his own family didn't support his views. They didn't have to agree, but they didn't have to make it seem as if he was so alone.

He brought out the earth mother in her. What was she going to do? She wanted him to know that she championed his ideas, not only because she cared so deeply for him, but because he was right.

She had to do something. He looked completely lost this time. What if she couldn't get him back to the Brandon of common sense, and he remained a man caught in self-doubt?

She loved him so. Oh, well. There was one thing she could do that would prove to him that she believed in him when no one else did. Millie slowly opened her purse and, knowing exactly where to look, reached two fingers inside and withdrew a small foil packet. It felt shiny and unfamiliar in her hand. "Millie," Brandon said on a gasp. "What have you been thinking about?" The surprise on his face shone in the moonlight. His eyes bore into hers with an intensity of pleading she hadn't seen before. He genuinely needed her, and that would be her undoing.

"I've been thinking about us. About you. I don't want to have a baby when I'm still a child myself. I bought these a few months ago just before we married."

He moved closer to her in the dark with awe in his heart and reverence in his fingertips as he touched the soft swells of her body. She shuddered with desire, sinking into his embrace.

"But why tonight, sweetheart?" he murmured, his warm lips over hers.

"Because you need me, and I love you," she answered, tasting him, reassuring him with her worried kiss.

##

Brandon dropped the unopened condom on the floor of the car as he eased away from Millie's spent body.

No use telling her he hadn't even bothered to open the packet. She'd find out soon enough.

If he'd been successful in giving her a baby, he figured she'd be furious with him at first, but then she'd understand that it wasn't a manipulation at all. It had been for her own good.

Okay, his own good, but she said she loved him many times, especially a few minutes before when he hesitated briefly, poised and nearly out of control.

Had she realized he didn't use the condom? Probably not. She didn't seem to notice. She'd been too caught up in the modesty he knew she possessed to be aware of the details.

Her soft cries of arousal had made him feel guilty. They had always previously used protection. But then the most disturbing of events had kept him steady on his course of action.

He'd heard his father's voice mocking him again, stealing his coming of age ritual even in the privacy of a car with steamed up windows in the middle of a deserted park.

If I stop now, he'd thought, my father wins. But if I carry through in at least this one act of love, then I win.

He hoped it would be a boy.

Chapter 8

"Mrs. Christiann, I'm here for our appointment about my thesis."

Lisa turned toward her, a fist load of plastic bandages in her hand. "Millie, you're very punctual, as usual. Please call me Lisa. I've collected more of the data you're going to need to analyze and also have some additional references that may be applicable. Did I ever tell you about the time I had gathered more medical literature references than anyone else in nursing school? Of course, I couldn't use all of them in the various papers I wrote, but the research experience I gained was invaluable."

Millie smiled and kept nodding. Lisa loved to talk. She'd heard that her husband never listened to her, so that was probably the reason.

"I appreciate your help with my paper," she said when Lisa stopped to catch her breath. "It's about incidence rates and statistics reported in epidemiological studies. I've been able to formulate a concise discussion of the historical background; however, there is one particular study that reports shingles incidence that presently makes no sense to me. I know I can ask my father any time. He's always willing to help me, but this time I want to try to work through the project on my own, completing the sections concerning the methodology, data, analyses, discussion and conclusions. Then I will ask him for his input to make certain I have everything clearly stated and properly formatted. I want him to be proud of me."

Lisa nodded. "I know he's already proud of you. He's always telling me how diligent and trustworthy you are; how you go to whatever lengths are necessary to insure a good job. How can I help you?"

"As I mentioned earlier, there is a specific shingles study authored by a local health department in cooperation with the CDC that I just can't seem to understand. I have the reference right here in my notes.[23] Here is a copy of the abstract."

"Yes, I am familiar with that abstract—your father has cited this in his research. Did you have a specific question about the reported incidence figures?"

"Yes, the problem seems to be that the CDC is reporting a shingles rate of 40 cases per 100,000 among children aged less than 10 years and a rate of 45 cases per 100,000 among individuals aged 10 to 19 years."

"I see your point Millie, the rates are nearly the same, differing by only 5 cases per 100,000."

"That is precisely what does not make sense to me. At least 80% or more of the children under the age of 10 years have been vaccinated in the study population, while virtually none of the 10 to 19 year-olds have been vaccinated. Shouldn't the rate of shingles be much lower among the vaccinated children compared to the rate in the older individuals—the majority of whom have had previous histories of natural chickenpox? In other words, based on earlier reports promoting varicella vaccination, should we not expect a much lower

---

[23] Civen RH, Maupin TJ, Xiao HL, Seward JF, Jumaan AO, Mascola L. A population-based study of herpes zoster (HZ) in children and adolescents post-varicella vaccine licensure 2000-2003. In: Proceedings of the 38th National Immunization Conference of CDC, Nashville, TN, May 11, 2004, Abstract #5427

rate of shingles among those who received the varicella vaccine relative to those who had a history of the natural disease? I just can't comprehend why these reported shingles rates are so similar among these two different age groups—the majority in the younger group having received the varicella vaccine and most all in the older group having had natural varicella?"

"Millie, this particular study is really no different from many other studies that have a predetermined agenda to present selective data in such a way so as to promote high vaccination rates and the associated monetary enrichment. While Dr. Leviticus often quotes these figures as the gospel truth, in reality they represent little more than positive propaganda that is disguised as pseudo-science. In this study, it appears the presentation of data has been carefully manipulated to mask the surfacing of flawed assumptions underlying the Universal Varicella Vaccination Program. Statistical methods have been applied in an erroneous manner leading to meaningless results and flawed conclusions. Failure to apply capture-recapture methods to adjust the incidence figures for under-reporting of cases is also another pertinent factor leading to grossly underestimated shingles incidence rates in the community. So multiple issues are involved here. Let's address them one at a time."

"I am glad you have the insight to sort out the issues here. Lisa, please, go slowly so I may add explanatory information to my notes.

"First, let me tell you that in Sycamore Springs, prior to licensure of the varicella vaccine, students normally contracted chickenpox upon school entry, around 5 years old. Shingles was relatively rare in children aged less than 5-years—since susceptible children are not candidates for shingles. Presently, however, all children at the age of 12-months are administered the chickenpox vaccine, so they harbor the attenuated live varicella-zoster virus that can later reactivate as shingles."

"Lisa, I think I understand… 1-year-olds now have been exposed to chickenpox through the universal varicella vaccination program, and any of these children that subsequently reactivate shingles within the next 4 years would contribute to a higher burden of shingles disease than existed previously in the less than 5 age group. The reason for this is that prior to the vaccine, there were many children in this age group that simply were not candidates for developing shingles since they had never had natural chickenpox."

"Your comprehension of this point is excellent."

"Thank you."

"Next, let's specifically look at the shingles rate that the CDC reports as 40 cases per 100,000 among children less than 10. This figure is meaningless since it represents the average or mean rate of shingles among the vaccinated children as well as among those who did not receive the varicella vaccination due to their previous history of natural chickenpox. If early reports are correct, we would expect a low shingles rate of about 18 cases per 100,000 among the majority of vaccinated children. Upon closer inspection, Craig has verified that the shingles rate is approaching 300 to 400 cases per 100,000 among those children who were not vaccinated due to their history of natural chickenpox."

"Lisa, isn't this the preliminary finding that worries my father and other researchers? That the rate of shingles among those children with a history of natural chickenpox is approaching the rate in older adults? This finding would tend to support the hypothesis that children previously received boosts to their immune system each time they were exposed to other children with active cases of chickenpox. These exposures helped to postpone reactivation of the latent varicella-zoster virus as shingles."

"Yes, you are right. And if the exposures to natural chickenpox helped children to suppress the reactivation of shingles, it is worrisome if the same boosting mechanism were true for adults as well. Craig has already seen one recent report from the CDC where a 90% increase in adult shingles has been reported from 1998 to 2003 during a time of increasing varicella vaccination. There also appears to be a statistically significant increase in cases of adult shingles from 200 to 2002 reported by the Varicella Active Surveillance Project (VASP)."

"Lisa, that seems logical—as cases of chickenpox have dramatically declined due to the universal varicella vaccination program, the potential exposures that previously boosted the immunity of children and adults has also declined."

"Getting back to the initial issue you raised—the fact that such a wide variation in shingles rates exists among vaccinated and unvaccinated children, it does not make sense to simply average both cohorts and report a single incidence rate. This is a misapplication of statistical methods when working with what is called a 'bimodal distribution'. Such averaging is misleading and reflects the rate of neither group well."

"Yes, I understand. My dad frequently talks about the need to stratify results according to vaccination status; otherwise the true trends can be masked. Lisa, what about this anomally that the incidence rate CDC reports in the older group (10 to 19), the majority of whom have had natural chickenpox, is similar to that reported among vaccinated children less than 10?

"Again, what the CDC has reported is a meaningless incidence rate that assumes 100% of all cases were reported to the VASP."

"Lisa, isn't that assumption almost always wrong? A study usually never achieves a complete count of all cases."

"Millie, again you are correct. Especially since the cases are reported voluntarily to the project, any shingles incidence rates computed, merely reflect the level of reporting completeness and are not the true incidence rates."

"Is this where capture-recapture techniques can be used to perform ascertainment correction, where there is a calculated adjustment of the number of shingles cases based on the level of under-reporting?"

"I see you have done your research well. Yes, it only makes sense to 'ascertainment correct' and adjust the reported counts of shingles cases so as to compensate for the percentage of under-reporting that is unique to the study. If all studies performed a capture-recapture analysis, then shingles rates could be compared across the different studies, regardless of the level of reporting completeness associated with each study. While capture-recapture does not produce exact rates, the options are (1) not to use capture-recapture and report shingles incidence rates that are uninterpretable, (2) try to count every case of shingles which is horrendously expensive and slow, or (3) utilize capture-recapture which, depending on the degree to which the assumptions are satisfied, can be a compromise, reasonably accurate, quick, and inexpensive approach."

"So, then, if capture-recapture were applied to the number of reported shingles cases, incidence rate figures estimated by the CDC could be compared with rates reported in other studies having nearly complete ascertainment of cases."

"Yes, Millie, that is correct. So if there was 50% under-reporting in these age groups as your father determined, which is typical of cases collected via active surveillance, doubling the reported rates should yield a closer estimate to the true rates in the community."

Having addressed the issues at hand, Lisa settled back in her chair.

"Thank you so much for helping me understand the confounding issues here."

"Millie, are you familiar with the principle of challenge-rechallenge. If a child is given a vaccine, and …."

Millie stared at her. She had never seen Lisa agitated before, no matter if she were lecturing an auditorium filled with high school seniors about the proper use of contraceptives, or applying direct pressure to a six-year-old's injuries before the paramedics arrived. When Millie had asked Lisa how she kept control, Lisa had replied that her training helped, but it was also her belief that others in her profession were skilled as well, and everything would be done in a logical and reasonable order to help the situation. What was bothering her about the chickenpox vaccine?

"Has something new developed?" she asked, ready to take additional notes.

Lisa shifted restlessly in her official chair. "Babies are generally born healthy to healthy parents. But from the age of one day, which is really only a few hours out the womb, the assault on every baby's tiny body begins. The Hep B vaccination is the first of some thirty shots[24] the infant will receive prior to school age. Not only do infants have to adjust to the basics of hot, cold, and sleeping through the lonely night, they have to cope with the preservatives and heavy metals in the shots, all of which are toxic or proven deadly in certain quantities. Add to this the fact that a certain low percentage of vaccines may become contaminated during the vaccine's preparation and administration or through some other human error in the manufacturing process. Some infants are bound to get sick and the sad part is there is currently no way to prescreen to see which children will or will not experience an adverse reaction."

"I know you're an honest person, Mrs. Christiann, and I can see that uncertainty about safety really bothers you. You've been a nurse for a long time in Sycamore, and people trust you. I trust you. Is their anything I can do to help? You seem worried."

Lisa took a shallow breath. It was all the oxygen she could force into her overstressed body. Yes, something was wrong, and maybe Millie was the person to help find out exactly what was happening.

---

[24] Counting MMR and DTaP which each contain 3 different components as one shot, and including the yearly influenza vaccine.

"Can I trust you?" Lisa asked quietly, without leaning closer until she was sure. "You can't tell anyone about this. I tried to tell Damon Leviticus, but he got furious at me. He can't be challenged, even if he's wrong. He's setting something up, and it's going to hurt a lot of people."

"On purpose?"

"No, his only intentional crime is excessive pride, but that trait makes him unreachable."

"You can trust me, Mrs. Christiann. You've been my friend since I started grade school."

Lisa couldn't smile, even at the instant memory of a scared little girl instead of the poised woman sitting in her office. "Then it's Lisa, because we're going to have a lot of work to do."

##

"I'm not speaking to you."

Millie wanted to hang up the phone and go back to her report. What was she supposed to say to the man she loved, after he may or may not have done something on purpose that she did not want him to do?

"Millie, come on. I got carried away. Don't hang up."

"I can't believe you'd do that to me," she whispered, hurt and angry, into the phone. "You tricked me."

Silence.

"Millie?"

"Who said there's going to be any more times?" she answered softly.

Silence.

"Because married people have sex on a regular basis," Brandon replied as firmly as he could with his voice shaking. He sounded upset.

Served him right. What if she couldn't go to college? What if she had to get a nothing job, or worse be dependent on Brandon for an income? A woman with her intelligence and high grades would resent him for the rest of her life.

"I should divorce you now. I apparently can't trust you."

Silence, and then the line went dead. Brandon had quietly hung up.

Millie stared at the phone in her hand. Had she gone too far?

Chapter 9

"Lisa, can I ask you a question?"

"Sure, Millie. Come in. You look worried. Don't you feel well? If you don't, we can postpone our meeting for a better day?"

Too many questions already, but that was part of her job. Why hadn't Lisa become a doctor? She knew more than most of them did anyway because of her years of experience seeing so many students from different walks of life.

"I'm fine. I must be coming down with a flu bug or something."

Lisa peered at her. "Plenty of liquids and bed rest." She turned and pulled out chairs for both of them around the small conference table in her office. More parents had been in her office than the principal's over the years. She took a personal interest in each and every student, from the youngest to the graduate, as if their health was her personal responsibility. Yet, she didn't pry.

Millie nodded, and a wave of unfamiliar nausea hit her hard. "It must be a stomach bug. I couldn't keep my lunch down."

Lisa stopped abruptly. She didn't turn around. "You know, Millie, if it was any other high school girl in this town with your symptoms, I'd know immediately what was wrong. But in your case, I'd bet on a stomach bug."

"What do you mean? It's probably from the cafeteria menu. I don't know what's in the food supply these days. Between the pesticides, fungicides, genetically altered food, and preservatives, it's a wonder everyone isn't sick to their stomachs all the time."

Lisa sat down slowly, averting her gaze from Millie's tummy, keeping it on her face. "That's true, and I know that's why you want to pursue a career as a medical journalist, to right all the medical wrongs against humanity."

Millie took the second chair and opened her notebook. "Yes, it's all about the collective good, don't you think? No one person or one group should profit on the backs or the health of another individual or group. It's so sad to see people on television telling their stories to the impersonal camera. Who is really listening at home? We have to be heard. What's worse, is that the stories are often edited and changed to fit the agendas of the program advertisers and sponsors. Drug companies will sponsor National Fill In The Blank Week, to 'accidentally' coincide with a new medication that just received FDA approval. People who would never think to have any symptoms of a disease or problem, begin to worry and turn up at doctor's offices all of a sudden after hearing about it, or after seeing a made-for-television movie about the same illness or disease sponsored by the drug companies, all for the hype and promotion of a new drug. The bottom line is money, not health. It's disgusting."

Lisa nodded. "And shocking, considering the manipulation of statistics and scare tactics that often go along with it. I've been grappling with some interesting data myself. The conclusions that I have formed have major implications that have been keeping me up nights. I had hoped that I would find some error in the analysis, some mistake in the calculation. But after repeatedly deriving the same results, I can't help but see some disturbing trends in my own office which likely would be reflected in other offices throughout the United States."

She ran her fingers through her short, straight hair. Millie figured she probably didn't have many opportunities to spend time in front of the mirror. Some people were dedicated to their jobs, and Lisa was one of those harassed, exhausted, and noble people. Lisa didn't wear make-up and dressed in generic, serviceable clothes, easily thrown in the washer instead of having to be dry-cleaned.

Lisa's home was neat and efficient. Millie had never seen Lisa employ outside cleaning services or gardeners. Lisa did everything herself, which was quite a contrast to Damon's house with its live-in housekeeper and two gardeners. Millie's parents also took care of the maintenance of their own home, which is why it was so comfortable and private.

Millie sat up straight, her reporter instincts on alert. "What kind of trends? Anything I can use?"

The lines in Lisa's forehead got deeper as she scanned the reports in front of her. She looked them over carefully, following some of the type with her finger.

"Shingles," she answered quietly. "Craig and I believe we are on the brink of a nationwide shingles epidemic."

Millie paused, the point of her pencil snapping off. "In children?"

Lisa nodded. "Potentially only for a short term in children, but a fairly long-term in adults. For the first time in kindergarten through the third grade we have seen some shingles cases among those who had been vaccinated against chickenpox and even more cases among those who were not vaccinated because they had a previous history of the natural chickenpox. Other doctors in the state have told me that at first, they were misdiagnosing these childhood cases of shingles because they had been so rare and unexpected. At least some of the children have suffered a great deal of pain because of misdiagnosis which caused a delayed their receipt of prescriptions for antiviral drugs. Most people think shingles is just a painful skin rash that occurs on the torso, neck, arm, or leg. But, shingles can affect the eyes and vision, cause facial paralysis, or attack any nerve throughout the head and body."

"That sounds miserable. Lisa, can you describe for me the actual characteristics of the shingles rash?" Millie took a pen from the cup on Lisa's desk.

"It's a fluid-filled vesicular rash along a dermatome usually on one side of the body. It is not uncommon, however, for two or three adjacent dermatomes to be affected; infrequently the shingles can disseminate over the entire body."

"What does vesicular mean?"

"A fluid-filled blister."

"Dermatome?"

"Basically this is a localized area of the skin that has sensation via a single nerve root of the spinal cord. Shingles most commonly affects an area of the skin supplied by sensory fibers from a spinal nerve. These are designated by a T1-T12 for the thoracic region on the torso; but, shingles can appear on dermatomes in the neck, designated C2-C8 for cervical region; or on other body parts, L1-L5 for lumbar region, or S1-S5 for sacral region. Shingles can also adversely affect the eyes (or vision), cause facial paralysis on one side of the face or affect other regions of the head, depending on which branch of the Trigeminal nerve that the virus attacks."

Millie's stomach lurched. She found that disturbing. She had never thrown up in her life. As a matter of fact, she had always considered herself to be quite steady in the digestion department.

"You, okay?" Lisa asked.

"Must be the scientific talk. It seems particularly gross today." *Hopefully, it won't get any grosser.*

"Words like 'skin' are not very scientific," Lisa reminded her. "Would you like a glass of water?"

The room spun without warning. The floor was on the ceiling, and the windows became the doors. To Millie, blisters were everywhere, like giant, nauseating spots before her eyes.

Before she could grip the arm of the chair to steady herself, suddenly, everything turned to a night sky.

##

"I want all the details, Nurse Lisa, and I want them now," Damon thundered over the phone. "Faith and Craig called to tell me Millie fainted in your office. I'm her doctor, and I want to know what happened."

Brandon hid in the shadow of the half-open door to the den. Something was wrong with Millie. Or something was right with his new family. He knew all about the signs of pregnancy from his friends, who discussed their latest girlfriends with undisguised detail.

"Forget the privileged communication and release authorizations," his father shouted. "You're a nurse, not a doctor. You are supposed to present to me."

Damon was breathing too hard and fast for normal conversation. Brandon didn't think he really cared about Millie as his patient as much as he cared about Lisa as his unofficial employee.

He yelled, "What happened and why?"

Damon's speech became clipped and professional. He couldn't hear the other side of the conversation, but apparently, Lisa was immune to intimidation, probably from years of working with difficult kids and their parents. "All right. Have it your way. I'll stop by their house and check on her myself."

Brandon pushed away from the wall and started for the back door, pulling the car keys from his jacket as he grabbed it off a chair.

Not if I get to her first, you won't.

##

"What are you doing here?" Millie whispered.

Brandon put the flat of his hand against the door before she could close it. She looked pale and tired. His feelings of guilt skyrocketed along with his worry about her. "My father's on his way, and if you don't want the first ob/gyn examination of your life, get in my car, and let me get you out of here."

Millie's eyes widened like saucers. She reached for her sweater and purse on the coat rack by her front door and followed him on a run to his car. He opened the door, guided her carefully inside, slammed it, ran around to his side, got in, and turned the key in the ignition as he saw his father's car round the corner. He backed quietly out of the driveway into the side street by the arroyo.

"Hurry," she whispered, panicked, glancing back and forth over her shoulder.

"No," he answered calmly. "He's too upset to look around at his surroundings. I know him really well when he gets like this. He doesn't see us."

"He'll recognize your car."

"We're out of his line of vision. If we move slowly and don't get his attention, he will continue to be as self-absorbed as he always is."

Millie watched in disbelief as Damon screeched to a full stop just short of the hedge bordering the empty arroyo. When the winter rains caused run-off in the valley, the ditch would catch the downpour and keep the area from flooding. She remembered when she and Brandon used to play in the dry ditch in the heated summers. She'd watch him show off on his skateboard, looping up onto the smooth concrete sides.

Now, he had come to rescue her from . . . .

Wait a minute. Had he said an OB/GYN exam?

"Brandon," she began, "why would your father dare to think I would . . . ." Her voice faded away to nothing.

"Not yet. Slouch down just in case."

She did.

"Is he in the house yet?" How long would it take him to get inside the foyer so she and Brandon could drive quietly away?

"Your father just opened the door for him." Brandon slid the gear shift into reverse and backed quietly away from the house. Where he would take them both, he wasn't sure. She wouldn't be safe in either of their homes. Who would take them in without question? A motel wouldn't work. Millie would never go for it. The Beaumont Inn was definitely out of the question. Travis Beaumont ran a third-class dump, catering to anyone with cash, looking the other way when kids his daughter's age signed in with phony IDs. Anything for the almighty dollar, that was Travis.

Damon liked money, too, and fame, power and glory. To what ends would he go to acquire them all exponentially? Would he resort to more force than usual? Perhaps, would he look the other way if his goal made people sicker than usual? Would he care if people died?

Silently, Millie turned toward him and touched his arm. He liked that. He loved her, and the sensation of her body anywhere near him made him happy. They were good together, and they were going to grow old in each other's arms.

"Would you please tell me what's going on?" she asked quietly. "I'm confused."

Brandon gunned the motor, and they sped out toward the boondocks. The landscape whirled by at a dizzying pace. "It's simple. You fainted in Lisa's office. Your parents called your doctor, who happens to be my father and they seemed to think Damon might have had something to do with it, perhaps some school program he might have initiated. Damon called Lisa asking her what happened. She, out of loyalty to you, refused to tell him. He stormed over to your house to discover the facts for himself."

"That's not simple. It's an invasion of privacy. Doesn't anyone have any secrets in this town?"

"No."

She looked out into the night. "I fainted. Big deal."

He pulled gently to a stop on the shoulder of the road and turned off the lights. The darkness enveloped them in the seclusion she craved. "The question is, Millie, why did you faint?"

Chapter 10

"I want you to have the volunteers move all the available tables outside my office building," Damon instructed, ignoring Barbara.

"Yes, Doctor," came the automatic response from Ricki, the nurse who had been with him since he opened his office.

Barbara didn't like her. Rumor had it that she had been in prison, but no one could prove it. She had been implicated in a scandal involving a drug salesman, but Damon had laughed it off at a party at the Spartacus Club when Travis said he could have sworn he saw her at his motel with some sleazy-looking, trashy man with a large briefcase. Speculation ran high as to what was in the briefcase.

From where she sat on the bleachers borrowed from the high school athletic department, Barbara didn't think Ricki was attractive enough to attract even a drug salesman, but she kept her opinions to herself, as usual, with a snicker that Damon consistently mistook for loud evidence of a sinus infection.

Barbara finished the last of her Tippy's Flavor Special cone and crumpled the paper wrapper into the trash. They hadn't had Boysenberry Punch, but the Apricot Dream wasn't a bad runner-up for a favorite.

They'd been up since the pre-dawn hours. She'd watched as the entire staff of Tippy's had prepared to keep their doors closed for Injection Day and set up shop on the street outside of Damon's office. She'd seen her overbearing husband write a substantial check to the owner of Tippy's, a morbidly obese woman with a mustache, hiring her, her company, and her inventory to give ice cream to every susceptible man, woman, and child who turned out and lined up to receive the Varivax® or varicella vaccine and any other they may have missed prior to this special Injection Day.

What had he done to the center of town? The preceding week had been an exercise in garish preparations. Damon had paid for huge American flags and had hung them on every street corner interspersed with flags in red, white, and blue emblazoned with the words *Injection Day* on one side and *Your Good Health courtesy of Dr. Damon Leviticus* blaring in red lettering on the other. His name and rank were double the height of the other letters, of course. She would expect that, given his ego and purpose to be the most important of all men on the face of the earth.

His plan, from what she could tell, was to line the street with tables covered with red, white, and blue cloths and bottles of vaccine. By running power lines to the frost-free -15°C (or +5°F) freezers behind the tables containing the vials of lyophilized or freeze-dried Varivax® inoculant, it was convenient to reconstitute the 0.5ml vaccine preparation with the diluent just prior to the injection so as to maximize the potency or number of plaque forming units (PFU) of the live varicella virus. He had spent the entire weekend gathering all the inventory he had stockpiled for every vaccination mandated by the state, because Injection Day, he had told her as she had tried to fall asleep during his tirade to escape the boredom, was also going serve as a catch-up day for all the citizens who had missed or could not afford their vaccinations in the past.

On each table, Damon had put a framed picture of himself next to a smaller picture of the President of the United States, alongside a loud and tasteless brochure detailing his education and awards.

Barbara snickered. Was she the only one who saw through his pomposity to the pompous man who was the self-proclaimed medical leader of the community?

"Barbara, did you hear me?" Was that Damon calling her? She blinked, shaking her head in an attempt to stay awake.

Was Damon talking at her again? What did he want this time?

"Are you going to be by my side when the line forms over here?" He gestured with a flourish to the sidewalk near the largest table with two of his pictures on it, on both sides of only one of the President's.

"Do you mean the way I do for your booth at Moonlight Fun and Madness Shoppers Incentive Night?" she asked, amused by the similarities. Every few months the Chamber of Commerce sponsored an evening carnival-type event with booths from the local merchants. They lined the streets with racks of outdated sale merchandise in a bait and switch attempt to draw customers into their stores. Inevitably, Damon sponsored a health fair at the same time with local doctors and drugstores on display, with a free blood pressure reading as the gimmick.

She hated closed communities that rarely went anywhere else for merchandise or health care. No competition, no new ideas, no freedom of choice. Just the same-old, same-old, recycled items on racks to make them look new, when in reality it was only a pathetic attempt to ring more money and health out of an already ailing society by a morally bankrupt health and merchant economy.

Damon glared at her. "If, for one minute, my dear wife, you would take your nose out of Tippy's and away from having your nails done with Aileen, you might remember that this is going to be the most important medical event since Joseph Lister discovered there was a reduction in mortality when doctors observed even the most simplest of antiseptic practices. He was vital to preventive medicine, and I applaud him and follow in his footsteps."

She shuddered before she sighed. *That was only one hundred years ago. Before Lister, no doctor even washed his hands before performing surgery, let alone sterilized the instruments.*

"Before Lister," Leviticus went on, "the problem in half of procedures, was that the surgery was successful, but the patient died. That's where I'm going to be just as important in the history books. My immunization program will be successful, and the patients are going to live."

Barbara looked at him for a long time as he straightened a tablecloth in an obsessive-compulsive manner she could easily dismiss as his way of doing things instead of the manipulative, purposeful ego-driven plans he carried out for his benefit. Over the years of their marriage, she had watched the traits that had once attracted her to him consistently turn to disbelief.

"Why do they call it 'immunization'? Breast-fed babies are immunized naturally; but children injected with dead or attenuated live viruses are vaccinated and vaccination doesn't usually stimulate the body in the natural ways via the nasal and respiratory routes. Varicella vaccination does not effectively boost cell-mediated immunity as thoroughly as does natural exposures to chickenpox in the community," she called.

Damon turned back to her, shaking his pointed finger in her direction. "Don't hold forth on subjects on which you know nothing about. We doctors express it as 'immunization', which seems to cause the body to produce antibodies that correlate with protection, so that the common Joe Schmo will understand."

She snorted. "Understand? You mean be manipulated, don't you?" She climbed down the bleachers and came closer, watching his face cloud with his anger and his fists clenched with suppressed violence. "Then why don't you call it what it is? If you withhold the actual evidence, then you are just as guilty of deceit as if you had told an outright lie. It's lying by omission."

His face twisted and turned with the building fury she knew from experience could explode at any minute. "You call me a liar? Your husband? A pillar of the medical community?"

Ricki looked up from her task of lining up the hypodermics in neat rows. She cocked her head closer, listening, an unnecessary gesture since Barbara and Damon were hardly whispering.

Barbara sighed. Why had she bothered? Questioning him was useless, even if her questions expressed genuine concern and interest. He hadn't heard any other voice but his own ever since he'd received the Outstanding Citizen of Sycamore Springs award when he'd organized the first well-baby clinic in the area. He told the populace that he was concerned that parents might be negligent, failing to bring their perfectly healthy babies in for their necessary immunizations. He'd frightened them all so much, that she'd overheard Lisa tell Lindsey that she'd never seen so many children walk into the doctor's office healthy and happy, and then walk out screaming, sometimes later reporting continued illness due to adverse reactions to shots and medications.

That day she and Lisa had discussed the issue of government mandates and government interference in the health decisions of the country. They'd come to the conclusion that the government had enlisted the medical and pharmaceutical complex through powerful lobbyists to create and enforce laws that gave doctors and drug companies free rein to essentially do whatever they wanted. By establishing a limit on compensation claims for vaccine-related injuries and providing immunity to both physicians and vaccine manufacturers themselves from litigation and class-action law suites, there are no incentives to conduct thorough safety studies and improve medical practice. In some communities, doctors and drug companies muscle the parents and caretakers by supporting children's services who use threats of court orders and jail time to any who think for themselves and don't stand in line for shots and pills that likely have some association and risk leading to illness, disease, and death. What exactly was a government mandate anyway? Was it blanket leeway that said that doctors ruled? Wasn't it, in reality, the fruit of the lobbyists labor which resulted in a carefully worded official ruling depriving parents of their rights to decide on issues of healthcare concerning their own children?

She and Lisa agreed that they could think of several words describing doctors and the medical industry, most of them quite obscene, yet one they could use in public was bullies. Another was cowards.

Who in their right mind would cower in front of a bully with scare tactics and slogans of positive propaganda, manipulated data generated by researchers with special interests, and two sets of pockets.

One filled with drugs.

And the other filled with the money from the sale of those drugs.

"Let's forget it, Damon. I can't discuss anything with you like we used to when we were first married. You closed your mind to new ideas, and you closed your heart to me, years ago."

He snickered. "You've been watching soap operas again, haven't you? How many times have I told you that the fictional media is no place to get your news."

Barbara stared at him. "And what you create isn't fiction? Don't your medical groups create casts of actors and give them the words to say, the props to use, and the legal backing to declare it all freedom of speech?"

"You need more replacement hormones," he said flatly, staring her down.

She watched his eyes. They were cold and empty. "It's not hormones. It's reality. You support your own, and defend your own. If one of you makes a mistake, and the patient dies, your cronies run to the witness stand and yell, 'Protocol—it was the accepted form of treatment and the outcome was an acceptable risk.' If one of your own gives a 16-month-old toddler an MMR shot, even though the measles component has been associated with both gut disorders and autism in children, the vaccine propagandists would like to have us believe this was some sort of genetic defect present at birth or early onset autism. But the reality is that these children could speak some words and had developed skills, but after vaccination regressed into what is now being called late-onset autism with a price tag of $2 million in costs to raise each such child. You say, 'That child was born that way. He was sick to begin with. He had underlying problems.' Surely, there may have been a genetic predisposition Damon, but it was an environmental trigger such as provided by the vaccine that caused a vaccine-induced injury. Certainly you must realize a genetic defect does not reasonably cause an illness that is now occurring in epidemic proportions of 10 new cases per day in California alone, and certainly you can't fool the parents of that toddler by telling them the child was autistic from birth! He was healthy. He was whole. You destroyed his brain for a few dollars of government funding."

Tears filled her eyes faster than usual when she was trapped by social obligation to talk to Damon. She had to get out. What was going on? Was she crazy? Why attack him after all these years for no stepped-up reason? He had always been a company man. Was something going to happen?

He advanced cautiously, as if she were some mental patient. "You've lost your mind, Barbara. Would you kindly tell me why you are attacking me and the profession that has made you a very wealthy woman?"

She looked up and down the cordoned off street and panicked. The people were going to be roped in—in more ways than one. Was it his "Injection Day" festival? Was it going to turn into something more tragic than the Moonlight Fun and Madness Shoppers Incentive Nights?

It was going to be a circus, but small communities like Sycamore and the surrounding areas were so isolated from larger cities like Los Angeles that they had to make everything into a carnival or die of boredom. The citizens were smart and educated, some were cynics like Lisa, some already knew more than they desired to know like Aileen. But they all had something in common. They didn't truly understand how far evil would go, how evil operated.

Barbara did. Evil had operated on her.

She patted her abdomen again and turned away from the man who had unnecessarily held the knife. He had ripped the future from her body along with her womb. The hysterectomy he performed had caused her premature hormonal imbalances. Why was she so frightened about the Injection Day model project?

"I don't want Brandon in this project, do you understand? He doesn't react well to either shots or medications."

"Baloney! He's a healthy young man because of the medical care I've given him. The sick children in town are the ones who have never stepped foot in my office. If you would have listened to what I've been trying to tell you, you'd know that Brandon is the poster boy for Injection Day."

Barbara gasped. "What are you saying? I don't want him near this project. He's my son, too. I say he's had enough shots and pills. Leave him alone."

Damon grabbed her by her wrist and pulled her around. "You be quiet. I'll not have you spoiling this media event for me. I'll not allow you to taint it with your fears. You are a hysterical woman, too old and unqualified to decide what a young man like Brandon needs. Let him speak for himself."

Barbara wrenched her hand away, obviously startling Damon with the hate she knew he must see in her eyes. "So you're going to validate Injection Day by making Brandon advertise it, as if he'd be a trained monkey?"

He leaned closer, towering over her. "Yes, my dear. But he won't be a monkey, he'll be a hero following in my footsteps as a man, instead of in yours as a weak, poor excuse for a woman. The way you've babied him all these years, sharing advice with him, when you should have been sending him to me. I'm his father. I'm the head of this household. When the line forms right here . . . ," he announced making a wide-sweeping gesture with both arms to the street in front of The Damon Leviticus Center for Medicine, "my son, Brandon will be the first to receive his injection."

Chapter 11

The drive out to the boondocks had taken only a few minutes at top speed with her heart racing faster than the motor.

Barbara knew she had to leave town. The thought of Brandon too young to say no to a vaccine he didn't need for a generally mild disease with fewer complications than Damon wanted the public to think was too much for her.

He was her only child.

She loved him with a devotion that she didn't think possible. If she would have had more children, if she would have been further blessed, she would have loved them all equally with as much intensity and power.

She was stunned. Was she going to be powerless to stop more unnecessary procedures on him? Her son, she was quite sure, wasn't even aware of how many times she had stepped in between him and his vicious father, how many times she had flushed medication she knew her husband was pushing as a result of some overpriced dinner, courtesy of the pharmaceutical company, the night before.

Her son wasn't an experiment, and he wasn't a pin-cushion either, or a repository for biological and chemical substances.

He was human, just like all the other children and adults in Sycamore and the rest of the world. No one was supposed to be sacrificed to make someone else rich. How was she going to stop Damon?

She pulled off the road into a clearing nearest to town, one she knew was a favorite make-out spot for the kids. She stepped out of her car and closed the door softly behind her. The breezes disturbed the tall grasses. She could hear the rustle of life, not in human form, but alive in the same sense of having a heart and soul. Smaller animals with complicated systems for survival abounded in the hills and valleys. How did they do it? How did they escape from the greed and misery of people?

They left. They knew better than to live near the Damon Leviticus' of the world. They populated the fields and rivers, the mountains and streams, with their own ways, undisturbed by shots and pills. They had inborn senses for healing, a plant here, a seed next. They instinctively knew what allowed them to live in health and solitude, and reveled in the joy of running free, trusting that their environment would support them and give them all they needed.

She wished she could take Brandon and escape with him as far away from Damon as they could get, and exist like the free and wild animals who had the privilege of living out their life spans, interrupted only by the natural order of things like predators and brushfires.

What would it mean to live a natural life? To be able to develop natural immunity to illness and disease through good nutrition and by living in balance with nature?

Maybe cows that were grass-fed in earlier days somehow produced milk that protected children from asthma and grass allergies? But when milk production began to be artificially stimulated through use of hormones, somehow this began compromising the health benefits that would have otherwise existed.

Barbara giggled. She was beginning to feel better. Coming to her private space outside the city always helped her put things in perspective.

She went back to her comforting thoughts, anything to get through her life with Damon.

What about all the hormones currently given to beef cattle. Could these hormones be causing girls to mature faster from children to adults? And could children's ingestion of the additive antibiotics be contributing to antibiotic resistant bacteria? This conjecture didn't seem far-fetched. Barbara knew that 100% of poultry, 90% of pigs and veal calves, and 60% of cattle have regular amounts of antibacterials added to their feed. Also, 70% of U.S. beef is from cattle fed on hormones to promote growth.[25] Without medical interference, species of animals and plants had existed since the first one-celled animal appeared on the face of the planet.

But take the animals away from their pasture land, out of their natural surroundings; take them to an artificial environment, and disrupt their normal diet and life-cycle—then watch what happens. Sure, a measured increase in milk and meat production is achieved. However, but due to man's intervention, complete with the homogenization process, the nutritional benefits inherent to the raw milk are compromised and the cows die prematurely.

I guess the same held true for horses. In their natural habitat, they graze all day long and travel miles on end. They live 40 or 50 years in the wild. But when they are maintained in a small box stall with their feet shod with iron shoes, it seems they live only about half their normal life span. It has been documented that horseshoes cut off about 50% of the circulation in the horse's legs, and prevent the naturally coned hooves from properly flexing and pumping the blood volume needed to maintain good health. While horseshoes appear to resolve any previous pain or disorder the horse might have experienced in its legs, this outcome is only superficial and due to diminished feeling in the horses legs caused by the lack of proper circulation.[26]

In captivity, unless frequently exercised by their owners, horses don't have a chance or the longevity they once enjoyed in their natural habitat with a varied diet. Normal daily living was what the medical profession called it. NDL. If a patient couldn't continue with NDL, well, they just needed pills and shots and operations to get them on with their lives.

If they lived.

But, how could their lives ever be normal again? They could only subsist with a new normal, fabricated and devised by the medical industry. Something would have to be lost once the chain of natural health and in-born immunization mechanisms were circumvented, dysregulated, or broken by chemicals and knives.

---

[25] Drugs in Livestock Feed, Volume 1, Technical Report, Office of Technology Assessment, Washington, D.C., June 1979, p. 3.

[26] Tomas G. Teskey. The unfettered foot: a paradigm change for equine podiatry. Medical Veritas 2005 April; 2(1):409-417.

Barbara moved slowly, walking around the car, studying the wild and free vegetation on the hills, trying to capture what was real around her from the hot California autumn sun to the cooling afternoon winds that sent hope in her direction. The natural wonders of life were her inspiration. They would continue to make her strong and renew her resolve. If she kept her goal in mind, which was to keep Brandon safe from harm, she could make sure he would be unavailable to take the shot. She knew him well, and she could manipulate him if she wanted to, especially for his own good.

A small creature scurried across her path, and she took a deep breath and looked around her, surprised she had walked away from the clearing. She'd left her car a half-mile behind her. What lay ahead?

##

Was that Brandon's voice?

Barbara spun in a complete circle, looking for him. What would he be doing way out here? Didn't he have a class?

Her first explanation, or guess, was that Damon must have said or done something again to drive him out of the house and into the lonely, empty space of what the teenage population called the boondocks. It wouldn't surprise her if her son knew the desolate hills around Sycamore Springs as intimately as he knew the young and nubile cheerleaders who followed him like lost puppies, waiting for any indication at all that he knew of their existence.

Just the way she had done with Lindsey.

But Brandon only had hot eyes for Millie, although she couldn't for the life of her see why. Millie was thin and pale and about as interesting as a flat soda, and nothing like her parents. Her mother, Faith, was vibrant and beautiful. And her father, Craig, was everything Damon was not, except for their doctorate degrees.

Craig was handsome, and his intelligence shone from the inside out. She'd recently listed to his hour-long interview on Varicella Vaccination on *Liberty Radio* and had read about his research in *Mothering Magazine* and *Nexus magazine*. His colleagues praised him as a genius, both in and out of his fields of research. She'd even read in *Popular Science and Mechanics* about his patented invention, a "Power Wheel," a microprogrammed-controlled electric motor inside a wheel that might someday benefit humanity by providing energy efficient electric vehicle transportation of the future.

Barbara felt the inner rankling of jealously. What had Damon ever invented? What had he ever done to benefit real people who came to him in their hours of pain and illness?

Nothing.

Strange, because Craig had chosen a non-medical path with a Ph.D. in computer science. Research meant more to him then anything else. She always thought that it was his intuitive understanding of mathematics, coupled with powers of observation and logical deduction that gave him the ability to formulate hypotheses that eventually were borne out in theories.

What would happen, she wondered, if Craig ever observed something in conflict with Damon's stranglehold on the community? Would the two men make good their frequent jibes at each other, and escalate them into something more than a conflict of ideologies? What if lives were at stake? Would they be crusaders or combatants?

Barbara jumped. There it was again, someone shouting in the distance who sounded like Brandon. She turned around again and saw her son, running up one of the hills, closing the distance between him and a young woman. From her attire, she wasn't a fashion follower.

It had to be Millie.

"Brandon," the fashion mistake turned and called, "you've got to understand. I didn't want to have a baby at this time."

Barbara looked for someplace to hide, to conceal herself so she could hear more without being seen. She never felt guilty about eavesdropping, even though she wouldn't admit it to anybody, because it was her only way to get information in a family as repressed as hers.

"Why not, Mil?" he shouted into the sunlight.

"Because you tricked me. You knew I didn't want a baby early in our marriage at this time, but you got me pregnant anyway," she yelled back.

Barbara felt her stomach pump a truckload of acid into her throat. She couldn't discern Millie's words clearly, especially the words "early in our marriage." Being unaware of Brandon and Millie's secret marriage, Barbara thought Millie was going to have Brandon's baby without the blessings of standard matrimonial procedure. As bad as that sounded, she knew what was going to be worse.

She was going to have to be the one to tell Damon.

"Millie, don't run away from me. I want you and the baby to be my family."

"I have a family," she said angrily, backtracking, closing the distance as he ran closer.

"I know you do, but I don't," Brandon said, his panting unable to hide his despair. "I need you, Millie. I don't have anyone to care about me except you."

He finally reached her and grabbed her in a hug that shook Barbara to her core. *You used to hug me like that. What happened? What made you run away from me to a child-woman?*

She watched in cold silence as her son plundered a skinny young girl's mouth. The salt of tears bit into her eyes, making her try to blink them away. Unable to watch anymore, she moved toward the direction of her car. What was the use of staying? She was no longer necessary.

##

She could hear the comforting beat of Brandon's heart as he held her close to him. "It's not working," she said. "I want a divorce right now, no matter how safe and secure you make me feel." She wasn't as sure about that as she sounded. Strangely enough, she felt sufficiently secure such that she had no desire to leave the car. Her parents kept her safe, but maybe that was the answer. Maybe content and thriving kids seek further security in relationships, while traumatized kids look for an escape from the trauma and resulting insecurity by seeking stable relationships. Yes, that would explain the differences in her own background and Brandon's, as well as why they both wanted to have a pain-free, hurt-free future. Each of them must understand the needs of the other and see that even though they are coming from different realities, they seek the common goal of a happy life.

He stroked her back. "Then I'll have to try harder. I always get what I want, as long as it doesn't have anything to do with my father. There's something wrong with him. He's twisted inside. His point of view is only his own. He's never seen another person's side of any story. As a matter of fact, for him, no other reality exists except his own."

She nodded. At least he knew who or what his own father was. "You know what?" she murmured into his shirt, "I think you're obsessed with him and his faults."

He snorted. "And you're not obsessed with your dad? How perfect he is, how much you want to be like him? How many articles you want to publish to emulate his achievements?"

She sat up straight and pulled away from him. The car was getting too small again to confine her feelings. "Those aren't faults. My father is great to me. He's taught me the value of observation and sticking up for my own truths. I want to be just like him in every way."

Brandon opened the door to the driver's side and got out. "Well, congratulations, Miss Manchester. You are like him. In every way."

He slammed the door and walked away in a direction headed toward town.

##

Dexter skidded to a halt on his motorcycle and straddled it. "What's up, Millie?"

She'd been leaning against Brandon's car waiting for him to return when she'd heard a bike rumbling closer. Her first impulse had been to get back into the car and lock the doors, but Dexter had appeared before she had the chance. As far as she was concerned, he was harmless. She wasn't his type. He didn't go for the smart girls with any grade higher than a C minus.

"Nothing. I felt like getting out of the city for a few hours."

"In your boyfriend's car?" he said with a smirk.

Dexter had blond hair slicked into spikes, accented with bright magenta gel. His dark blue eyes bore into hers with an intensity that would have both attracted and frightened her if she didn't think he was a jerk and a half.

"He's not my boyfriend." She assumed she could get away with denying it. Who would date her? She dressed like a librarian and had the moral reputation of a naïve dork who wasn't worth the trouble, because underneath her bulky clothes she was really a walking encyclopedia.

"Whatever you say, but that's not the way I heard it."

"You heard wrong. What do you want?"

"Just stopping by to say hello. I saw you standing out in the middle of nowhere, and I figured you must need something."

"Like what?" she asked suspiciously. If Dex was anything, it wasn't considerate.

"Tire changed, motor started, lube job." He rubbed the stubble on his chin.

"Don't be gross."

He chuckled. "I was talking cars."

"Sure you were. Go home, Dexter. You don't know what you're talking about when it comes to women."

He howled with laughter, scaring her more than she wanted to admit. He had a reputation as a thick-headed moron on a bike with parents who were unsupportive and who were not good role models.

Maybe she would have been safer inside the car.

She scanned the horizon. Where was Brandon? Had he gone far? Would he hear her if she yelled for help?

"Looking for your boyfriend?" He smiled like a self-assured shark.

"I told you he's not . . . ."

". . . your boyfriend. I remember." He took a comb out of his pocket and slid it easily through his hair before putting it back carefully, as if it were the most expensive possession he owned next to his bike. "Then what is he? A casual acquaintance?"

Her muscles tensed. Even with her limited experience with men, she knew something had changed, even though she didn't know what that could be. He wasn't flirting. He wasn't even fishing. He knew something, and whatever it was, it made her too vulnerable, especially alone and miles from town. But what was it?

"Get out of here, Dexter. Brandon will be back any minute, and you don't want to make trouble." May as well take the offense. That's what Brandon played on the team.

"Ooo. I'm scared. The big football player coming after me, the troublemaker back from detention." He got off his bike and stared at her.

"I mean it. He's coming back right now."

Millie gasped. Dexter must know about the pregnancy. But how? Only she and Brandon knew for sure. But she better make sure before she approached Brandon insisting that she wanted a divorce. She shoved hard on Dexter's chest, catching him off balance. He landed on his backside in the dirt.

"What are you talking about, Dexter? You better tell me." Was that her voice? She sounded distant and furious.

It put him off. He sat on the ground, tense and sneering. "Easy, Millie. I know the truth. Your boyfriend came to me for advice and a phone number. I gave him both. Don't worry. That quack comes highly recommended by most of your friends."

The implications of what he was saying shocked her. Had Brandon really told a moron like Dexter about their baby? Did he ask for an abortion doctor?

Had she misjudged the father of her child?

She dug the toe of her shoe into the loose gravel and kicked a splattering of rocks and sod into his face. "You're a liar."

He didn't move. "Lots of lying goes on in this town. You better be careful who you trust."

Without another word, Millie yanked open the car door, huffed her way inside, and slammed and locked it a few seconds before she saw Brandon appear over the hill. It only took him a few seconds to take in the picture.

"Did you touch her?" he shouted at Dexter before he reached him on the run and jerked him to his feet.

"Not worth the trouble, my man. You can have her." He snickered.

Millie had never seen Brandon violent off the football field, so she didn't expect him to slam his fist into Dexter's stomach. She didn't think a tough loser like Aileen's son would crumble, curled up into a fetal ball.

She didn't think she'd smile.

Chapter 12

"Is there a way to test first if a child is allergic to vaccine ingredients or will have an adverse reaction to a vaccine?" Millie asked Lisa. "With so much at stake, it seems irresponsible to inoculate an entire population without first determining who is at high risk and which individuals should not be vaccinated at all."

"I agree, but no one does preliminary testing because it isn't cost effective. Medicine is an assembly line. Once someone gets on it, they can't get off. Each medication, inoculation, or procedure either has or usually leads to a side effect that might trigger a chronic illness or in some cases prove deadly. Does that surprise you?"

"Not really. It's logical that just as vaccinations are supposed to produce long-lasting immunity, we should not ignore the potential for long-term detrimental effects. This is especially true today since vaccines are aimed at preventing diseases that are no longer prevalent."

Lisa nodded. "You're intelligent."

Millie smiled proudly. "My father says I am, too."

"Your dad has written many significant articles and contributed consistently to the community. He's told me on several occasions that he's pleased you're following his example by questioning and researching all information, even if it appears to come from a reliable source."

"That's because he's taught me that money rules the world, and a reliable source usually means a funded source."

Lisa laughed. "You sound just like him. He's right. That's what makes my job so difficult. I'm on a salary, and I need to keep my job, but I've seen things that make it impossible to keep quiet. Like for example . . . ." Her voice trailed off as she checked through the folder tucked away, almost secretly, in between the row of others. Her office was an example of organized clutter. Every inch of available space was used to its greatest potential. She must have had records on every child who ever enrolled in the Sycamore School District since the town began. Yet, she knew where everything was, and she could find it at a moments notice.

"Have you found something important?" Millie asked, her voice rising.

Lisa nodded conspiratorially and checked to be sure the door was closed tightly and no one was standing outside, at least anyone observable through the glass panes. It was early, and no one was loitering in the halls, but Lisa was a careful person. She didn't like to leave anything to chance. Anyone could come by and overhear their conversation, even though most people were on the streets of Sycamore entertained by clowns and mimes, guzzled free soft drinks and people clogging their arteries with Tippy's full-fat ice cream in anticipation of the appearance of the poster boy for Injection Day as he kicked off the mass inoculation program by receiving the first Varivax® shot of the day.

Poor Brandon. A victim of his own life.

"Certainly, Millie, in recent years you have noticed the classrooms in Sycamore Springs' schools just overflowing with students who require special education services. At one extreme end of the spectrum, children were developing late-onset autism (with boys being affected 4 times that of girls), while at the other end, many were being diagnosed as having ADD (Attention Deficit Disorder) and ADHD (Attention Deficit and Hyperactivity Disorder). Since the CDC at least suspected that mercury toxicity might play a role in increasing neurodevelopmental disorders, they suggested that by 2000, pharmaceutical companies voluntarily remove the Thimerosal "preservative", about 50% mercury by weight, that was present in the Hepatitis B and other vaccines.[27] Unfortunately, just as autism spectrum disorders were found to be decreasing in 2006 due to the compliance by some pharmaceuticals to remove the Thimerosal or use only trace amounts, the CDC again authorized use of a yearly Thimerosal-containing influenza vaccine in children aged 6-months and older.[28] This restored approximately 60% of the Thimerosal dosing that had previously and voluntarily been removed or replaced by only trace amounts by 2000.

"Lisa, when year 2000 rolled around, were any remaining Thimerosal-containing vaccines recalled from the healthcare and medical facilities?"

"Unfortunately, no. Instead of pulling these particular vaccines from the shelves, physicians continued to administer them to children until their supply was exhausted. This action was apparently taken to minimize the vaccine maker's financial loses due to recalled vaccines at the sacrifice of patients' health."

"Why wasn't the public fully informed about all of this?

"Millie, a secret meeting was convened by the CDC and representatives of the pharmaceutical industry at a convention held June 7-8, 2000 at the Simpsonwood Retreat Center in Norcross, Georgia. The transcript of this meeting was finally obtained through the Freedom of Information Act, despite the fact that each page of the transcript was stamped 'DO NOT COPY OR RELEASE' and 'CONFIDENTIAL.' The CDC initially investigated the possible link between increasing neurological developmental disorders and the dose response to Thimerosal."

"Lisa, what is the meaning of 'dose response'?"

"This means that as the quantity of mercury from Thimerosal-containing vaccines increased, the likelihood of autism or other neurological disorders among children correspondingly increased.[29]

"Now I understand. So what findings did the CDC present at Simpsonwood?"

"Prior to the meeting at Simpsonwood, Dr. Thomas Verstraeten, using a CDC database, initially found that the risk of autism was over 7 times greater among children

---

[27] Appendix II. Summary of Highlights of Simpsonwood Meeting; and Appendix III. Mercury Toxicity: Genetic Susceptibility and Synergistic Effects.

[28] Appendix IV. Mercury in Vaccines: Institutional Malfeasance and the Department of Health and Human Services; also see Appendix VII. Interview with Dr. Mark Geier and David Geier: Decreasing Trends in Autism and Neurodevelopmental Disorders following Decreasing Use of Thimerosal-Containing Vaccines.

[29] Appendix II. Summary of Highlights of the Simpsonwood Meeting.

receiving Thimerosal-containing vaccines compared to those not exposed to Thimerosal. However, later, after a reanalysis of the data, the relative risk dropped to about 2.5 times greater. By the time the Simpsonwood meeting was convened, the relative risk dropped again to about 1.7. President Bush actually tried to protect the pharmaceutical industry by secretly including a rider in the Homeland Security Bill to dismiss lawsuits against Eli Lilly and prevent civil lawsuits against this pharmaceutical firm. Interestingly, George Bush Sr. sat on the Board of Directors of Eli Lilly for many years and other Eli Lilly company officials have been appointed to different Homeland Security advisory panels."

"Lisa, this Simpsonwood meeting seems to have revealed a great scandal in healthcare."

"Yes, indeed, Millie. After diluting the data still further by using data available from other healthcare institutions that demonstrated poorer reporting, the CDC finally published a study that concluded no link existed between Thimerosal and neurological developmental disorders. Other independent researchers and scientists simply could not understand this gross discrepancy between the initial and final report conclusions. A congressman and physician, Dr. Dave Weldon, initiated an investigation to discern the true facts. It was learned that the initial datasets that CDC had used, had been 'lost' (or destroyed) so that it was not possible to duplicate the figures CDC initially reported. Later, a research team consisting of Dr. Mark Geier and David Geier were allowed access to the Vaccine Safety Datalink (VSD) database. They spent 1½ years attempting to access this database. The Geier's compared data for one vaccine, the DTaP with Thimerosal as a preservative and the same vaccine by another manufacturer using an alternative preservative, 2-Phenoxyethanol. When their preliminary analysis demonstrated that the rate of autism was six times higher in the group that received the Thimerosal-containing DTaP, the CDC denied the Geier's further access to VSD. CDC charged that the independent research team was violating patient confidentiality by accessing personal data;[30] however, the Geier's reported that no such personal data were available in the dataset they were analyzing."

Lisa stopped the rush of words to look around again, obviously worried she'd said too much. "This is just between us, okay, Millie? Most people in the pharmaceutical industries know this and more. Some time ago, countries such as Denmark and Russia took the initiative to halt the use of Thimerosal-containing vaccines. Today, both these countries have significantly lower autism rates than those in the U.S. Public health officials have a huge dilemma—if they report the deleterious effects of vaccines accurately, this will instill lack of public confidence in vaccines and negatively impact vaccination rates. This could also trigger class-action law suits involving billions of dollars. I won't be able to help if I'm discredited before I have more detailed studies and documentation."

Lisa, after checking again to see that nobody else was eavesdropping on their conversation, continued. "SIDS or Sudden Infant Death Syndrome is the diagnosis given when an infant death appears to have no underlying cause or explanation. Recently, under

[30] Appendix VI. Interview with Dr. Mark Geier and David Geier concerning Thimerosal, Testosterone, and Autism Treatment Hypothesis.

further scrutiny, at least some instances of SIDS have been found to be vaccine-related deaths. Especially tragic have been arrests for what has been termed Shaken Baby Syndrome (SBS) where the parent or caretaker last in charge of an infant who died, was accused of shaking the baby to death. In one case, parents concerned about the health status of their newborn made some twenty visits to the pediatrician before their child suddenly died and they were charged with SBS and imprisoned. Additional investigation found the physician had vaccinated a premature, underweight infant—which was contraindicated. Additional toxicological analysis of the subdural bleeding in the child's tissue found bleeding that was not consistent with shaking.[31]

"Lisa, I recall hearing a news special where the reporter told of a father who was arrested—I think his last name was Yurko—for killing his own baby. This was totally out of character for this caring parent and a real tragedy for all affected. I can't imagine how his wife endured the pain and injustice of it all."

Millie's eyes were as wide as saucers. She had never seen Lisa lose her low-key, nurse demeanor before. She must have come across still more disturbing information to get so upset.

"Why don't they do anything about it if they know?"

"Because they'll lose money and if the negative outcomes are exposed, the public will lose their trust and confidence in what currently appears to be trusted medical institutions. Also, the public health authorities adopted a position that allowed vaccines that are not acceptable to the United States, to be sold and shipped overseas to unsuspecting countries."

"Poor people," Millie said quietly.

"When children suffering from malnutrition are given these vaccines, they become sick."

"Don't these public health officials have a conscience?"

"No," Lisa said angrily. "I don't know how these people sleep at night. As long as their own children and other loved ones are healthy, they don't care how many people they kill or maim or destroy for the saike of their money and retirement funds. Someday, I hope it all blows up in their faces and huge corporations fall with their CEO's taking the losses for a change."

"It will never happen, Lisa. They have too much money and too much power. They're not even in the same mindset as the rest of humanity. They have too many zeros in their salaries and bonuses."

"That's true. But there is always a greater evil. One of their own could be hurt. It won't make a difference to humanity, but at least they would know what it means to suffer the loss of a family member through medical and pharmaceutical negligence. It's bound to happen, just from the sheer numbers alone. Do you know what it means to be 'hoisted by one's own petard,' Millie?"

"Yes. It is an old English expression used for someone who finds themselves hurt by the very device intended for others."

---

[31] Appendix V. Shaken Baby Syndrome (SBS): General Commentary

"That's exactly right. It happens all the time, because people without a conscience also think they are invincible. Yes, they can do or allow things that harm others, but that they will somehow escape being harmed. For most in the medical profession that is probably true, but not for all; when they do fall, however, they will never be whole again."

Millie sat silently. What was going on? Lisa, like her father and perhaps a few others, knew the flaws in the system. They must have had this awareness for a long time. Why were these flaws being revealed at this particular moment?

When Lisa had driven Millie home after she passed out, and after she'd begged her not to call the paramedics, Lisa had asked her point blank if she was pregnant.

Millie had been evasive, but she had answered the question to Lisa's satisfaction. She'd said that the only reason she would have fainted would have been that she was going to have a baby. Lisa had looked after her for a long time, checked her blood pressure, and asked her when her last period had been.

Then she asked her if the father of the baby knew of her pregnancy.

Millie had looked out the window for a brief second, and Lisa had correctly read that as the answer to the pregnancy question and had driven her home with only one sentence of advice. She'd told her not to do anything on the spur of the moment without talking to her parents and, if she wanted to, to her as well.

When they'd gotten to her house, Lisa spoke to her father and mother right in front of her, telling them only the facts. Millie appreciated that. Lisa respected her and trusted her to tell her parents.

Her father and mother exchanged a look she didn't recognize. It frightened her that they would know without her saying a word. Her dad made a big deal about her seeking prenatal care, and she noticed her mom's forehead had an extra crease or two during dinner, which Millie couldn't keep in her stomach.

Funny, no further explanation had been necessary.

Then Brandon had shown up, and things had moved to a new level of existence – for the three of them. She had a family, a career, and was still a senior, about to graduate high school in a next few months..

"Lisa," she began tentatively, "remember when you said I could talk to you whenever I'd like? Well, since you know what's going on, I was wondering if you'd tell me what you know about the actual birthing and which vaccine that the physician will first want to inject in my newborn. I want to do all I can to insure that I have the best chance for a smooth delivery and a healthy child."

Lisa slowly put her research files aside. "Your parents will be able to tell you more on that when you're ready to openly talk with them, but I'll tell you what I know. With regard to birthing, an example of a poor practice that has become standard protocol/procedure is the flat on-the-back or semi-sitting birthing positions. While such a position is convenient for the attending physician, it unfortunately restricts the birth canal opening by as much as 30%, necessitating more episiotomies and C-section deliveries than a natural arched-back or squatting position that fully opens the birth canal and also takes advantage of natural gravity to aid delivery.[32] You have plenty of time to investigate the birthing positions further and in areas outside of Sycamore Springs, some hospitals are starting to allow mothers to specify a birth contract, allowing birthing to take place in a comforting warm water pool.

"Previously, I guess because I was not pregnant, I didn't question the standard birthing position as being problematic. What you have shared is most helpful."

"Millie, often it is the case that problematic practices are disguised as standard protocols or standard medical procedures. One glaring example of this is the current medical practice of instant or early cord clamping (ICC/ECC). A nine-pound (4.1 kg) newborn has approximately 10 ounces (300 ml) of blood. At birth, usually within 30 seconds or so, the umbilical cord is clamped and subsequently cut, preventing as much as 60% of the newborn's blood volume from traveling from the placenta to the newborn.[33] This 'standard' protocol, which saves the attending physician's precious time, deprives the newborn of the volume of blood necessary to properly expand his or her heart and lungs. The newborn is also deprived of important stem cells, enzymes, hormones, proteins, nutrients, and iron reserves that would have otherwise transferred from the placenta to the newborn.[34] While the newborn appears alive and healthy, closer inspection often reveals that the newborn actually has suffered brain damage that does not manifest itself until later years when the child starts to develop higher-level language and math skills. Further, the newborn must recover from an anemic condition (which takes up to two months to resolve) and may require resuscitation and/or blood transfusions that were all induced unnecessarily by the ICC/ECC procedure. The damage from ICC/ECC makes the newborn more vulnerable to infant diseases (because of lost maternal antibodies) and probably predisposes ICC/ECC infants to asthma and other disorders. In this weakened state, the child may be more susceptible to serious adverse reactions to any vaccines and their adjuvants (consisting of heavy metals and other associated chemical/biological products mixed with the vaccine). Medical persons have long known the facts concerning improper handling of the umbilical cord and the injurious affects. In 1801, Erasmus Darwin wrote, 'Another thing very injurious to the child, is the tying and cutting of the navel string too soon; which should always be left till the child has not only repeatedly breathed but till all pulsation in the cord ceases. As otherwise the child is much weaker than it ought to be, a portion of the blood being left in the placenta, which ought to have been in the child.'"[35]

"Lisa, again, I never knew about this procedure. How tragic to think that sometimes the attending physician will initiate the ICC/ECC procedure by having the husband participate in doing the immediate clamping and cutting of the cord! Again, if only more couples knew of the inherent danger this procedure is causing newborns.

---

[32] De Jonge A, Teunissen TA, Largo-Janssen AL. Supine position compared to other positions during the second stage of labor: a meta-analysis review. *J. Psychosom. Obstet. Gynaelcol.*, 2004 Mar;25:35-45.

[33] *The Lippincott Manual of Nursing Practice,* 7th edition, Chapter 38. J.B. Lippincott Company, Philadelphia-Toronto.

[34] Reproduction, The Cycle of Life. K. Jensen. U.S. News Books. ISBN 0-89193-606-8, 1983, page 98.

[35] Zoonomia, Volume 3, page 302.

"As far as your question regarding the first vaccine… that would be the Hep B, given to newborns just 1-day old. Dr. Jane Orient, director of the Association of American Physicians & Surgeons, writes, 'Doctors reported only about 10,000 hepatitis B cases in the U.S. in 1997 with only 306 occurring in children under 14. The only babies at risk are those born to hepatitis B-infected mothers. In 1996, only 54 cases of the disease were reported to the Centers for Disease Control and Prevention (CDC) in the 0 to 1 age group. There were 3.9 million births that year, so the observed incidence of hepatitis B in the 0 to 1 age group was just 0.001 percent. In the Vaccine Adverse Event Reporting System (VAERS) there were 1,080 total reports of adverse reactions from hepatitis B vaccine in 1996 alone in the 0 to 1 age group, with 47 deaths reported.' For most children, the risk of a serious vaccine reaction may be 100 times greater than the risk of hepatitis B. Overall, the incidence of hepatitis B in the U.S. is currently about 4 per 100,000. The risk for most young children is far less; hepatitis B is heavily concentrated in groups at high risk due to occupation, sexual promiscuity, or drug abuse."

"Lisa, it just doesn't make sense to unnecessarily expose the newborn to a vaccine that has more potential risk associated with it than contracting the actual disease itself."

"You're right. The U.S. tends to specify more vaccinations on the childhood immunization schedule combined with earlier dates of administration than any other country. That is, in part, why it is believed the U.S. has one of the highest rates of autism spectrum disorder diagnoses. According to the CDC's own statistics, in 2004, the rate was 1 in 166—with 1 in 6 children manifesting some type of neurodevelopmental or behavioral disorder. So prior to your giving birth, be certain to discuss these concerns, including your exemption from having the Hep B vaccine unnecessarily administered. From my years of experience, and based on the vaccination schedules in other countries, children have experienced healthier outcomes when their parents either filed an exemption from vaccines or at least postponed vaccinations until their children were older and their immune systems better able to tolerate them. There are many other deleterious effects that I won't mention right now. Do you know why they exist?"

Millie shook her head, frightened by the intensity in Lisa's voice. "No, why?"

"Money and greed. Greed and money."

Whew. Millie had never heard Lisa so angry. What was going on in Sycamore Springs?

##

"Autism, a Figment of the Mind."

Barbara had looked up from her book two months before Injection Day. She had known she needed time to prepare what she was going to say to Brandon to dissuade him from taking the vaccine. Usually, Damon didn't bother her when she was reading, so she'd opened a book to the middle and pretended to read while she formulated her plan. "What did you say, Damon?"

"It's the title of my article on vaccine-linked autism. What do you think of it? I think it's brilliant," he said smugly from his desk chair.

She frowned. The title didn't make sense. "How can autism be imagined? It's either there or it isn't."

Damon snorted. "Again, you don't know what you're talking about. My profession is being questioned. Someone, using improper statistical methods, is going around saying that children who received Thimerosal-containing vaccines are at greater risk for autism and other attention deficit problems than those receiving Thimerosal-free vaccines. That's malarkey. Our profession always does its due diligence. No shot or medication goes out to the public unless it is safe." He scribbled a few additions to his paper.

"Damon, please I'm not in the mood for comments like that. Nothing can be 100% safe. It's statistically impossible. Surely you have noticed that the pharmaceutical companies themselves disclose serious adverse reaction on their product inserts. There is associated with all estimates, a ninety-five percent confidence interval—a range of values that account for random variation that is based on statistics usually assuming a normal distribution of events. The public health officials will say anything they want to back themselves up for an unsuspecting public that trusts anyone on television. It's a good thing we don't listen to the pharmaceutical ads on TV and radio, but most of the population does and they can be classified as addicts waiting for their next commercial fix."

"You're crazy. Drug ads in the media make this great country of ours even healthier. They bring more health issues to the fore and more people into doctor's offices demanding what they saw on television, they also . . . ."

He stopped abruptly. "Barbara, that's it. I've just had another outstanding idea. We'll advertise Injection Day on television. Of course, it is going to make the news, but we'll buy advertising time and link it to everything from political campaigns to supermarket openings. We'll get it on milk cartons. We'll get banners at football half-times. We'll pay for it, and they'll do it. Sycamore Springs Injection Day will become the model for all Injection Days to follow across this great land. Now we need a slogan, something catchy, something with a hint of intimidation for the timid." He laughed. "Look at that, will you? Timid is part of intimidation. That's great. It means we have to make people follow us."

He sat down next to her and took her hands, causing her book to fall to the floor. "Okay, how about this slogan for the chickenpox vaccine. 'Don't be chicken! Get your shot!'"

She cringed. "That's horrible. How about, 'Be informed. Chick it out.' It's corny, but at least it implies people have a choice."

His face turned to stone. "What choice? We don't want them to have a choice, except the ones we give them. We're not lying. They trust us to have shuffled through the dissident voices of choice. We know what's best. That's why we went to medical school. We'll tell them what they need to do."

Barbara looked him in his cold eyes. "Craig attended a university, too. But he knows that his education and training by no means makes him always right, and he does not constitute himself a god."

Damon shook his head. "I can't believe you actually bite the wealthy hand that feeds you."

Something turned over in Barbara's stomach. Damon believed every word he said. How different would her life had been if she had married Lindsey. "And I can't believe you follow misguided logic that if you shine the light of panic and fear in someone's eyes you can prevent them from seeing the truth. Are you blind yourself, Damon? Can't you understand that there is more than one way to do something?"

"There is only one right way."

"Your way? What if by some infinitesimally small chance you're wrong? What if there are adverse, long-term consequences that you simply do not have the foresight to understand at this time?"

"Don't try to argue this point. It doesn't become you."

Barbara rose slowly to her feet. "Is that what you think? That a word or a phrase taints the picture you've painted? What if I tell you that some in your profession are frauds? What if I tell you that in 1993 when doctors were on strike in a foreign country for a month, there were half as many funerals?"

Damon snorted. "I'd respond by saying it was a coincidence. Doctors save lives, they don't take them."

"What about Sarah Perkins."

"An accident. They mixed up a couple of hoses. It's surprising it doesn't happen more often considering the amount of surgeries performed in this country. As a matter of fact, it happens much more than the public knows."

Barbara's eyes filled with tears as she remembered the confidences she had share with her friend. "How can you be so callous? Sarah was a human life. She had beauty and feelings. She gave love to her family and support to her friends. She didn't even need the surgery, but you needed more money for the wing on the hospital with your name. She trusted you."

"Are you taking her side against me? You vowed your devotion to me as a husband."

"But not as a man. Do you know that it would not be possible for me to hold you in greater contempt?"

"I can't believe you're saying these things. I want you in my office for a complete checkup and a full panel of tests. We'll get to the bottom of this and make you well."

Barbara pushed her way closer to him in the thick air between them. "I am not sick. You are. Your profession is. You have a manipulative fraternity of lies with your secret drug company information that states how many people really die from the use of a drug, and your guarantee of reimbursement from the insurance companies whether you kill the patient or not. You have a sweet deal, Damon, but I don't want to be part of it anymore. While I still have any part of my body left, I want a divorce, and I'm going to get one."

##

"A divorce?" Aileen's eyes were wider than her cheap make-up as she refilled Barbara's coffee mug. "You can't mean it. Damon will never allow that. He'll come after you."

Barbara unpacked the last of her overnight bag. "No, he won't. He'll be too busy denying it to his friends and colleagues and then end up blaming me for everything. And with Injection Day coming up, he'll have only that on his mind. I'll only show up to stop Brandon. Damon is a master when it comes to cover-ups. No one will ever know I left him. He'll say he threw me out, because I didn't support his Injection Day."

"You don't," Aileen confirmed softly. "I know you think it's dangerous."

"Don't you agree? You should have a talk with Craig. He says that chickenpox is a mild disease. Instead of the chickenpox vaccine reducing medical costs by protecting against chickenpox disease, the vaccine will actually increase medical costs due to corresponding increases in shingles cases. Did you know the shot had been available for ten years in the U.S., but the drug companies couldn't push its approval through until recently?"

"No, I didn't know that." Aileen sounded worried.

"Yes, they finally justified its use when they considered societal costs, that is, time parents lost from work taking care of children with chickenpox. You know Wayne Porter, Helen's son?"

"Of course. He's a wild kid, even crazier than my son. There's something not quite right with him."

"Do you know why?" Barbara asked rhetorically. "He had encephalitis shortly following an MMR booster vaccine."

Aileen stopped suddenly and stared at her. "I didn't know that. It wasn't in the gossip or in the local news."

Barbara's legs felt weak, the way they usually did when she thought about people being hurt in secret, like a military police that butchered and maimed without a word about it ever appearing in the newspapers. "That's because Damon made sure not a word got out. He and the vaccine manufacturer had dinner, and the next day Dr. Leviticus had a new car."

Aileen turned even paler. "I don't believe you. No one is that powerful."

"The legal pushers are. They rule more than you know."

"Why didn't you tell me before?"

"I couldn't. Damon said he'd make me pay if I ever betrayed him in his profession."

Aileen grabbed her arm. "Aren't you a little worried he's going to make you pay for leaving him in front of the whole city, in front of the American Medical Association, just before Injection Day?"

"You must mean the American Murder Association. I'm going to do much more than leave him. You know the Internet? It may be relatively new, and everyone may not yet be online with an Internet provider, but it's still a powerful tool for truth. Someday soon, it may be the only place intelligence and freedom of speech will exist, depending on the political climate and media manipulation by powerful conglomerates. Millie has a computer. I'm going to put messages all over the net about the real concerns parents should have about inoculating their children. For every pro-shot message and slogan Damon and his cronies are going to get on television and radio and newspapers by paying for ads, I'm going to post messages that contain the balanced truth all over the net. I wish I could reach everyone who doesn't have a computer, too, but the real truths will be shared, and the pharmaceutical profession will be held accountable for what they do, and will do, in the name of good medicine."

"Not to mention the effect you're going to have on the new-car-for-bribes industry," Aileen added, a slow smile on her face.

"That as well."

##

"You moved out on Dad?" Brandon stopped chewing on the massive hamburger in his hand. "Why?"

"He said things to me I could no longer tolerate."

"And that only bothered you now? He's always said and done things that made you upset. I've seen it since I was old enough to understand what was going on. What's different about this time?"

The fast-food junkies hadn't yet arrived for their afternoon get-together, and Barbara had asked Brandon to meet her for a talk. She wanted to tell him personally what was going on so he didn't hear it first through local gossip.

He looked very adult to her, especially strong and healthy. He was doing well in school and scoring touchdowns for the Sycamore Saints as well as overtime with every cheerleader on the squad, those hefty, corn-fed, bleach-blond, pom-pom waving distractions that worked the stadium from the beginning to the end of the game.

Damon watched the cheerleaders with more than a passing glance. Then, he's watched Paul approach the girls and tell them what a great job they were doing, how they made him proud to be at the game. Then, Paul would turn away and lick his lips. Damon always smiled at that part.

Unfortunately, Damon's furtive glances at the young women made her stomach hurt. Would he never be honest about any of his feelings, even personal, physical ones? Now, Barbara was going to divorce him, and he could have his fun.

Barbara pushed her lunch away. She hadn't felt like eating even though she'd bought the food, because she didn't have an appetite for more intrigue and deception. Would she ever be rid of the plagues of her life?

"You don't understand, Brandon. This time Damon's actions have gone too far. Not only do they encompass his family and the select people who are stuck in this burg—because of the limited choice of medical care, either sanctioned or alternative—but his plans will affect everyone who can be reached by the intimidation of his voice and his face."

Brandon snickered like all kids his age who hadn't lived long enough to think before voicing their opinions. "How can that happen? Is he going on network television?"

She stared him down, making him uncomfortable. She could tell because he squirmed in his seat. "Yes," she answered.

Brandon paled. "Great. Now all my friends, instead of the few of them unlucky enough to have medical care forced on them, will know him for the dork he is. They'll see how he acts in public, they'll hear him and the way he talks. What am I going to do?"

She sighed. Her son got his rebelliousness from her, but he inherited his self-centered personality from his father. "This isn't about you. You're not the only person who is going to be affected here. This is about Craig's study."

Brandon blinked. "What are you talking about? What's Millie's father got to do with my father being an embarrassment?"

Barbara took a deep breath before she answered, because the stakes were high enough for her to be dramatic. "To be humiliated is one thing, but to be murdered is another."

He looked away at two carloads of his friends making their way to the take-out line. Barbara knew he was considering bolting, anything for the swaggering football star not to be seen with his mother.

"Make it quick, Mom, I gotta pick up Millie. She's been feeling a little funny lately."

I'll bet.

"I can't hurry through the explanation, Brandon. This is important. Let me go with you to get Millie, and we can talk on the way."

He looked at her as if she were certifiably insane. "You can tell me later, okay?"

"But, Brandon, I . . . ."

He disappeared quickly along with his uneaten burger and fries.

##

"Barbara, great to see you, as always.

Craig greeted her with a hug. He was one of the few genuine people she had ever met. Everything about him inspired trust and security. Barbara began to think, maybe it would be good to have Millie as a daughter-in-law. Her parents were good, honest people who put themselves after their family, friends, and community – the complete antithesis of prioritizing that her husband followed.

Craig and Faith's home was warm and welcoming. Instead of overpriced, worthless copies of valuable art and musty antiques like the ones that Damon had insisted on buying in her own home, Craig and Faith had decorated with taste, space, and tranquility. Plants abounded, and chimes caught the friendly breezes.

They lived in harmony with nature. Instead of altering the balance of life in the ecosystem of Sycamore Springs, they respected all living things and worked for environmental balance. Craig was involved in volunteer community service activities and lent his abilities to furthering the common good of mankind.

Theirs was the only family she had ever met that was completely unselfish.

Quite a contrast to her home, where nature had been replaced by laboratory versions of life.

The Manchester household was a haven for strength. Craig himself was tall and rugged. He didn't talk about his athletic abilities, but everyone in town knew he had built his house from the foundation to the roof. Ironically, it had been his unexpected experience with installing roofing *shingles* in 115°F Sycamore Springs heat, that had lowered his immunity and resulted in his agonizing experience with herpes zoster, also called shingles. Barbara admired him for seeking help for reoccurring post herpetic neuralgia (PHN) despite the inadequacies of the medical industry to produce any truly effective treatment and then turning around to give the benefit of his research to the public. He was a generous and caring man, and everything Damon was not.

"I want to talk to you about the shingles study," she said firmly. "Don't ask how I know about it."

Craig smiled. "Between Faith and Lisa, who both echo my concerns, I came to the conclusion long ago that valid research should be made public immediately, and even faster when it involves vaccine or other public health and safety issues. Which one told you?"

"Both."

"Figures. Sit down and we'll talk."

He closed the door to his office, the entire top floor of his home. From the spacious windows, Barbara could see much of Sycamore Springs and the surrounding boondocks. Sometimes she forgot how isolated they really were. The daily living with an egomaniac like the power-hungry Doctor Leviticus left her drained and angry at the end of the day and lonely in the morning.

How grateful she was that she no longer had to portray the wife to his poorly played partner's role.

"What do you know so far, Barbara? I don't want to bore you."

"You couldn't possibly bore me, Craig. You're one of the few reasonable men in town. I don't know very much, just that you see a disturbing trend in the incidence of shingles."

"Yes, that is correct. I observed an anomaly in the data that stood out against being just a chance or transient occurrence. The incidence rate of shingles among children was higher—much higher—than the rate among adolescents and young adults, and virtually all historical studies have reported the reverse—incidence rates of shingles increase with advancing age. At first, I wondered if it was an erroneous result, but after scrutinizing over the calculations, I have come to a better understanding of the biological mechanisms involved. I believe we have a problem of epidemic proportion with the chickenpox vaccine. The varicella vaccine certainly is not new, but the U.S. is the first country to recommend a Universal Vaccination Program, whereby all healthy susceptible children are vaccinated. This amounts to a human experiment on a grand scale because studies indicate that adults receive a boost to their immune systems each time they are exposed to children infected with chickenpox. This exposure produces an immunologic boost that helps to postpone the reactivation of the varicella-zoster virus as shingles. There is a need to exercise caution since if the vaccine dramatically reduces natural chickenpox, outside or exogenous boosting will be reduced as well. Thus, I and other researchers expect that shingles incidence rates among adults could be higher than they were prior to licensure of the varicella vaccine for the next 30 to 50 years."

"So, Craig, this is the heated controversy that is going on behind the medical scenes."

"Yes, there are additional concerns as well. This varicella vaccine is a live-virus vaccine that is injected into each child that is 12-months or older. This manner of inducing immunity via injection, is not a natural route that the virus would normally take. When the varicella virus is acquired naturally through a respiratory path, breathing droplets containing the virus through the nasal or throat passages, a strong cell-mediated immune response is elicited. This is not the case when the virus is injected. Then there is the cost/benefit analysis for the vaccine. If one considers the deleterious effects of the vaccine, it does not take many serious adverse reactions and their associated medical costs to offset any relatively minor savings associated with preventing cases of chickenpox. Since 75% of medical costs associated with the varicella-zoster virus are due to shingles (and not chickenpox), a relatively small increase in shingles could more than offset the savings associated with chickenpox vaccination. Many medical professionals have questioned whether or not it is better to leave an at-risk population alone when it comes to a disease that is usually benign. When I wrote to a researcher at Merck, I expected him to disagree with my analysis."

"Craig, what did he say?"

"I have the e-mail right here. He wrote, 'You are not the first to ask this question, and it is valid. Merck and managed care will have to figure it out.'"

"But didn't the CDC commission a study that showed that no increase in shingles had occurred?"[36]

"Yes, the CDC has previously cited two rather small studies with a study population of only 3,000 to 4,000, as well as a larger study that showed no increase in shingles had yet occurred. However, an editor of the journal that published the larger study, commented that varicella vaccination coverage was not widespread in the community, therefore, he questioned the purpose and value of such a study. So when the CDC states 'there has been no statistically significant increase in shingles,' this statement is misleading and is based on either (1) studies with too small a sample size and therefore they have insufficient statistical power to detect increases, or (2) studies in communities where adults are still receiving exogenous (outside) boosts from children with natural varicella, since vaccination coverage has not reached a moderate to widespread level (with at least 50% or more of the children

---

[36] [1] Jumaan AO, Yu O, Jackson LA, Bohlke K, Galil K, Seward JF. Incidence of herpes zoster, before and after varicella-vaccination-associated decreases in the incidence of varicella, 1992-2002. J Infect Dis. 2005 Jun 15;191(12):1999-2001; [2] Roche P, Blumer C, Spencer J. Surveillance of viral pathogens in Australia—Varicella-zoster virus. Commun. Dis. Intell. 2002;26:576-580; and [3] Burgess M. National Center for Immunisation Research and Surveillance of Vaccine Preventable Diseases, NCIRS Newsletter, Dec. 3, 2002.

under the age of 10-years-old vaccinated). Recently the CDC conducted a large study and found adult shingles increased 90% from 1998 to 2003 during a period of increasing varicella vaccination."[37]

"Craig, after Lisa filled me in on some details, I had many remaining questions: If the vaccine efficacy or protection eventually declines, as studies currently indicate is happening, will children, as they reach adulthood, be at increased risk of chickenpox[38] at a time when the disease presents with more complications? Also, if pregnant mothers no longer have varicella immunity, will antibodies fail to be transferred to their infants such that babies will be at increased risk of varicella prior to the age they can be vaccinated? Will new VZV strains derive as a result of the live, Japanese Oka-strain in the varicella vaccine genetically combining with natural wild-type strains[39] that circulate in the United States?"

"Barbara, the answer to all of your excellent questions is 'Yes!' I should also mention there are other deleterious scenarios. If a vaccinated child is exposed to an adult with shingles or another child with the natural disease, the vaccinated child could harbor both the vaccine strain and natural strain viruses. After such an exposure, the vaccinee may experience a breakthrough case of chickenpox consisting of less than 50 lesions or may not manifest any clinical symptoms of chickenpox at all. However, the natural strain would dominate over the attenuated vaccine strain. Such a vaccinee would be subject to the same increased risk of shingles as a child who had a previous history of natural chickenpox. Furthermore, there is a delicate balance in nature and marvelous wisdom beyond man's comprehension when we consider the intriguing possibility that adults who failed to contract chickenpox were at significantly higher risk for the formation of gliomas (fast growing brain tumors) than those who had contracted chickenpox.[40] Interestingly, a different study conducted in Germany did not support this association.[41] In any case, if varicella did play some protective role with respect to other harmful viruses that may have shared one or more common characteristics, the question remains: will varicella vaccine elicit the same protective response?"

"Barbara, you are correct in concluding that the effectiveness of a single dose is questionable. After about 10 years of varicella vaccine experience in the U.S., it appears the recommendation is going to change from one to two doses of varicella given in the quadravalent MMRV (measles, mumps, rubella, and varicella) vaccine. The children receiving one dose, as well as those receiving a booster dose, will lose the protective effect

---

[37] Yih WK, Brooks DR, Lett SM, Jumaan AO, Zhang Z, Clements KM, Seward JF. The incidence of varicella and herpes zoster in Massachusetts as measured by the Behavioral Risk Factor Surveillance System (BRFSS) during a period of increasing varicella vaccine coverage, 1998-2003. BMC Public Health. 2005 Jun 16;5(1):68.
[38] Arvin A, Gershon A. Control of varicella: Why is a two-dose schedule necessary? Pediatr. Infect.Dis. J. 2006;25:475-476.
[39] Grossberg R, Harpaz R, Rubtcova E, Loparev V, Seward JF, Schmid DS. Secondary transmission of varicella vaccine virus in a chronic care facility for children. J. Pediatr. 2006;148:842-844.
[40] Wrensch M, Weinberg A, Wiencke J, Miike R, Barger B, Kelsey K. Prevalence of Antibodies to Four Herpesviruses among Adults with Glioma [Brain Tumor] and Controls. Am. J. Epidem. 2001;154:161-165.
[41] Poltermann S, Schlehofer B, Steindorf K, Schnitzler P, Geletneky K, Schlehofer JR. Lack of association of herpesviruses with brain tumors. J Neurovirol. 2006 Apr;12(2):90-99.

and become susceptible to chickenpox at an older age when there is greater likelihood of complications."

He continued, caught up in reporting his research to her. "Following some vaccinations, especially attributed to the Pertussis component of the trivalent DTaP vaccine, parents reported their child's so-called innocent fever and agitation, including shrill screaming. Sadly, these can be indicators of neurological damage occurring due to swelling of the brain and the body's attempt to cope with the assault.[42]

When a death subsequently occurs, the medical profession calls it SIDS or sudden-infant-death syndrome, when in reality a vaccine-related death has occurred."

"Craig, could you please backtrack and explain to me again why naturally acquired varicella immunity is better?"

"Many reasons. As I indicated earlier, each time an adult is exposed to children with chickenpox, the adult experiences an immune boost that helps to suppress the reactivation of shingles. Once the chickenpox vaccine becomes widespread, there will be few opportunities for these immune boosts. Shingles in adults will likely double and the public health agencies will come to the 'rescue' by providing a shingles vaccine to provide the immunologic boosting that previously occurred naturally in the community during chickenpox outbreaks in the community. Likely public health officials will claim that this shingles vaccine reduces shingles by 50%; what they won't admit is that the varicella vaccine caused a 100% increase in shingles to begin with; therefore, the net effect of costly mass chickenpox and shingles vaccination campaigns will be zero. For the first time in history, a 'shingles' vaccine will be required to offset the deleterious effects of the varicella vaccine."

"Craig, I have also heard that the CDC's Advisory Committee on Immunization Practice (ACIP) has recently recommended an influenza vaccination during pregnancy. I know my husband has administered this vaccine to a few pregnant women already, but plans to vaccinate many more on Injection Day."

"Yes, this presents another problem. Most formulations of the influenza vaccine contain Thimerosal."[43]

"Craig, I already know this Thimerosal is used as a preservative and that it contains mercury."

"Yes, but the problem is that Thimerosal has been implicated in human neurodevelopmental disorders ranging from autism to ADD/ADHD. What is worse, the substance is considered a teratogen."

"What is that?"

---

[42] Berkovic SF, Harkin L, McMahon JM, Pelekanos JT, Zuberi SM, Wirrell BC, Gill DS, Iona X, Mulley JC, Scheffer IE. De-novo mutations of the sodium channel gene SCN1A in alleged vaccine encephalopathy: a retrospective study. Lancet Neurol. 2006 Jun;5(6):488-492.

[43] Ayoub DM, Yazbak FE. Influenza vaccination during pregnancy: a critical assessment of the recommendations of the Advisory Committee on Immunization Practices (ACIP). Journal of American Physicians and Surgeons 2006 Summer; 11(2):41-49.

"A teratogen (pronounced ter-ra'-tə-gen), similar to a mutagen, is a substance than can cause mutations and genetic problems. On the Manufacturer's Safety Data Sheet (MSDS), it states that Thimerosal 'exposure in-utero can cause mild to severe mental retardation and motor coordination impairment.' It also states, Thimerosal 'is known to cause birth defects and other reproductive harm.'"

"Craig, Now I am really worried. My best friend, who is pregnant, plans to have the flu vaccine on Injection Day."

"Barbara, it's still not too late to warn her. You and I know that when we consider (1) the flu vaccine only protects against 3 strains and (2) the chances of one actually contracting the flu virus, the average vaccine effectiveness is only 7.2%. In some years the flu vaccine offered no protection! I don't want you to scare your friend, but my research uncovered a paper that discussed 4 patients, who all filed VAERS reports on the same day in North Carolina,[44] 2 of the 4 involved the same vaccine lot, and all experienced a stillbirth within 30 days of receipt of the flu vaccine. Their viable babies ranged in gestational age from 27 to 39 weeks at demise. These adverse outcomes were biologically plausible since a fetus of 1 kg (2.2 pounds) weight could have been exposed to 25 micrograms of mercury from the flu vaccine. This is over 200 times the 0.01 microgram amount daily allowable by the Environmental Protection Agency (EPA) and based on a 4.1 preferential accumulation of mercury in cord blood. So far, I have not heard of any stillbirths occurring in Sycamore Springs, but then again, the ACIP recommendation to vaccinate during all trimesters is new and therefore more similar tragedies should be expected. Unfortunately, Dr. L's Injection Day, combined with his misplaced confidence in the safety of this recommendation, could contribute to these death statistics."

Craig continued, "I have also come across the statistic that after the receipt of five consecutive flu vaccines, an adult is at ten times greater risk for developing Alzheimer's."

"Craig, it seems the CDC is getting more and more brazen with its vaccination policies and these play right into my husband's hands."

"What's next?"

"Fluoridated water."

Barbara furrowed her brow, and he leaned closer.

"The practice of adding fluoride compounds to the U.S. water supply as a 'safe and effective' preventive for fighting tooth decay began in 1950. Sycamore Springs, as in other communities maintains a concentration of fluoride of 1 part per million. Interestingly, most countries worldwide have chosen to reject the practice of water fluoridation, recognizing that fluoride in the concentration provided, is a highly toxic poison."[45]

Barbara gasped. "I never knew that."

"Not many people do. Please let me elaborate. Studies conducted since the 1950s have shown there was a difference in improvement of less than 1 of 128 tooth surfaces in children in fluoridated versus unfluoridated water areas. The CDC's findings, based on many

---

[44] VAERS ID #249829, 249831-3

[45] See Appendix I. Fifty Reasons to Oppose Fluoridation

dental researchers, indicate that *topical* fluoride has benefits so that systemic fluoride via the water supply is unnecessary. Furthermore, fluoride exposure has been associated with lowering of I.Q. Again, just as Public Health Officials cannot admit Thimerosal-containing vaccines (including the flu vaccine) play a role in higher risk of autism due to significant legal liabilities and loss of public confidence in vaccines, so too, governmental officials defend water fluoridation as a healthy practice rather than acknowledge its contribution to increases in hip fractures, arthritis, bone cancer, brain disorders, and underactive thyroid.[46] Landfills and toxic waste disposal are big, political, hot potatoes. No one knows what to do with fluoride, so people should drink it. Makes perfect sense to them."

"Is there any way to remove the fluoride from our drinking water?"

"Perhaps the simplest way to remove 90% or more of the fluoride is through the use of a reverse osmosis filter."

"I am glad that I've always used such a filter for my drinking water. But can we put a stop to the use of fluoride?"

"Probably not. There are enough people who can lie and say that fluoride is harmless—even propaganda indicating water fluoridation is beneficial for teeth. Therefore, the industry makes a fortune selling the fluoride, instead of paying a fortune trying to dump it, and the worst part is that completely innocent people are adversely affected. This, in turn, creates a steady flow of monetary enrichment to healthcare facilities from patients seeking medical attention to treat the wide diversity of problems caused by their drinking fluoridated water."

She sighed. "So it's not only in medicine."

"It's everywhere, but medicine is the worst. Defective study methodology and flawed statistics are combined to yield virtually any effect desired. And if that doesn't work, the doctors and pharmaceutical companies lie outright and pump their mutual funds with the bodies of people who died for nothing, beautiful, healthy people who were in the wrong place at the wrong time."

"Which is?"

"The doctor's office."

Barbara took a deep breath to force clean air into her lungs. Craig echoed her thoughts, but it was still difficult to digest everything after all she had gone through and witnessed.

"What are we going to do, Craig? Damon is moving his doctor's office into the street in front of his medical building. He's going to blitz the media with scare tactics and lies about the chickenpox vaccine. People will be shot full of every vaccine they are currently lacking, and who knows what long-term consequences will follow?"

"I know," Craig stated grimly. "I know exactly what will happen."

---

[46] See Appendix I. Fifty Reasons to Oppose Fluoridation.

Chapter 13

Barbara always liked autumn in Sycamore Springs. She remembered the first time she'd seen the awesome orange and yellow hues of leaves on the many limbs of Sycamore tress glistening in the sun. It was the only season having a moderate temperature with a light breeze that made one especially comfortably in the midst of a rural, but developing town. The scenery was against a backdrop of the San Bernadino mountain range with glorious cumulus cloud formations visible in the distance. From the beginning, she had seen what a small town could do with the coming of greater darkness, and she felt a kinship with her new neighbors. Most of the time, things went smoothly. Hyperactive kids out of control on their post Halloween sugar high soon dressed as pilgrims in Thanksgiving pageants at their schools, their proud parents commenting on how quickly time went by, and how happy the lucky ones were to have healthy, intelligent children.

So, why did she feel impending doom? What was going to go wrong this year? It had to be something. She'd observed Craig pacing in front of his own house, and she'd seen Lisa in the antacid section of the supermarket. What disaster was it going to be? The town had suffered through fires set carelessly or intentionally, earthquakes from their unenviable position right about the major San Andreas Fault, the spill-over of race riots from the turmoil of Los Angeles. But those events had been out of her control. Why did she feel that this year's coming disaster was something she might have prevented?

No, this year it was going to be something personal and close to home. Why did she know that? Because she was irrevocably divorcing Dr. Leviticus, a decision reinforced by her disbelief of seeing her son's picture all over town advertising Injection Day.

The most tasteless display was in front of the medical building, where the streets had been cordoned off as if a mass murder had taken place. Tables lined the streets, and as Barbara turned her car into the supermarket lot blocks away, she could hear a band playing "The Star Spangled Banner" as the day began.

How ingenuous of Damon to link vaccines and patriotism. One of his slogans was, "It's Un-American to Say No Today."

The fall air was colder than usual, and she pulled her sweater on over her head, unable to do it smoothly in her state of mind. It caught on her sunglasses, and she sighed in exasperation. Unnerved by what she considered to be a signal of coming events, she shuddered knowing that by nightfall she should be in total chaos with an uncontrollable level of stress.

"Need help?" a voice behind her asked.

Brandon. He was always there when she needed him, even if she embarrassed him. "Yes," she mumbled, muffled by the wool.

She could hear him chuckling as he freed her from the tight collar.

"Seems like you used to do this for me," he said softly, and her heart turned over. She loved him so. She had to stop him from being a puppet again.

"Now we help each other," she replied, a catch in her voice. "Did you have to park all the way over here, too?" she asked.

He nodded. "They've got all kinds of security over there, and an ice cream truck from Tippy's, you know the one that circled the neighborhoods all summer. Dad has a sign up saying all frozen treats courtesy of Injection Day. But then he has a disclaimer in the corner, saying that to be served, the parents must present a proof sticker indicating their children under the age of 12 have their immunizations up to date. Those children under the age 12 will be served if they either have a documented history of chickenpox or have received the chickenpox vaccine.

Barbara wasn't surprised he had made it even more slanted to his side, requiring people to turn over their first born to get an ice cream cone. Yet, in effect, wasn't that what he was saying? *Give me your children, and I will do whatever I want with them for my personal profit and ego?*

Barbara linked her arm with Brandon's. "Speaking of immunizations, I want you to do something for me."

"Anything."

He hadn't heard what she wanted yet. Once he did, she wasn't sure if he'd agree. He had to have the approval of all his friends, and deep down he wanted to please his father no matter what his mom said.

How was she going to tell him that Damon was ignoring Craig's research? How was she going to tell him that his own father had been, and would be, responsible for bringing long-term illness, suffering, and possibly death to his friends and neighbors in a small community like Sycamore that was too isolated by distance and ignorance for people to seek healthcare elsewhere beyond the county boundaries?

Barbara recalled the words of Dr. John R. Lee, "Most over-the-counter and almost all prescribed drug treatments merely mask symptoms or control health problems, or in some way alter the way organs or systems such as the circulatory system work. Drugs almost never deal with the reasons why these problems exist, while they frequently create new health problems as side effects of their activities." She wondered how many other towns, cities, and neighborhoods were blinded to the truth. She was sure that Sycamore Springs wasn't the only city duped by medical and pharmaceutical politics. She was certain that Dr. Damon Leviticus wasn't the only despotic cog in the wheel of health care deception, intentional or unintentional.

Barbara took Brandon's hands in hers and looked directly into his guileless eyes. "I want you to refuse the vaccine."

"What?" he asked with disbelief, backing up, pulling his hands away, and shielding his eyes from her request.

"I want you to refuse to take the vaccine, and I want you to make a statement to the press that you are not entirely convinced the chickenpox vaccine is needed or is safe."

He sat down hard on the pavement. "Do you understand what you're asking me to do? Not only would I be humiliated as a crybaby who didn't want his doctor daddy to give him a shot, but I'd be opening the door to all the yelling and misery that my father heaps on his family whenever he doesn't get his way. I'd be the one accused of having a tantrum. Instead, if I go through with his stupid Injection Day, we'll prevent him from throwing a tantrum in front of the entire world, thanks to the media. Why are you asking me to do something like that?"

Barbara advanced on her cub. "Didn't you hear me? Because the vaccine isn't safe," she repeated, her anger rising. "Craig has some preliminary evidence that eliminating chickenpox will increase shingles incidence among adults for an entire generation. Even though the chickenpox vaccine is not new, no country has ever vaccinated all healthy children. So the universal varicella vaccination program is essentially a huge experiment with the entire U.S. population as the guinea pigs. Lisa has also seen some disturbing trends in school children with shingles. But the most important personal reason is that you've had a history of bad reactions to vaccines before, and I don't want you to take a chance with this one. Chickenpox is a minor problem. Shingles is a bigger one. If you've never had chickenpox or the chickenpox vaccine, you can't get shingles since shingles occurs when the dormant chickenpox virus reactivates. Even though the CDC recommends the vaccine to all susceptible adolescents who believe they have never had a previous history of chickenpox or their history is unknown, studies indicate that as many as 80% of such adolescents actually demonstrate titers indicating a previous chickenpox infection, perhaps a case that was so mild that it went unnoticed, undetected, or mistaken for insect bites or some other rash. Since two doses four to eight weeks apart are necessary to protect children aged 13 years and older, it is actually more cost effective to do the laboratory testing on adolescents first to determine whether or not they already have antibody titers to the varicella-zoster virus. People should not take as many drugs and shots as they do, just because they're intimidated by medical industry and their medical insurance reimburses for such interventions."

"You mean medical profession," he corrected wearily.

"No, I mean medical industry," she said firmly, spitting out the words. "It's a business, dependent on profit for survival, and don't you ever forget it." She fumbled in her pocket. "Here, I've written out what you should say to the media. Craig and Lisa assisted me with the words."

Brandon backed away as if he'd been bitten by the snake of maternal madness. "In front of my friends? The team? The cheerleaders? They'll say I'm afraid."

She snorted. "I don't think they're going to think you're scared of a needle after being tackled by Dexter last year. He nearly took your head off. Here, look over your speech with me, and read it aloud at least once."

He pushed the paper back into her hands. "Take it. I'm going to get the shot. Big deal. What difference is one vaccine more or less going to make?"

Barbara felt a sob rise in her throat. Pure panic kicked her adrenaline supply into overkill. "Please don't do this to me. You're my only child. You may be a strong athlete, but you're still a human subject to potential ill-effects of medical interventions. Your example can influence a lot of people, not just those in Sycamore Springs, but those throughout the nation watching CNN, to reflect more seriously on vaccine safety issues rather than give *carte blanche* support to medical mandates. Please don't take the shot."

Brandon's eyes filled with tears. "I don't want to take anything from Dad – not a dime, not a pill, not a shot. But if I don't do this, they'll say I'm chicken. Also Dexter, who was previously living with his father, does not remember ever having chickenpox, so he plans to follow me in the vaccine lineup." He turned and ran across the parking lot to the circus in front of Damon's office.

Barbara felt the waves of anxiety turn the world white with fear. Impending doom flooded her. She knew there was generally no cause for concern if a typical adolescent who had had a previous history of chickenpox was needlessly administered the Varivax® vaccine. But Brandon was a special case with a history of some type of adverse reaction to almost every vaccine he had every received throughout childhood. Although extremely rare, Brandon might be just the one to have an anaphylatic reaction to the trace neomycin antibiotic contained in the vaccine. Barbara also did not know if Brandon perhaps had a life-threatening allergy to the gelatin that was also present in the vaccine. Then there was always the potential for human error resulting in a contaminated vaccine dose. What if something happened to the only person in life who mattered to her?

"Oh my, what have you done, Damon? You're going to sacrifice your only son on the altar of greed."

Barbara couldn't stop her legs from shaking, hoping Brandon would tolerate this vaccine better than he had tolerated others in the past. She leaned against her newly-detailed car, the worst slogan of the batch resounding in her mind: "Don't be chicken. Don't get chickenpox".

Chapter 14

"Over here, Son," Damon shouted as soon as he saw him turn the corner.

Brandon rounded the edge of his father's medical complex and gasped. Barnum and Bailey had come to town. Flags adorned the tops of the buildings. The high school band faced a grandstand set of bleachers that overlooked an elaborate set of tables laced to form a giant "I". His father's nurse, wearing her customary, phony, plastic smile as far as he was concerned, handed out pep rally tags in the shape of giant hypodermic needles.

His mother was right. He shouldn't be a part of the sham any longer. She got out, but who was going to give him the guts he needed to walk away in front of his friends, with Dexter next in line? If he were alone with his father, he would bolt like a caged wild animal whose captor had unknowingly left the door open. Even though just a few of his friends were actually getting the shot (because they or their parents could not recall their ever having a previous history of chickenpox), most of his other friends were in attendance and watching since their younger siblings were brought to Injection Day to be vaccinated, except for the lucky ones like Rochelle, who had a family emergency out of town.

He heard a male voice yell his name and turned around. Dexter was only a few feet from him. "Hey, Poster Boy," he called with a smirk longer than Main Street. "They got your ugly face plastered all over CNN. You got connections?"

Brandon shook free of his rival's grip on his arm. "You know I hate this," he muttered.

Dexter laughed. "Good thing he isn't my old man. My father's a loser, but he's not a moron."

Out of the mouth of the son-of-a-loser, came the truth. Maybe in front of Dexter, he could call his father on his project, announce his opposition to the crowd, ruin the House of Leviticus, and leave, still in possession of some shred of his pride. But what about Dexter and the others? Did they understand the real risks of varicella vaccination—both short term and long term? Did the cheerleaders know despite their youth and rebellious morals?

Where were his morals? Prisoners of his pride, that's where.

He slouched forward into the waiting embrace of his father, who crushed him with an elaborate show of pride against his official white coat and stethoscope hanging around his neck.

Why would this shot hurt more than the others?

Why should this shot make a difference?

Chapter 15

An ambulance siren.

Barbara sat upright on Aileen's couch and fumbled for the light switch. She hated that sound, especially in the middle of the night. It meant someone was in deep trouble.

And it meant that Damon would make it worse.

She stepped into her slippers and started for the front window. She hadn't had a good night's sleep since she moved to Sycamore Springs with Damon. None of her old friends could understand why. Sycamore was a small town with little outside interference, basically a closed community. When they pulled up the sidewalks early in the evening, the adults went home and the kids left the city limits. Yet, sleep had eluded her, as if she had taken on the guilt her husband should have claimed as his own.

She turned at a sound from the bedroom and saw Aileen switch on the bed lamp behind her and begin tying her robe together.

Barbara turned away toward the kitchen, hoping to give her privacy. How had Aileen gotten by her without awakening her from sleep on the sofa? Either Barbara was sleeping more soundly now that she didn't have to lay next to Damon, or Aileen was just exceptionally quiet.

"You okay?" Aileen asked.

"Fine, just shaken by the sound. You okay?"

Aileen replied, "Yes, the siren broke my sleep too."

Now that Barbara would soon be single again, she had no idea what she would do in the near future.

"Barbara. Just because you're going to be divorced, doesn't mean our friendship is going to change. We've been too much together to change the basis for our friendship now. I've always given you the ins and outs of my relationships, and now I expect to hear all about yours. So what's bothering you?"

"I didn't know you could tell. I'm uncomfortable with everything these days. Since Injection Day last week, I'm more upset than I've ever been."

Aileen pushed the blankets aside and sat down on the sofa. "What's worrying you?"

"Brandon. He took the shot after I begged him not to. He's sensitive, maybe hypersensitive to one of the components of the vaccine. What if something happens to him?"

Aileen stared at her. "Unfortunately, against my wishes, I heard that my son Dexter also took the vaccine following Brandon. Likely he saw this as an opportunity to showoff to the cheerleaders. Since he was over 18, no parental permission was required. What could happen? He's young and strong. Only babies have side effects, and these are supposed to be normal and expected. A little crying, a little temper tantrum, a high fever... Typical baby stuff."

Barbara watched her own hands shake. "That's not what Craig says. He tells me that in a safety report concerning varicella vaccine, some adults experienced serious side effects.[47] By comparison to the large number of children reported on in the chickenpox vaccine safety study, only relatively few adolescents and adults received the vaccine. The adverse reports among the older aged individuals, combined with the fact that few were vaccinated, demonstrate a potential for greater risk of deleterious effects among older persons. Despite the adverse reactions occurring in adult recipients of the chickenpox vaccine, the report conclusion summarizes that there were too few reported adverse events among adults to present a statistically significant trend at this time and that the chickenpox vaccine is generally well tolerated and found to be safe. Of course this conclusion is carefully constructed and is more pro-vaccine propaganda than actual scientific fact based on the available data presented." Barbara continued, "Unlike babies, adolescents and adults can frequently verbalize their distress. Unfortunately most patients, including many physicians, don't think to consider that a vaccine can trigger an adverse event. So the statistics on adverse reactions are grossly under-reported. Babies either live or die. Adults may be able to verbalize their need for help."

Aileen patted her hand. "Well, then, that's the answer, isn't it? Should Brandon or Dexter feel sick, they'll call for help. Let's go back to sleep."

##

A pounding on the door woke Barbara again. Was that Damon's voice?

Outside, Damon shouted, "Aileen? Are you in there?"

Barbara switched on the lamp by the sofa again. What would her soon-to-be ex-husband be doing knocking on Aileen's door in the middle of the night? Certainly he couldn't be there for entertainment purposes, could he?

Aileen appeared in the dark doorway to her room again. "Is someone here?"

Barbara swung her legs onto the floor. "It sounds like Damon," she replied doing her best to keep the suspicion out of her voice.

Aileen detected it anyway. "Well, that would be a first. I'm not his type, and he's definitely not mine." She knotted the belt on her robe.

Barbara snorted. "You can say that again."

Aileen glanced up, hurt in her eyes. "I guess I don't have your taste in imported crystal."

Oh, no. What was she doing to their friendship, which was probably the only good one in Sycamore Springs. She'd have to mend it before it shattered.

"I'm sorry. I didn't mean that the way it sounded. You're too good for Damon, and if he was coming on to you, I'd share even more of his hideous traits."

"Aileen," Damon yelled in his most professional tone, "open this door at once."

---

[47] Wise RP, Salve ME, Braun MM, Mootrey GT, Seward JF, Rider LG, Krause PR. Postlicensure safety surveillance for varicella vaccine. JAMA 2000 Sep. 13;284(10):1271-1279.

"I better open it," she muttered, "before he breaks it down. Do you want to hide in my room?"

Barbara's eyes widened. "What would Damon say if he found me in there?" She moved closer to the dark bedroom. She'd be safe, and hidden; she would have a few minutes reaction time to figure out what was going on. It would be best if Damon didn't see her at Aileen's. She wanted him to think she had gone to Los Angeles to get as far away from him as she could get.

She ran for the bedroom and closed the door, leaving it open a few inches so she could hear what was happening.

Aileen smoothed her robe and her hair in practiced gestures Barbara found enviable.

She watched silently as Aileen opened the front door just as Damon had changed his tactics to jiggling the door knob with alternating open-palmed slams onto the door itself.

"At last," he exclaimed, lurching into the room, catching his balance before he fell. "Didn't you hear me? I've got news, and I want you to remain calm."

Aileen backed up. "Is something wrong?"

Her voice shook, and the sound of the fear and panic in it, instead of the stability and common sense she had learned to rely on, sent a chill of fear up Barbara's spine.

Damon grabbed Aileen by her shoulders and shook her hard. "Calm, do you hear me? Nothing could have been done for him. It was one of those unexplained events that we, as professionals, have no way to prevent."

"What in the world are you talking about, Damon? What's going on? You're scaring me."

Damon took a deep and practiced breath. "Dexter is paralyzed."

With those words finally expressed, Aileen's legs began to fail.

##

Barbara closed the door to Aileen's bedroom. Aileen lay on the rumpled sheets, ashen, drugged from a heavy sedative. The news had sent her into hysterics. She'd loved Dexter. No matter who the father had been, it didn't matter to Aileen, as long as she was the mother. Aileen and Dexter seemed to understand each other, both a little too wild for normal society.

What had gone wrong? How could a healthy eighteen-year-old man suddenly become paralyzed? Damon said they'd get to the bottom of it, and that he suspected street drugs were the cause.

Barbara doubted it. Dexter didn't use drugs according to Brandon. Young girls were his addiction, and he nurtured it at every opportunity.

It had to be directly linked to the varicella vaccination Dexter had received from the hand of Leviticus on Injection Day. What would make a healthy man collapse waiting for a burger?

Her chest was tight and her breathing was shallow. What if the same thing happened to Brandon? She'd read too much, and she knew too much. Anything could have gone wrong, from some undisclosed contamination in the vaccine manufacturer's production lot to some rare neurological problem that would not have been detected in vaccine trials conducted largely among younger children.

To add to the tragedy, chickenpox was considered a benign disease with very low rates of morbidity and mortality prior to the FDA's licensing the vaccine. Crippling even a few healthy individuals could certainly more than offset any benefit attributed to preventing many cases of chickenpox.

##

Craig leaned forward in his dimly lit office. Lisa noticed the tension in his expression. It would have been hard to miss. How many nights hadn't he slept since Dexter was stricken?

"The advertised benefit of the chickenpox vaccination is this," he began. "The children that are vaccinated, at least at this time, seem to have a lower incidence of shingles than children who acquire natural chickenpox. The more significant, long-term problem already in its first stages of development is this: those children and adults with a previous history of chickenpox, who did not receive the chickenpox vaccination for this very reason (i.e., they previously had a natural case of chickenpox), will continue to experience a higher risk of shingles, relative to the risk in the prelicensure era, for at least the next 30 to 50 years. I do not think that such a precedent for increased pain and suffering has ever occurred in vaccine history. This is the first time that universal vaccination has been adopted to try to eradicate one disease—chickenpox—which is closely related to shingles—both primary and secondary diseases caused by VZV (varicella-zoster virus). When the incidence of chickenpox is low, the incidence of shingles is high and vice-versa."

"That's because they share a common origin, right?" she asked.

"Yes, other diseases do not have a primary disease, in this case chickenpox, and a secondary disease, shingles." He moved his desk chair over a few feet and reached for a copy of his latest articles in a large file on a second desk.

"So, Craig, what you're saying is that chickenpox and shingles are linked together no matter if the patient has had a vaccine or not. That those who were inoculated with the live chickenpox (or varicella) vaccine virus can break out in shingles, just as can those who acquired the natural chickenpox disease."

"That's correct; however, it is suspected that since the vaccine strain, or Oka-strain as it is called, is a weaker, attenuated strain, any resulting shingles among vaccinees may be more mild compared to the shingles that reactivates from those who have experienced the natural or wild-type disease. There is a complication, however, worth mentioning. A benefit promoted by the public health officials is that the incidence rate of shingles among vaccinees is lower than the rate among those having natural chickenpox. However, when a vaccinee is exposed to either an adult with shingles or a child contagious with natural chickenpox, that vaccinee contracts the natural or wild-type strain of the virus. At this point some vaccinees demonstrate a breakthrough chickenpox rash which is mild and usually consists of less than 50 lesions. However, it is also possible that the resulting infection may be subclinical—meaning there are no outward or noticeable signs of illness. So regardless of whether or not the vaccinee manifests a rash, he or she now harbors both the vaccine and natural strains. Since the natural strain dominates, the vaccinee is then subject to the higher risk and greater severity of shingles that is associated with the natural strain."

"What are the implications of this for the greater population?" Lisa asked, writing her notes quickly. Things were moving faster than she had anticipated, while Craig was not surprised, but intensely dismayed, by the reactions of the public health officials who were observing these breakthrough cases and yet making recommendations for administration of a booster vaccine. This booster would be formulated to contain higher potency viral components or more plaque-forming units (PFUs) than the first vaccine. Likely, it would be given as the quadravalent, or four-in-one, MMRV (measles, mumps, rubella, and varicella) vaccine.[48]

"Good question, because you know large populations are made up of individuals. About 95% of all adults in the U.S. population that have already had chickenpox (usually during their childhood) will no longer receive periodic natural exposures (boosts) to their immunity—especially as the universal varicella vaccination program becomes more widespread and there become fewer cases of natural chickenpox. For example, you were never vaccinated for chickenpox because you had chickenpox when you were a child. You have a career that previously put you in frequent contact with children. Every time a child with chickenpox came into your office, you were re-exposed, and, therefore, your immune system received a boost. Because of those periodic exposures and boosts to your immune system, you were less likely to come down with shingles than other adults your age who had no contact with children."

"Craig, that seems to be a key point. I will highlight that in my notes. The more exposures to natural chickenpox that an adult has, the lower their risk of shingles."

"Lisa, there are still other more horrific scenarios that are possible. For example, brain tumors. According to a recent study, those who do not have chickenpox are more prone to gliomas, fast-growing brain tumors. It is unknown precisely how this mechanism works and whether the varicella vaccine will offer the same protection against gliomas as the natural disease.[49] But I should also mention that a German study[50] did not find such an association."

"That's amazing how nature works to keep a healthy balance in the environment."

---

[48] Arvin A, Gershon A. Control of varicella: Why is a two-dose schedule necessary? Pediatr. Infect.Dis. J. 2006;25:475–476.

[49] Wrensch M, Weinberg A, Wiencke J, Miike R, Sison J, Wiemels J, Barger G, DeLorenze G, Aldape K, Kelsey K. History of chickenpox and shingles and prevalence of antibodies to varicella-zoster virus and three other herpesviruses among adults with glioma and controls. Am J Epidemiol. 2005 May 15;161(10):929-938.

[50] Poltermann S, Schlehofer B, Steindorf K, Schnitzler P, Geletneky K, Schlehofer JR. Lack of association of herpesviruses with brain tumors. J Neurovirol. 2006 Apr;12(2):90-99.

He nodded. "I agree. Now, let's change the balance. Let's interfere. Let's vaccinate all healthy children so they no longer get chickenpox, which means, of course, that the community no longer has a high incidence of chickenpox or the annual epidemics that used to occur in March or April. Where are your outside or exogenous boosts due to periodic exposures going to come from?[51] How is your immune system going to be boosted to suppress the reactivation of shingles?"

"For argument's sake, if I don't get that boost, wouldn't the chance of my getting shingles decrease?" she asked.

"No, it's the opposite. If you don't get that boost, the chance of shingles is greater. The reason for this is that your cell-mediated immunity to VZV, varicella-zoster virus, begins to wane or gradually diminish over time. In children less than 10-years-old this waning of immunity occurs in just a few years; in adults a good exposure to a child with chickenpox can yield a protective effect to suppress shingles for about 15 years."

A shudder went through Lisa. "Wait a minute. So, if the varicella vaccine nearly wipes out chickenpox, then...."

"We're in for a nationwide shingles epidemic that will only end when the entire adult generation dies out." Craig finished her sentence for her and slammed his open hand down on his desk for emphasis. "Shingles can be excruciatingly painful, often causing scarring. It is estimated that shingles produces two to three times the morbidity as chickenpox and four to five times the mortality. Also, shingles doesn't always go away once the rash has healed. It can manifest residual painful effects known as post herpetic neuralgia or PHN in 20% of adults who have shingles. In some patients, it can and does reactivate even a second or multiple times with painful episodes. What if shingles occurs in highly vulnerable and sensitive places, such as the eyes? It has been known to cause blindness. What if it becomes disseminated and spreads all over the skin? Yes, shingles can manifest a wide variety of complications, affecting virtually any specific nerve in the body."

Lisa put down the pad of paper covered with her notes. "What are we going to do? Damon has used Sycamore Springs as an example to the world, an ideal model of successful vaccination compliance. He's decided the destiny of so many children and adults. We're too late."

Craig checked the clock. "For some things in the past, maybe. But we're just in time for the future."

##

"How long has he been like this, Travis?"

Damon took the stethoscope out of his ears and thumped on Lyle's chest.

"Don't know, Dr. L. Michelle went shopping with Pammi, and I heard Lyle crying, but he didn't seem to respond to me."

---

[51] See Appendix VIII. A Summary of Scientific Literature Supporting the Exogenous Boosting Hypothesis

Damon peered into Lyle's eyes, moving his finger slowly from side to side. "Hmm. He doesn't seem to be tracking any of my movements. How old is he now?" He pulled the chart from under the examining table.

"He's going on to two and a half and has met all developmental milestones on his previous checkups. Pammi's a good mom. We've been good parents to her, and she's a good mom," he repeated.

Damon ignored the worry lines on Travis' forehead. Probably nothing. Probably a temper tantrum. "He was fine before I gave him his catch-up booster MMR vaccination. Probably still angry about that needle." He grinned. Children always had to be held down for a vaccination. Good thing his office nurse was strong and could turn a deaf ear to the kids' crying and the parents' fears. Even grandparents like Michelle and Travis worried too much. He hated putting up with parents. He told them many times, only half joking, that he'd enjoy practicing medicine so much more if he could just ignore the parents of his pediatric patients.

"Know what he's been doing, Dr. L?" Travis asked.

"Acting like a child that didn't like getting a shot? We had to have two assistants hold him down."

Travis' face turned dark. "I didn't like that, Dr. L, and neither did my wife or my daughter. "I don't want you to do that again and because of this reaction, we will not consent to him getting any additional booster vaccinations."

Damon snorted. "I know best. I'm the doctor. I've spent years in training and in clinical practice. If a child squirms at the wrong moment, he could get hurt."

"You were already hurting him, Dr. L."

Damon brushed the comment aside. Travis didn't even finish high school. What could he know? "So, tell me, Travis," he said with mock patience, "what's our little Lyle been doing?"

Travis held up his grandson's arm. "See? Didn't you see this?" He pointed to red and angry looking welts on Lyle's wrist. "He's begun chewing on himself. Like an injured dog chews himself."

Damon turned the nearby lamp closer and examined the gnaw marks. "Yes, it looks that way." A warning bell went off. Autistic children sometimes manifest this awkward behavior—biting themselves on their wrists. "How long has he been doing this?"

"Since that awful shot, Dr. L."

Damon flinched. He hated to be called Dr. L. His name was Dr. Damon Leviticus. Why did the less educated citizens make up little pet names for him, as if they were equals? He and Travis would never be on the same social level, no matter how his motel-owning friend had forced his way into the Spartacus Club. Must be because he knew the down-and-dirty of everyone in town. That had to be it. And now this nobody was implying Injection Day had something to do with the appearance of autism.

"That's not possible, Travis. What Lyle may have, doesn't just appear out of nowhere. There has to be a reason for it, something that triggers it, but doesn't necessarily cause it on its own. Perhaps a genetic pre-disposition that a child is born with. Some events may appear coincidental, but if Lyle had or had not had the MMR vaccine, likely he still would be in the state he is in now."

"And, what's that, Dr. L?"

"It's probably autism or a milder form called Asperger's Syndrome, which is a high-functioning autism without the retardation or extremely low I.Q."

Travis' eyes widened to saucer size. "You're calling my grand-kid retarded?"

"Of course not. That's not a medical or clinical term we professionals like to use."

"So what do you 'professionals' use?"

Was that contempt in the voice of a low life?

"Impaired. We prefer to say the individual is impaired in come capacity."

"I don't know what *that* word means, Dr. L., but if you put something in that shot that made my grand-child retarded, I'm going to take you down."

Damon flinched at the menace in the voice of his usually calm, though ignorant, friend. First of all, no one could prove the shot did anything, even though he, as a medical insider, was aware of the research. But he knew that special interest groups who solicited the proper funding could carry out a study that "proved" just about any conclusion desired by manipulating selective data. He preferred to side with the funding and spending sanctioned by the American Medical Association and every pharmaceutical company that turned a profit. He was perfectly comfortable with those judgments and values. They wouldn't make all that money if they weren't right, now would they? They must have done their due diligence of safety testing before they put the drugs and shots on the market to minimize their lawsuits. Besides, they were hedging their bets, was how he looked at it. If the media hype was strong enough, if even people with access to lawyers could be convinced, and rightly so, that doctors and drug companies knew best and were working for the good of humanity, then where was the problem? A few disgruntled patients or survivors of patients? That did not matter. For the most part, physicians were automatically protected and given immunity against vaccine-injury claims as were the vaccine manufacturers. How convenient. That did not matter, the AMA and the drug companies had more power and better lawyers than any motel owner could ever find. At best, under the National Vaccine Injury Compensation Program (NVICP) based on an act of 1986 (PL-99-660), a maximum settlement of $250,000 could be awarded for a vaccine-associated death. Unreimbursed medical expenses and custodial and nursing care were also covered by the program.[52]

He was safe. He was untouchable.

He was Dr. Damon Leviticus.

"Did you hear me, Dr. L? If anything is wrong with Lyle and it's your fault, I will hunt you down like the deliberate liar you are."

Damon drew himself up as coldly as he could. No one spoke to him like that. "Are you threatening me? How dare you talk to me like that? If we weren't members of the same club I'd call the police and have you thrown out of my office."

[52] See Appendix XV. Filing for Vaccine Injury Compensation

Travis moved in on him until they were nose to nose. Damon hated that. He needed the space he had earned in medical school.

"Consider it the biggest threat you've ever had. No one could stop me for standing up for the health of my grandson. I'll repeat myself, just in case your medical degree got in the way of your understanding." His voice moved an octave lower on the scale but a significant number of decibels louder in volume. "If you've hurt my grandson, your fancy life won't be worth a plugged nickel."

##

Millie looked at Sylvia with a mixture of dislike and surprise.

She'd been on her way to Lisa with a folder of articles from Craig when Sylvia cornered her outside the drugstore. After a few minutes of annoying conversation about soap operas, cigarettes, and hair mousse, the topic had turned suddenly to a serious vein, surprising Millie, who thought that girls like Sylvia had a totally different agenda than anyone else that dealt only with the least important things in life unless they benefited her directly.

"You're what, Sylvia?"

"Preggers. And I'm keeping the baby."

"Whose is it?" Millie prompted, annoyed at the way Sylvia drew out every verbal encounter to her advantage, at least keeping the listener corralled until she had her manipulative say.

"Dexter's." Sylvia replied with a grin, showing cigarette-stained teeth.

"Are you crazy? Dexter is paralyzed."

Sylvia snorted and adjusted her cheap stretch skirt that left nothing to the imagination, much to Millie's discomfort. "He wasn't always paralyzed. As a matter of fact, the night before Injection Day, we were in the boondocks having a party."

Millie's eyes narrowed as she thought of the last encounter with Dexter she had herself. What girl in her right mind would marry him, much less stay married to him? He was rude, obnoxious, condescending, and probably unfaithful.

A smile replaced her frown. Of course. Sylvia was the female counterpart of Dexter. No wonder they got along, if they had. She could understand their attraction to each other, but it would appall Dexter, if he still had the mental capacity to understand that his wife would actually go through with the process of having his baby. He certainly was not ready to settle into family life and devote the time necessary to raise a child.

"Yes," Sylvia continued in her whiny voice. "He was something."

I might throw up. Millie found her impulse to turn and walk away. Hearing about Dexter wasn't what she had in mind. She stared at Sylvia in her trashy attire. Who ever told a woman she would be attractive dressed like that? Her tank top was too tight, and the colors of her garish make-up screamed thrift shop Saturday specials.

Millie stared down at her own outfit, right out of *Boring and Dull*, the fashion magazine for women who put the power of their minds over the unimportance of their clothes and physical looks. What was wrong with Ivy League loafers and long pleated skirts that covered rather than revealed? What was wrong with a blouse that fit instead of a stretch tank top two sizes too small?

Sylvia watched her. Millie hated that because she knew the next words her classmate would utter would be aimed at bettering her position at the expense of everyone around her. Sylvia always knew what everyone else was thinking, probably because she imposed the lowest standards on the people around her by pushing them around. She always wanted something, and one day Millie figured she'd get more than she bargained for in the flea market of manipulations.

"Yeah, Mil, if you dressed like a girl instead of a dork, men would take an interest, want to marry you and have children, and then you could live off *them* the rest of your life, just like I'm going to do."

If you only knew how pregnant I am, Sylvia. I'd love to tell you and wipe that superior look off your dime store made up face. But I can't. Brandon is far more of a husband than Dexter. He supported my pregnancy and wanted to raise a child. But I'm not going to sponge off him for the rest of my life. I'm going to go to college, become an investigative journalist, and write books that not only contain startling conclusions but transcendent implications. My child will be proud of me.

"Them?" she asked instead. "You said live off *them*, meaning more than one. Only one biological father per child, Syl."

Sylvia popped the top on another beer. "Depends. Dexter is paralyzed. He can't do anything. His mother is going to either sue the drug company and Dr. Leviticus personally or accept the maximum award allowable under the National Vaccine Injury Compensation Program. Dexter is going to be a rich, helpless man. He can't tie his shoes, he can't raise a spoon to his mouth. Someone is going to have to look after him by hiring people to look after him."

Something twisted in Millie's stomach. What had happened to Dexter? He had been young and healthy, and now he was young and doomed. She'd heard about Epstein-Barr, a paralysis that could occur after vaccines, like after the swine flu vaccine fiasco a couple of decades before. After attending a convention on July 26, 1976 at a hotel in Philadelphia, 221 people contracted a disease and 34 died. The disease was later identified as a form of pneumonia and given the name Legionnaires Disease which was spread through the hotel's air conditioning and ventilation systems. Much research funds were devoted to ascertaining the origin of the disease which was advertised as being similar to the Spanish Flu of 1918 which was responsible for the loss of 20 million lives. Scare tactics? Manipulation of public fears? The illogical tying in of one event to the other to secure huge sums of money in research grants?

Yes, yes, and yes.

What could the general public do against such an assault of the common senses? Blind trust obviously didn't work in a system constructed of selective funding, selective reporting of results, intrinsic cover-ups, and the shocking acceptance of an arbitrarily high number of allowable "casualties" for every drug. The pharmaceutical houses decree that it is okay with them if a base number of people die or suffer irreparable loses and lifelong pain by taking a drug or vaccine. What about their families, the people who love them and want them to be alive to kiss and love and invite to family get-togethers?

Tears filled Millie's eyes. What right did a drug company mogul have to have time off and go on vacations with his family when he had deprived thousands of people the right to ever see members of their families again? What gave that CEO the right to decide who would live and who would die? Was there no justice in the world? Was it all greed and lies, deceit and cover-ups?

Why couldn't her father get his articles to the public? What would it take to give the victims their rights before they were unexpectedly given their last rites or their final good-byes. Her father was a brilliant man who had carefully observed and recorded data from studies and experiments, but he had received everything from threats to orders to cease and desist publication from attorneys prompted by the public health department. Why were certain individuals at the CDC and in the public health department so intent on keeping his research out of medical journals and inaccessible by the public and other researchers?

How did those people sleep at night?

It would only take the death of one of their own to bring the point home to them.

Humanity is a collective group of people, and their weakest link shouldn't be the very inhuman people who run the health care system.

"Are you crying, Mil?" Sylvia asked, her beer can in the air. "I've never seen you cry before."

Millie turned away and wiped her eyes. Good journalists didn't cry, no matter how disgusting and disgraceful their opponents were. The only way she knew to discredit them was with facts.

That was why she was going to assist her father and help him achieve publication of every single abstract and article he had written and would write. She loved him. She believed in him. He represented the truth in the face of adversity. It was one thing to tell the truth in a vacuum, but to stand up for what he believed despite the hardships —

That's what made him a hero.

##

"You wanted to see me?" Brandon asked coldly.

Damon pushed his glasses farther down his nose. "Yes, son. Sit down." He pointed to the chair his patients sat in on the other side of his antique desk.

Brandon sighed and obeyed, looking out the window of his father's office for relief from the oppressive sense of illness and disease ever present in the medical building. Even if no one walked in sick, they always left with alleged problems and real worries about them.

Hoping to at least mentally escape, he concentrated on the fact that winter had come to Sycamore Springs, bringing with it the chill of indifference for the changing of the seasons by the people who ignored all of life's more colorful passages anyway. The snow clung to the far away mountains; the desert floor was a ringing, flowering valley with fields of natural poppies. The Joshua trees were constantly green, always turning the sunlight into life. Nature was the complete antithesis of medicine, which, to him, always turned life into the darkness of fear and ignorance through intimidation.

With any luck, Damon should be through with him in a matter of minutes, and he could go back to football practice.

"What is this all about? You usually don't summon me to the Oval Office."

His sarcasm was lost on Damon.

"Son, how have you been feeling since Injection Day?"

"Besides humiliated by having been turned into a lab animal by my own father? Good, and how are you?"

Damon stared at him. "Don't act like the child you are. Do you feel sick in any way?"

"You're the doctor. Do I?"

Damon resisted the urge to smack him, something he had never done, because Barbara, such a weakling, forbade him from doing so. "I need to know, to follow up on my patients. Did you have a fever? Did you feel disoriented?" He paused. Now for the difficult question. "Did you have any muscle weakness or feel any tingling or lack of feeling in any part of your body?"

Brandon sat very still. "You mean did your precious shot turn me into a vegetable like Dexter?" he asked quietly.

Damon snorted. "Dexter is far from a vegetable. His thinking is clear, and he is going to rehab."

"When I talked to him, he didn't seem to hear me, and he can't go to the bathroom by himself, or brush his teeth, or ride his bike. You've ruined his life."

Damon shuffled through the papers on his desk, and then stacked them into a neat pile. "You better be careful what you say to me. I and my colleagues will back me up on this point: know that there are going to be people who are adversely affected by any drug, vaccine, or procedure. I accept that. In fact, this rare adverse condition suffered among vaccinated individuals is no different than the background incidence suffered in those not vaccinated in the general population. Why can't you accept this?"

The anger in Brandon's chest burst into a wave of nausea. He lurched to his feet, startling the pen out of Damon's hand.

"Because these people are real," he shouted. "They're not pawns. They're not statistics. They have hearts that beat and minds that think. If you honestly believe that you can destroy their ability to walk and form sentences and that they are merely statistical casualties, then you're evil and your pledge to do no harm is a sham and a crime."

"You're ridiculous," Damon interrupted. "Of course people are statistics. What else makes up the numbers? People and their lives," he finished flatly with no emotion Brandon could detect other than disgust.

A faint siren on the poorer side of town sounded in the sudden quiet of the office. Did his father really believe that? Were his own suspicions of Damon finally out in the open as an undeniable truth, that the Hero Doctor was a criminal who used people up like paper bags at Jamboree?

"Brandon, my boy, do you hear that?" Damon gestured toward the window. "That's an ambulance, probably taking one of my patients to the hospital. Soon, I'll get a call, and I'll go over there and see what I can do. If I didn't do it, someone else would. If I didn't administer the shot, if I didn't perform the surgery, if I didn't prescribe the drug, another doctor would. People want me, because I do it better. It doesn't mean I do it right. I'm not evil. I'm a doctor. It's a job, not a religion, but people believe in me, because I have more education than they do, I possess more skill, and I have the education and experience to back it up. There is built-in room for error, because medicine is an art, not a science."

Brandon's heart rate tripled. It had to be one hundred and eighty by now. "What do you mean by that? Medicine better be a science. People come to you because you're supposed to know where their nerves are, not because you're going to paint their portrait. Why are you trying to justify your mistakes? You're not playing with inanimate objects. These are people. They were born to parents who loved them. They have children who want them to last as long as a higher power will allow them to live. You're not that higher power. You're mortal just like they are. If you get sick, and you go to a doctor, would you want to be treated with the same callous contempt you give your own patients?"

Damon jumped to his feet. "Enough! I've heard too much from a whelp like you. You're not even dry behind the ears yet. I've saved more lives than I've lost, and that's the best statistic I can give you."

He kicked over the wastebasket with a vicious punctuation to his words and marched out of his office, his head held high, his eyes blazing, curses flowing from his lips.

Brandon listened as his father slammed the door to the building, escaping from the confrontation he believed he won. "Great, Dad. Any shred of respect I possibly had remaining for you is gone. It's too late for Dexter and people like Sarah Perkins, but it's not too late for me. I'm going to take Millie and get as far away from you as I can get."

##

Lisa closed her office door. "I can't prescribe anything for you. I'm not a doctor."

Aileen felt the blood rushing around her head. Why couldn't she calm down? There was nothing she could do to help Dexter. He had been destroyed by one shot. "Damon won't give me anything stronger than the tranquilizers. I need something to make me forget I'm alive."

Lisa leaned closer and put steadying hands on her shoulders. Her emotions showed in her own tears. "I know how you must feel, but you're not going to be able to help Dexter if you don't get a grip."

Aileen brushed her hands away. "I thought you were my friend. I thought I could come to you, but you're going to side with your cronies in the American Murder Association. They paralyzed my son. If it had been someone in your family, you would be just as desperate as I am to have the grief go away."

Lisa looked at the floor. "It has frequently been people in my family. My mother was murdered by a medical mistake. They were testing a new drug on elderly patients. The permission to administer this drug was slipped in somewhere on some consent form when she was admitted to the hospital. It happens all the time. Patients are always victims of the medical industry. They are parts of studies without their full knowledge of the deleterious outcomes. The last time I went for a pap smear, the doctor told me it would be a month before I got the results, because she was sending it to a friend of hers in the East who was doing a study. She didn't tell me beforehand, and she said she didn't have to because it was only a pap I was getting anyway. But she was wrong, because she took away my freedom of choice. I wanted the results right away. I didn't go to her to be a guinea pig, and she was the head of OB/GYN at a big Los Angeles hospital. Then, she had the contempt to tell me that all women should have every test available to preserve their freedom of choice. When I said that the more tests, especially unnecessary tests, one takes, the more likelihood of there being a false positive result, she lied right to my face and said I was wrong."

Keep talking, Lisa, keep talking. If you can't help Aileen through this soon, her nervous breakdown will be complete and she'll be getting into the mental health industry. No one comes out of that one the same way they went in, any more than they do from the base medical industry.

"I know you don't believe me, but you still have a choice if you keep your head. That's why I push alternative medicine so hard. That's why I read between the lines of every piece of data, every paper, and every article of the ruling medical class regarding topics of concern to me. They will often say flat out that everyone has to take a shot or a pill. This, however, is not a mandate. I heard a newscaster say that it's time for everyone to get their flu shots. Isn't the news supposed to be unbiased and report conditions? When were they given the right to push drugs on people, who will think it is common, an everyday occurrence, for people to get a flu shot. It's a choice."

Aileen tried to focus on Lisa through the tranquilizer haze. "You're crazy. My choices were taken away from me."

"That's what the head of OB/GYN told me would happen if I did not do what she said. As vicious, manipulative, and greedy as she was, she was still wrong. She shined the light of fear in my face, hoping I wouldn't see any alternatives. You can help Dexter if you'll only listen to me."

"I can't take away the paralysis."

"You can't be sure of that. The first thing we have to do is shine a big, big light on the situation. Damon used the media to get Dexter into this, let's use the media to try to get him some help."

Aileen shook her head. Lisa was offering her a lifeline, but she was too drugged to take it. "I don't understand you. I want to, but the drugs are taking my mind." She felt the tears she had been holding back burst like a dam, and she put her head down on Lisa's desk and sobbed.

Lisa held her hand. "I want you to give me the bottle of pills, and I'm going to help you withdraw from them. Then, we're going to enlist Craig and Millie, and get Dexter some attention. This is one case that isn't going to be swallowed up and swept under the rug by the medical profession."

##

Sylvia pulled Dexter's car out of the truck stop parking lot. This stop had served many purposes. She'd had a good lunch and used the ladies room several times. She checked the map and headed toward Los Angeles. The day was warm and she had worn her favorite shorts and tank top. The truckers at the diner had made some filthy comments about her, but she ignored them. She was a mom, and moms didn't have to talk to gross men.

Aileen had let Sylvia drive Dexter's precious motorcycle as soon as she learned that Sylvia and Dexter had recently married and shortly thereafter, she became pregnant by her son. Sylvia seemed a little out of it, probably from the shock of seeing Dex unable to move.

If Sylvia had to admit it, she'd say she was shocked herself. She and Dex had spent many a night enjoying each other's company. They understood each other. They both didn't do well in school. They both liked doing forbidden things, yet they both agreed drugs were lame. Dex had taken an extra summer job to pay for their small private wedding and honeymoon trip. Earlier, she'd helped him move back to Sycamore when his father threw him out, reassuring him that not everybody in town was looking at him when he walked down the street. She liked to ride his motorcycle, and he told her he liked it when she put her arms around him when they rode.

One night last month, he had told her he loved her, and she'd choked on her drink and asked him if he really meant it. He looked sorry he'd said it, and now she supposed she'd never know if he cared about her or not.

Sylvia felt a sprinkling of water on her naked legs where her shorts ended. She blinked. Was she crying? Over Dex? Because he didn't recognize her when she went to see him in the hospital?

A sob escaped her throat. She was crying, and it was over Dexter. Well, she wasn't surprised.

She loved him.

What was she going to do? He would never be able to ride with her on his motorcycle, or open her drinks for her, or tell her how beautiful she was. The worst part was that he'd probably never recognize his own child, but even if he did, he wouldn't be able to be a typical dad, shooting hoops and yelling at his son. Poor Dex.

She wiped her eyes, trying to keep her attention on the road.

Los Angeles was only an hour further, and she needed to get away and find a place to live far away from the people who knew her. Things were going well. She didn't want to admit it, because it wouldn't work with her tough-girl image, but she was thrilled to be pregnant. A baby of her own, someone to love and take care of, would make her feel wanted and loved herself.

"I'm going to be a great mom, better than my own. I'm not going to let my kid get into any trouble. If I can find a place to live in L.A. with my aunt, the one who will do anything for me because she thinks family loyalty is a good thing, then I can make a new start. Dexter will be in Sycamore with his mother, so she can send me money, and as soon as he's better, he can come to our new home. I'm going to make it nice, a real safe place for my baby to live. Will you listen to me," she said with a laugh while keeping the motorcycle steady in the freeway slow lane. "I'm starting to sound like a real mom. That dumb Millie doesn't know anything. She thinks I don't have feelings, but I do. I love Dex. He's the father of my baby."

She squirmed in her seat. "Oh, no, it feels like I have to use the restroom again." She scanned the freeway for another rest stop. "I'll find one soon. I want everything to be perfect for the baby. I want it to be healthy. Nothing's going to go wrong. I don't know anything about how to be pregnant, or what the stages are, but I'm...."

A sudden rush of sensation sent her heart rate soaring into the sky. She looked down and saw her lap was filled with liquid. The seat was drenched.

"Oh, my God," she cried out, "I'm going to lose my baby."

She had to find a place to stop, somewhere she could hold her body together so the baby wouldn't come out, too.

The world turned white with fear and she starting losing control of her steering. The oncoming traffic wasn't staying in its lane. She had to swerve to the right to miss a truck coming right for her. She turned the wheel as hard as she could coming down the long incline. She was too close to the divider. She wanted to turn the wheel back. Her hands were shaking too violently to keep a grip. She saw her hands leave the steering wheel, she saw the wall of the mountain pass beyond the concrete barrier guarding the edge of the gorge. She heard the frightening loud sound of Dex's motorcycle crumpling against the concrete. The sky was blue, the clouds were white, and then the darkness took her out of her agony.

Chapter 16

"You know how to shoot this thing, Travis?"

"Of course I do, Sam."

"What do you want it for again?"

"A little skeet shooting, that's all. I'm not going to kill anything that deserves to be alive."

"I thought you had a gun. Why don't you use your own?"

"Sights are bent. Gotta take it to the shop on the highway. Won't get it back in time." Travis tried to keep his voice from shaking. He'd been a hunter all his life, over the protests of his family, but he'd never gone out to kill a man. He was lying about the sights on the gun he owned and kept hidden in the far reaches of his closet. He didn't lie much, except maybe to turn away when couples came into his motel to use the facilities using false identification. This time was different. Someone had lied to him, and that lie had hurt his grandson.

Sam nodded. "Would you like me to take a look at it? I know a lot about guns. When Sarah was alive, she didn't like me having them, so I had them locked up, but now I take them out once in awhile."

Poor Sam. He never got over Sarah. She was a nice lady. He remembered how she always said hello to him, even before he had a legitimate business. Sam always suspected that Damon had something to do with the operation going bad. That's why Travis thought of using Sam's gun to kill Damon. May as well serve justice in the names of two victims—Lyle and Sarah.

Travis didn't want to use his own gun. As soon as Damon was dead, he intended to leave Sycamore and head for Mexico, or any place that would be far enough away. He couldn't help Pammi and Lyle, but he'd at least have done the right thing.

An eye for an eye.

No one would trace the murder to him. He'd dump Sam's gun over the border. Maybe years later he'd come back and see how his family was doing. It would be too painful to watch his grandson now that he was retarded. Lisa had explained autism to him after he found out for sure. He'd cried like a young child in front of her, but he figured she'd understand, since she was a school nurse.

She told him that Lyle would need constant care, but that Pammi was young and would probably be with him for many years.

He'd asked her what was in the MMR shot that hurt Lyle. She'd told him it could have been many things. Since the MMR vaccine did not contain the preservative Thimerosal, an overdose or accumulation of mercury, which produces symptoms very similar to autism was unlikely in this case. However, unlike some vaccines that contain just one virus component, the MMR was a trivalent vaccine, designed to protect against three different viruses—measles, mumps, and rubella. Some experienced physicians held that instead of doing one vaccine to stimulate immunity against three different diseases, it was safer to administer three separate vaccines in different office visits, each stimulating immunity against a single disease; however, doing so was costly in terms of time and inconvenient to healthcare professionals in terms of the extra storage requirements. Of the three components in the MMR vaccine, the measles component had been implicated in late-onset autism, being present both in the cerebral spinal fluid (CSF) and in the guts of autistic children.

The word twisted in his gut. He considered using a knife on Damon to tear out his insides, so his gut would hurt, too, but he didn't want to get that close. He didn't want to leave his fingerprints around Dr. L's neck or leave any of his DNA at the murder scene. He watched television. He knew what was going on, maybe not in doctors' offices, but he had watched lots of crime shows.

It had to be quick, and it had to be clean. Dr. L would never know what hit him, but he wanted him to know who had hit him. He wanted him to know that really bad.

##

"So that there was no loss of profits, physicians were permitted to use up all remaining stocks of vaccines that contained Thimerosal, even after the decision by public health officials in 2000 to remove Thimerosal from new lots of vaccines," Craig said, refilling the coffee cup in front of Lisa.

He continued, "The late-onset autism in Travis' grandson, however, is linked to MMR vaccination and is similar to another case he studied where a laboratory confirmed that measles RNA was present in the gut—and that explained why many autistic children also experience digestion and bowel-related problems.[53,54] The pharmaceutical firms would have you believe that his autism was a genetic disorder present from birth. The facts are to the contrary—after the grandson had gained several skills and could speak some words, he regressed and lost eye contact with his parents and grandparents. This outcome, referred to as late-onset autism, is different from early onset or congenital autism that may have a genetic basis and which is easily recognized by both the physician and parent within the first few months following birth.

"Perhaps, the first MMR vaccination caused the autism and the second MMR vaccination caused further problems involving the bowel or gut."

Lisa had been ignorant regarding this background concerning the MMR vaccine. She was now curious about the recent enrollments of children in the special education classes.

---

[53] Wakefield AJ, Murch SH, Anthony A, Linnell J, Casson DM, Malik M, Berelowitz M, Dillon AP, Thomson MA, Harvey P, Valentine A, Davies SE. Ileal-lymphoid hyperplasia, non-specific colitis, and pervasive developmental disorder in children. Lancet 1998 Feb. 28;351(9103):637-641. (Note, most authors, except Wakefield, Linnell, and Harvey, later retracted the findings in this manuscript—see Lancet 2004 Mar 6;363(9411):756).

[54] Research presented at the International Meeting for Autism in Montreal (June, 2006). Study led by Arthur Krigsman of New York University School of Medicine involved 275 children with findings repeating those of A. J. Wakefield. Dr. Stephen Walker, assistant professor at Wake Forest University Medical Centre in North Carolina, analyzed the gut samples and found a strong association between measles and autistic children with bowel disease.

Out of concern, Lisa explained, "We are seeing many more children in special education classes as well as an increase in those having ADD and ADHD. The parents seem to recall noticing changes in their children following booster doses of Hep B or other Thimerosal-containing vaccines. Craig, is their any validity to these parental observations?

"In the studies I have seen, infants received on a single day, a dose of Thimerosal, that contained a quantity of mercury that far exceeded the maximum allowable dose established by public health agencies. Such an overdose that the infant received, referred to as a 'bolus' dose, would have been safe in a person weighing 200 to 300 pounds, which of course, was significantly greater than the weight of any vaccinated infant! In one particular study, parents saved hair from their child's first haircut. Upon analysis it was demonstrated that autistic children had only minor amounts of mercury present in their hair samples.[55] By contrast, normal children exhibited high amounts of mercury, indicating these children were able to eliminate the mercury from the brain. Those having autism, somehow are unable to eliminate the mercury from their brains."

Lisa shook her head in disbelief. "Do you mean that the doctors knew or should have known that they were giving vaccines with a mercury preservative whose accumulation in the brain and body tissues could cause autism especially to babies, toddlers, and young children, yet they administered them anyway?"

"That's exactly what I mean. It's shocking but true.[56] These details are available through a transcript obtained through the Freedom of Information Act. Citizens can read about the secret meeting that the CDC convened at the Simpsonwood Retreat Center with representatives from the pharmaceutical industry.[57] In fact, it has been estimated that some two million or more children may have been affected." He looked angrier than usual.

Lisa had called and asked if Craig had time to help her with a report she wanted to make to parents at the next Ask Your School Nurse Afternoon she decided to implement without any of Damon's help. She had to start a dialogue with the families who had not received full disclosure concerning the vaccines they had been coerced into receiving along with the free ice cream on an historic day in Sycamore Springs.

"That makes them murderers. It's premeditated, don't you think?" she asked, knowing the answer. The fury she had kept bottled up inside had exploded the night before at Paul, when he made some remark about Aileen looking unusually tired and severely depressed. Her husband was a philanderer and an insensitive moron, but making comments about Aileen during a time of great trial for her was a new low, even for him.

She worried about Aileen whose depression was getting deeper. Lisa figured that her friend had more than one bottle of pills to dull her mind, even though Aileen swore she had

---

[55] Holmes AS, Blaxill MF, Haley BE. Reduced levels of mercury in first baby haircuts of autistic children. Int. J. Toxicol. 2003 Jul-aug;22(4):277-285.

[56] See Appendix IV. Mercury in Vaccines: Institutional Malfeasance and The Department of Health and Human Services.

[57] See Appendix II. Summary of Highlights of the Simpsonwood Meeting.

given Lisa all her supply. Damon wasn't the only doctor in town, and she could have gotten whatever she wanted if she went to enough of them and paid cash at different pharmacies.

"Not one of them will see it that way," Craig answered. "They will say everything from 'they were not informed', or 'they were following the approved guidelines and accepted practices', or anything else that will exonerate them, make them blameless."

"And the drug companies that made the shot, how do they get out of the blame?"

"They lie."

"Outright?"

"Outright and on camera. They say that it is not harmful—that any studies reporting deleterious effects and adverse reactions are nearly always flawed."

Lisa flinched. "How do they get away with that?"

"They say that rare adverse reactions are too few in number to be statistically significant. They say the incidence of some negative outcome is no different than the incidence of that outcome in the general population. Yet, their databases contain only a small proportion of the true number of adverse reactions that occur. Vaccine safety studies are often limited to only a 3 to 45-day follow up period. They publish only positive outcomes because they don't want the truth to be investigated. They don't want their invalid assumptions to be questioned. Soon people believe the deception of the positive propaganda, because no one is balancing the falsehoods with the truth. The truth of the matter is: only a very small proportion of deleterious effects are ever reported because physicians and their patients are not trained to regard a recently given vaccine as a suspect cause."

"You are an exception in understanding these details," Aileen said with a sigh.

"Yes, I and a few others like me are exceptions because we have high ethical standards and morals. We don't care if we're ostracized or must leave employers who don't appreciate objectivity in research. Many methodologically sound studies exist that are not published in the mainstream medical literature because editors with conflicts of interests as well as the pharmaceutical-medical complex will do everything in their powers to keep the truth from reaching the public. Think of the money they would lose."

"Think of the Thimerosal-laden vaccines they would have had to destroy."

"Or send to third-world countries. They do that, too."

"What kind of people are they, to do immoral things like that?" she asked, her voice shaking.

"People with no conscience. People with no heart. People with no principles. People with no fear," he answered, trying to keep calm.

Lisa took the last sip out of her cup. "You mean the medical and pharmaceutical industries."

"Exactly," Craig said and poured another round.

##

"I haven't seen you for awhile, Millie. Are you mad at me?" Brandon kissed her before she could turn away. Tracking her down hadn't been easy. Her father said she was at the library, and he searched it completely before he found her hidden away in a corner, reading.

"Of course not. I've been busy," she whispered.

"Too busy for your husband, the father of your child?" he asked, nuzzling her neck. Someone smirked behind a floor-to-ceiling row of books.

"Our child," she corrected.

Brandon took her hand. She was rounder than before and even more lovely. "I want to ask you a question."

She looked a little wary to him, as if she knew what the question was going to be. He knew she thought he was going to ask her to abandon some of her higher education goals in view of the child they were now expecting. She would eventually. No need to nag her. That would only upset her and then he would become worried that he might drive her away from him, and that would crush him. He loved her more every day.

"Go ahead. Ask me," she said.

He cleared his throat. "Will you move away from here with me?" he asked.

She gasped. "From Sycamore Springs? I've lived her all my life. How can I leave?"

"Easy, give me your hand, and we're outta here."

She looked at his upturned palm. How easy it would be to leave the city with the man she loved and their baby. "Why do you want to go?"

"I need a fresh start. I want to get away from everything that stops me from growing old by making me old before my time. I want to be young with you, Millie. I don't want to be part of what kills people. I want to be part of what makes life grow."

She furrowed her brow and stared at him, patting her tummy. "Life can grow anywhere."

He patted over her hand. "You don't understand. We have to keep our child away from my father."

Oh. Now she understood. He didn't want the doctors and drugs near their baby. Neither did she.

"I'm not sure what to say. I love my parents, and I want our family to live near them, but I understand how you feel. We can live in Sycamore and never see your father."

"How can we do that? This town is so small, I practically know the middle name of everyone in it."

Millie laughed. "It isn't the biggest city in California. Let me think about it. Where would we go?"

He hugged her, and they heard more snickering from behind the wall of books.

"Anywhere, Millie. We can do anything we want. We have our whole lives together to grow old and watch our children grow old. Come with me. I love you."

Chapter 17

"I know what happened to Sylvia. The autopsy report came in," Lisa said.

"Drunk, right?" Millie guessed the obvious, considering Sylvia's reputation as an uneducated girl with a drinking problem.

"Sober, not a drop of alcohol. She had shingles."

Millie's jaw dropped. "She drove off the road because she had shingles? How can one be related to the other?"

"No she didn't drive off the road because of the shingles, but because of a chain reaction that was initiated by a symptom of shingles. This is a very bizarre set of circumstances. People usually assume that events follow a singular pattern, that a death is caused by one event. However, most of the time it is a series of events that could have been helped at many points along the line, before an irreversible tragedy occurs. That appears to have been the case with Sylvia's death. The best that can be determined was that she lost control of her bladder sensation, a possible and documented complication of shingles[58,59] which can attack the nerves in virtually any part of the body. At that point, and this is conjecture, she might have thought she was having a miscarriage and panicked. Then she drove into the barrier and was killed."

Millie felt the tears on her face and wiped her eyes. "How could something like that have happened? You know what this means? Damon Leviticus and the drug companies have claimed two more victims, this time a pregnant woman and her unborn child. It's murder. They have so much blood on their hands, it defies human understanding. Why doesn't someone stop them? This can't be the first time something like this has happened? They murder men, women, and children in cold blood. Lisa, these are calculated killings. They know the odds, and they know they will occur."

Lisa patted her arm. "I know. It's tragic and shocking. We can't help Sylvia or her baby, but we can warn others."

Millie paced, agitated beyond her usual ability to keep under control. She wanted to rub her tummy to reassure her unborn child, but she couldn't in front of Lisa. "It's really premeditated murder," she repeated, "because the medical and pharmaceutical industries know this, and other events, are going to happen to a certain number of people, and they think that's okay. Just because they don't know the exact names of their victims, doesn't make it any less premeditated."

Lisa nodded. "I agree. Now we have to make sure that people come out of the dark and become truly informed. Your father is right. The varicella vaccination which effectively decreases the incidence of chickenpox paradoxically is linked to a higher incidence of shingles. Recently, I'm seeing more and more students in my office with clear cases of

---

[58] Jellinek FH, Tulloch WS. Herpes zoster with dysfunction of bladder and anus. Lancet 1976 Dec. 4;2(7997):1219-1222.

[59] Julia JJ, Cholhan HJ. Herpes zoster-associated acute urinary retention: a case report. Int. Urogynecol. J Pelvic Floor Dysfunct. 2006 Mar. 7 [E-publication].

shingles. Although usually a mild disease in children, some are suffering excruciating pain and many end up with scarring. Consider cases like Sylvia's that will never be publicly linked to the shot unless we tell the story to the media or publish a case history. We need more people like your father in the fight against medically motivated murder in the name of healthcare. The real motivation is greed."

Millie forced herself to sit down. She had to keep calm. Sylvia hadn't, and look what happened to her. Millie had to find a refuge in her mind from the people she was investigating and researching. It didn't mean she had to be less involved, but she had to distance herself far enough to maintain her logic.

Lisa looked at her intently. "You have to remember something, Millie. Organized greed has been in business for a long time. It has tricks and shams and subterfuge that the rest of us have never heard about. Good renews itself with each generation in the promise of the future in the hearts and minds of everyone young and free. Organized greed knows smart people aren't going to be within their demographic. It's harder to fool smart people, unless they're carried in on an ambulance stretcher and can't speak for themselves. Then, with no one to question every medical procedure, routine or otherwise, they are lost from the start. The medical and pharmaceutical industries love people like that. They wait for them. They want their victims helpless, or else where will they find them? Anyone smart and strong enough to walk out of a doctor's office can do so if they don't like what's going on. The demographic that both the AMA and drug companies want is the uninformed, the trusting, the brainwashed. We can't be any of those if we want to help Dexter and prevent what's happening as a consequence of Injection Day from happening again in other counties throughout the U.S."

"What if we can't save Dexter?"

Lisa looked grim but ready to put her idea into action. "We sure are going to save somebody."

##

Lisa smiled sweetly at Damon. "So what do you think of my idea, Doctor?"

He beamed back. "It's outstanding. A follow-up media event praising Injection Day. National television, did you say?"

"Every channel that will carry it. International coverage as well."

Damon puffed out his chest as if she had pinned a medal on it. Everybody had their weak spots, and for him it was his pride. He lived for attention, no matter the cost.

Lisa didn't believe he ever thought about what he did. He religiously followed his training and the updates of his mentors. He was a pawn, but he had power, and that made him dangerous. He'd used that power to intimidate people into getting varicella as well as all other "necessary" vaccinations, but he still refused to believe that he had done anything wrong, or that he was in any way guilty of neglect.

She wondered what he was going to do with the lawsuit Aileen was bringing against him. She'd bet he'd dismiss it as a nuisance case that lacked any merit and keep rolling along until someone figured out how to stop him.

"Do you think I should wear a suit, Lisa, or my white coat? People like the professionalism of the white coat, but maybe a suit would make me look more human, more one of them." He paused, probably not because he was waiting for her response. He didn't care about that. He was, no doubt, listening to his own mind. Taking his own mental temperature. How was he feeling? How did he look? What should he wear on television? What should he say?

She nearly smiled. She had a question of her own.

Why had she never seen the answer to Damon's pride until that very minute?

##

"How is Dexter progressing?" Millie asked, hoping for some good news. She'd heard Aileen was having a difficult time making it through the day, and the nights for her were impossible.

Lisa pulled the door shut. "He can't walk. He can't move, but he's been trying to speak."

Millie nodded. "That's good. Any response might be a signal he has a good chance for recovering more of his motor skills, right?"

"Not necessarily. Everything is connected in the body, but some skills are isolated, and others are interdependent. If the damage is severe enough, it could be irreversible."

Millie flinched. "How could something like this slip through the alleged safety trials the drug companies are supposed to have conducted? Didn't they know?"

"I told you, they knew. They just didn't care. Dexter isn't the only one to experience paralysis or to be paralyzed after a vaccine. If the general public knew the *actual* cases, and I don't mean only the *reported* cases, then the drug makers know that a vast majority of people would think twice about inoculations. It's keeping people in the dark that works, but remember our plan, we're staging a Renaissance of knowledge and information. For every "Don't Be Chicken – Get Your Shot" button that Damon has in his office, I'm going to have a "Don't Be A Lemming – Be Informed" button available in my office."

Millie's eyes widened. "You could get fired, Lisa."

"I know that. But I don't care anymore. I saw Dexter grow up. He deserved the chance to grow old. It could have happened to any of the kids in town. Besides, it will take Damon awhile to figure out the counter-slogan buttons are against his campaign. If he asks, I'm going to tell him that it is an educational button, which is true, encouraging students to learn all they can before making a decision. This is also a good rule for everybody about everything."

"So they won't be lemmings, right?"

"That's right. Lemmings are a metaphor for the little animals that act as a group and don't think individually. Every year for no reason they all run to the edge of a cliff and jump off."

"Just like people who blindly follow any collective event without thinking."

"Exactly. You're smart, Millie. You're going to go far in your profession."

She glowed with pride. Lisa was an independent thinker. She carefully considered every skinned knee and elbow that found her office after playground mishaps. Everyone got special attention, because Lisa said that while many injuries only looked superficial, they could actually be more serious. A bloody elbow could be the signal for a chipped bone as well. Consequently, every student was given a personalized brief note of obvious problems and those to watch out for.

Lisa was the best-loved nurse in town.

Too bad about the gossip about her husband. Apparently, he has been seen with Aileen, and since she'd been distraught, he hadn't been home on a regular basis. Lisa pretended to ignore the whole situation for her son, Richard's, sake, but Millie had heard about the Paul-sightings. The rumors were all over town. Sycamore Springs had a grapevine that rivaled cell phones.

What kind of a person was Lisa that she could overlook the behavior of her own husband to help the son of the woman he had been seen with?

A very good person. Millie was sure of that.

Lisa was staring at her. "Something on your mind, Millie?" She glanced quickly at her pregnant tummy and then back up to her face.

"No, I'm fine. I was just thinking about how fast news travels in Sycamore by our famous grapevine."

Lisa smiled. "You mean, 'Tell Helen Porter, Tell The World'."

Millie laughed. "That's the one."

"Have you heard the latest gossip? Barbara Leviticus is supposedly back in L.A. visiting her old flame, Lindsey Fellows? And Lindsey's daughter, Beverly, is not happy about it? As a matter of fact, Lindsey's wife is ready to throw him out if he sees Barbara again?"

Millie shook her head. "How can that be? Barbara was staying with Aileen, and now I thought she'd found a small apartment in town. Brandon tells me she wants to move away, somewhere in the Midwest where Damon can't find her." Frankly, Millie had been surprised by Barbara's reaction to the whole Injection Day project. After so many years of supporting her husband, what had made her finally snap?

"For one thing, she was very scared that Brandon would have a reaction to the varicella shot similar to reactions he had had in the past with other vaccines. She was well aware of the liars and cheats in Damon's world, but she hadn't spoken up before."

"I know. Not only was she concerned about Brandon, she had read several vaccine journal articles Damon tried to suppress, and she worried that the effects of the vaccine would wear off and that without ongoing booster vaccines, children would be more susceptible to chickenpox as adults with more serious complications. Also, she expected that adults, whose immunity would no longer be boosted by exposures to natural disease, would experience the impact of increasing shingles. This impact would be long-term—maybe 30 to 50 years. The effects wouldn't be anything like the usually mild and benign disease of chickenpox There would be a shingles epidemic with untold morbidity and mortality of disease that one can only imagine. In some serious cases, adults would prefer death over the agonizing pain of shingles that was relentless and caused sleeplessness for endless nights.

"Those are all such good arguments against the varicella vaccination given on Injection Day. Why did Brandon go against his mother's pleading? He's a nice person. He gets along with his mother. I don't understand. Didn't he trust her to tell him the truth?"

"He did it because of his pride in front of his friends," Millie said. "It doesn't surprise me that he would do that.

"He gets his pride from his father. But Damon's pride is excessive, an obsession. It will bring death with it one day. "

How strange was that for her to say? Lisa was so level-headed that Millie relied on her responses to be logical. Something in Craig's research was too disquieting to accept anything logical about Damon's nightmare, Injection Day.

"But Brandon's fine, right? So Barbara can stop worrying." *Please God in heaven, let him be fine. I need him. We need him.*

Lisa looked away. "No one is fine when a program of universal varicella vaccination is implemented."

Millie's eyes misted over. "I know. I've read my father's original research as well as supporting research from the United Kingdom. He says that 95% of adults that had chickenpox when they were school age will now all be at a higher risk for shingles."

"He's right. Your father not only has the facts and figures, but he understands the biological mechanism of how adults are boosted by exogenous or outside exposures to children with chickenpox. Few who got a Varivax® vaccine and a free ice cream cone on Injection Day will develop chickenpox. This, in turn, will reduce the amount of outside exposures that occur in the community. Children who did not receive the varicella vaccine because they had previously contracted chickenpox will be at greater risk for shingles. Also, adults will be at greater risk due to the fact they currently receive less periodic boosts than were previously naturally available from the yearly epidemics of chickenpox that occurred in the community. You know recently in the school district, I've seen a few cases of shingles among vaccinated children, but an unexpectedly high incidence in shingles among students that were not vaccinated. I've also heard reports of more adults being diagnosed with shingles. Something's going on, and your father knows what it is." Lisa smoothed her shirt and tapped her fingers nervously on her desk.

Something was missing. Something was wrong. Why couldn't Craig get his research manuscripts published? Who was responsible for keeping his work out of the mainstream U.S. medical journals?

"Perhaps because his manuscripts were as yet unpublished, that is why vaccine reviews continually ignored the concerns he objectively highlighted. Why was his research not being published?" Millie persistently asked.

"Money," they both said in unison, but neither of them laughed.

##

"You got the time of day, Dr. L?"

Damon looked up and regarded Travis coldly. What did he want now, especially dressed like that? He had his hunting garb on.

"I'm busy, Travis. I'm writing a speech to deliver to my television audience. Lisa has me on a national news program. Let's talk another time," he said delivering his sentences in rapid succession, hoping to chase his unannounced visitor out the door before he was roped into any conversation dealing with the wholesale cost of motel pillows.

Travis closed the door behind him slowly, quietly. "I don't think so," he said, his voice deliberate in the silent room.

A shiver of fear ran up Damon's spine. He'd heard the click of the tumblers. Had Travis locked the door? He'd never liked Travis, and he certainly didn't trust him. What an afternoon for his nurse to have taken off. She was in such a rush to leave, she had forgotten her reading glasses. He could see them lying on her desk outside his door through the glass panes. He was alone in his office. Had Travis known that?

He had better take the friendly offensive. He had to deal with people less intelligent than Travis all the time. It was an annoyance that came with his profession, but he accepted it much in the same way he accepted taxes and convoluted health care systems that didn't allow him to make as much money as he had originally intended to make when he first started his practice.

Damon smiled broadly and put a speech he had been working on to the side. "Well, then, I'll make time to talk. That's what fellow members of the Spartacus Club are for. What can I do for you?"

Travis pulled a chair typically reserved for patients around and straddled it. He leaned forward and stared at Damon. "It's more what I can do for you, now isn't it, Dr. L? Seems like you've done plenty for me and my family already."

That didn't sound good. His vast training in the fields of psychology stepped in. He'd better evaluate the situation. Travis had a look on his face he hadn't worn before. Damon couldn't decide if it was disgust, or superiority, maybe even dislike.

Without warning, Travis dropped whatever control he had over his expression, and Damon recognized the now complete emotion immediately.

It was hate. Pure, undulating hate.

Stunned, Damon grinned even more widely. "No thanks necessary, my friend. I'm your doctor and your family's doctor. I do my job because I believe in my work and I do my darndest for you people."

Darndest. When was the last time he used a word like that? Why did Damon always feel the need to talk down to some of his patients, possibly most of them. True, he believed he was smarter than they were, but usually he had to hurry them along so he could get to everyone who needed him that day or night. Damon once got it out of Lisa that people said he always had his eye on the clock, and that might have been true. Not because he was rushing his patients, but because he didn't want anyone to be shortchanged. Patients didn't understand him. At least some thought Damon to be the most conscientious doctor they had ever met.

"That's not the way I see it, Dr. L."

"No? Well, how do you see it, Travis. I'd really like to know. You're a special friend, probably the best I have in this town." *Was he getting nervous? Was his voice shaking?* "You and I have never had a chance to have a talk like this."

"I know, and if I have anything to say about it, we're never going to have this chance again," Travis said grimly.

Was that sweat Damon felt breaking out across the back of his own neck? Strange, he'd never allowed himself to be intimidated before.

How many people are left in this building at this hour? It's late afternoon. If I yelled for help would anybody hear me?

"Something wrong?" Travis asked, his face back to its usual blank, except this time, Damon thought his practiced and skillful powers of observation detected something that went along with the hate he was concealing.

Travis was hiding something else.

Damon was sure of it. Whatever it was had to be tangible, because every muscle in Travis' body was tensed. If he were only hiding mental thoughts, if he ever had any, he would exhibit cardiovascular and respiratory signs of increased stress, like rapid breathing and jerky movements, just the way he felt at that moment. But, no, Travis was calm, almost calculating. He was hiding something physical. It could be anywhere on him, from somewhere inside his bulky hunting pants to the thick red vest he wore. What could it be? Nothing dangerous, probably. Travis wasn't stupid. Damon had seen Travis lose in games for charity at events sponsored by the Spartacus Club many times, and Travis always accepted defeat gracefully. As a matter of fact, Damon would bet a month of patients that Travis wouldn't harm a bug, hunting aside, of course.

Damon leaned back in his chair, momentarily pleased with himself. He was an expert at diagnosis. All his superiors in medical school always confirmed that he could tell what was wrong with a patient just from the way that a man or woman presented from the beginning, from the way he or she walked in the door or asked to see the doctor.

Travis cleared his throat and waited.

Damon stared at him. *What does the moron want now?*

Travis coughed.

"Coming down with something, Travis?" Damon asked, suddenly getting an idea. If he could get him to take off his shirt so he could listen to his heart, then he might be able to see if he had anything significant hidden in his clothes.

"No, I feel fine physically."

"That's good. Can't have any of my patients getting sick on me."

Travis gave him a cutting look that went through him more thoroughly than any scalpel could have done. The silence in the room grew deeper and more ominous.

Suddenly, Travis spoke. "So, Dr. L, what are you going to do about Lyle?"

Damon breathed a sigh of relief. The reason for Travis' unannounced and disturbing visit was out in the open. No need to worry. He'd handled distraught relatives of injured patients before.

"We're going to be sure he gets the finest medical care possible, including therapists, psychologists, and teachers," Damon answered.

Travis' eyes narrowed. "Is that going to fix him?"

Damon flinched. "It will manage him."

"Like he'd be retarded."

"Well, in a manner of speaking," Damon began trying to judge how to phrase Lyle's autism in a way that would not enrage Travis even further, "he is impaired."

"Retarded."

"Impaired," Damon repeated emphatically.

Travis touched the outside of his red hunting vest, directly over his heart. "I love that child, Damon. He's my own flesh and blood. Suppose the same thing were to happen to Brandon? How would you feel about that?"

Damon paused in his thinking. Brandon. *His own. How would he feel? Not that Brandon would ever suffer a neurodevelopmental disorder, because he was a doctor, and he saw Brandon every day, and he gave him the benefit of every medical advance, pill, and shot.*

A small, nagging thought twisted in his gut, just a little, just enough to make him rub his stomach. He did recall some studies, some of which were conducted by the CDC, which he and others dismissed as invalid. These studies demonstrated increases in autism incidence as the dose of Thimerosal increased. This mercury preservative had been definitely present in most of the vaccines that were administered to Lyle. Although vaccines manufacturers had formulated Thimerosal-free vaccines after 2000 when it was decided by medical authorities this was in the best interest of the children, doctors were allowed to use up their remaining supplies of vaccines that still contained it.

That couldn't have been what happened to Lyle, could it? Could Thimerosal used in many of the vaccines on Injection Day have caused a mercury overdose that impaired a child for the rest of his life, even if some studies said it didn't? Lyle's last injection, however, did not contain Thimerosal. It was the MMR vaccine.

"Travis, if the same thing happened to Brandon, I'd be just as upset as you are, but I would understand that these are rare and unusual events and you must understand the statistical implications and causalities of any medical procedure. Reliable studies confirm that the medical profession and the pharmaceutical industry save lives. That's the bottom line. We make people live longer. That's why we're here. That's what the numbers tell us."

Travis' voice was flat and cold. "What do the numbers tell you about autism?"

Damon stood up and tried to walk around his desk. Maybe he could get to Ricki's desk and then out the door.

He couldn't. Travis stood a second later and gestured with a pointed finger that Damon return to his seat.

Damon did. No use pretending to himself any longer. He was in deep trouble.

"That's a very good question," he said shakily, trying to keep his composure. "I'm glad you asked. I'm always happy to see my patients interested in what the professionals have to say about their health. The numbers say that vaccines do not cause autism. So, you can put your mind to rest that the somewhat sudden and severe autism that Lyle experienced in close proximity to the administration of his MMR vaccine was only coincidental and would have likely occurred even if he had not received the MMR vaccine."

Travis grunted. "Huh. Yeah. Well, I'm going to put something to rest all right."

Damon nodded approvingly. "That's a very wise decision, Travis. Now, if you don't mind, I'll get back to my speech. The world is waiting." He rustled the papers on his desk as a signal for Travis to take his annoying questions and leave the building. Travis didn't move. Damon cleared his throat once and then again. "Is there something else I can do for you?"

Travis put his open palms on his knees and stood slowly, keeping his hard gaze on Damon's face. "Yeah, I guess there is."

A sick silence filled the tense space between them. Damon blinked across the dryness in his own eyes. What was that moron looking at? "And what would that be?" he prompted, hoping to help his slow-witted intruder along.

Travis reached into his vest, and took out something shiny. "You could die, Dr. L."

Damon squinted into the afternoon sunlight streaming into the room. His heartbeat went from slightly elevated to a full-run gallop in the time it took the realization to hit him.

Travis had a gun, and it was pointed directly at his head.

"What do you think you're doing?" he yelled, jumping to his feet in the throes of panic.

Travis edged the gun closer. "I wouldn't move too fast if I were you. I think you're life is pretty useless right now, you going around turning kids into retards just so you can buy your own kid the fanciest car Sycamore Springs has ever seen. But, you see, you're wrong, Dr. L, and do you know why you're wrong?"

Damon sat back down slowly, hoping he could out-think the distraught relative. He'd done it before, but no one had ever held a gun on him. Usually, he all he had to do was call hospital security to have any upset people removed when one of his patients died. It wasn't his fault they'd died. He always had full consent before he operated, including consent for any administered drugs or medications.

This was the first time since Sam Perkins that he feared for his physical safety. Fortunately, the guards had managed to subdue Sam, and Damon had magnanimously refused to press charges, saying Sam was grief stricken.

Now what was he going to do? No private police in sight. He'd have to rely on his training in psychology to calm Travis down.

"Take it easy, Travis. We've lived almost side-by-side in Sycamore Springs for years. We belong to the Spartacus Club. Why, I remember that it was Barbara that put you up for membership. I even voted for you. Remember the time I blocked the City Council declaring the land around your motel a plant life sanctuary for the poppy? That would have cut into your business if you had had to give up your parking lot. Remember that? We've been friends for a long time."

"We're not friends now," Travis said, his voice as iced as the animal carcasses he kept in his freezer.

The room lurched forward with a jolt of adrenaline meant to move an animal out of the way of its predator. "I know it doesn't seem that way, but that's only because we have a small problem with communication, but we can fix it. You have to believe me when I tell you that I had no knowledge of anything contained in the varicella vaccine, MMR, DTaP, Hep B, Hib, PCV, IPV or flu vaccines on Injection Day that would have hurt Lyle or anybody else. You do understand that, don't you? I've never been one of those doctors who put their golf game in front of their patients' health. I've always kept my priorities straight."

He heard Travis pull the hammer back on the old gun, and he stared at it.

Is this how an animal feels when it knows it is seconds away from death at the hands of hunters like Travis?

"Recognize this, Dr. L? I borrowed it off Sam Perkins. Old Sam doesn't know what I'm going to use this for, to blow your brains all over your office, but I thought you might like to know, as the murderer of his wife, that he's part of the execution that's about to take place here."

"Travis, you can't be serious." Was that his voice? It was shaking like a flag in a hurricane.

"Know why I'm going to shoot you in the head? Because you shot my grandson full of viruses that went to his head."

"That's a lie," Damon shouted.

Travis leaned forward. "I wouldn't be yelling if I were you. I'm awfully upset, and if you don't want to have a few extra minutes of life, I'll be glad to oblige you."

"If you shoot me, the police will find you," Damon said, his voice a pathetic whine to his own ears.

"No, they won't. I've made some pretty good plans. They won't even know where to look, and do you know why? Because I've been watching you all these years, lie and cheat and steal your way into the Spartacus Club, into the country club, into every club a wealthy doctor with no conscience goes. I have watched your effect on the lives and the health of the people who trusted you. Like me. Like Pammi. Like Lyle. We trusted you, three generations of us. And do you know what we got in return?"

"Travis, I...."

"Murdered, ruined, destroyed. You've ruined my family. Now, I'm going to ruin yours."

"I'm sure we can talk this out. I'm sure I can explain that I had nothing to do with this." Was he begging for his life? "Doctors don't always know what the drug companies know. Sometimes they are selective about the testing and statistics. We all know that, and we accept it, because we rely on the pharmaceutical industry to do their own safety trials with due diligence. We take it for granted that they will give us reliable products. We rarely look beyond the product inserts they give us. Did you know that doctors get different ones than patients?" he babbled on stalling for time, dragging more minutes out of his life. "Patients get ones that don't tell them much, just a little information like dosage, basic cautions and adverse reactions, and maybe a coupon. The pharmacies don't share the ones they get with the patients. Most of the time they take them out of prepared preparations that are self-packaged, so as not to confuse the patient, not to worry them over details, like side effects that don't happen frequently, or insufficient testing and studies with only partial or inconclusive results. However, doctors get more in-depth ones. Most of the time we don't take the time to even read them, because we know the drug companies have done their homework. Do you understand? If there was a mistake, it wasn't made by me. It was made by the pharmaceutical companies that made the varicella vaccine, MMR, DTaP, Hep B, Hib, PCV, IPV and flu vaccines. It wasn't my fault. You've got to believe me," he finished, his voice trailing off.

"You gave him the shot," Travis accused with deadly calm.

"Yes, but I didn't know what was in the shot."

Travis snorted extra loud. "Good one, Dr. L. Maybe you're the one who is retarded. I know who's in my motel. How come you don't know what's in the vaccines you give your patients?"

"I didn't mean I don't know. I meant I didn't know the vaccine would be harmful since it previously had been approved by the U.S. Food and Drug Administration (FDA). The drug companies perform several tests to insure safety. They don't want to hurt anybody."

"That's not the way Craig and Millie and Lisa tell it. They say the drug pushing companies know exactly how many people and more their vaccine is going to harm or kill, but they don't care, because they will market the vaccine until such time that legal costs offset the profits. Have you already forgotten about all the cases concerning Vioxx®? After 2 million received this anti-arthritis drug, Merck withdrew it from the market since it greatly increased the risk of heart attacks, strokes, blood clots, and other side effects."

He moved even closer. Damon could see that his hand was shaking. The gun jerked back and forth in front of his eyes.

"Please be careful with the gun, Travis. You don't want to do anything you'll regret."

Travis sneered. "The only thing I'm going to regret is if you live to think clearly and my Lyle will never know what it means to fall in love, to have a job, to go hunting with his grandfather. That's what I'd regret."

Things were not going well. Travis wasn't backing down the way his patients usually did. Where had his power to control and intimidate gone? Had it been scared away by the threat of bodily harm? Did his patients ever feel that same threat when he approached them with medical care?

Damon shook his head to clear it, but Travis never wavered. The gun remained pointed directly at his forehead.

"Scared, Dr. L? Like the way Sarah Perkins was scared when you talked her into the operation she didn't need. That's the way Sam tells it. They were a nice couple. They loved each other. Sam's never been the same, and you may have not noticed it, but no one's seen Sarah for a long time. Know why? She's dead, Dr. L. You killed her."

"You're crazy. They mixed up the hoses in the operating room. They sprayed the open cavity with the wrong medication."

Travis shook his head. "She wouldn't have been there if it hadn't been for you. You even testified, defending the hospital. You didn't care. I heard the insurance company paid you off. That true?"

Damon could feel a noose of revelation tighten around his neck. He better do something or that crazy Travis might actually pull the trigger. He took a deep breath and slammed his fists down on the desk, ready to stand up again, and he watched Travis' eyes for an opening, a split second when he might let his iron guard down.

"Kinda noisy, aren't you, Dr. L?" Travis asked, menace in his voice that chilled Damon to his aging bones. "I wouldn't do that again, if I were you. I don't like loud noises. Makes me want to kill something."

Damon gulped and folded his hands obediently on the top of his desk.

"That's better," Travis said, unmoving.

"Why don't you put that down, and let's talk," Damon suggested weakly.

"Can't. Time's running out. I've got a plane to catch."

Anything to buy time. "Taking a vacation? Maybe I should come along." He attempted to laugh.

"No way, Dr. L.," Travis said with a sneer. "You're going to stay right here." He pointed to the floor with his free hand. "You've got your choice. I can kill you here, or I can kill you here."

"What kind of a choice is that?"

"The same kind you gave Lyle."

"Now, wait a minute...."

Damon heard a whimper, and he wondered if it came from him. He'd always been such a brave man. In Nam he'd been right up to the action and could have been killed at any time, but he'd never been held accountable before by a patient's relative with a gun. It was personal this time, and he didn't think he would be able to talk his way out. His only choice was to lunge for the gun, but Travis had kept the desk between them.

"Too late," Travis said. "Remember all those stupid slogans you made up for Injection Day? Well, I've got one for today. 'Dr. L — Go To H#**!'"

Damon heard a loud click. Was he dead?

"Doctor?" a woman's voice took a bite out of the fog of fear after she must have opened the outer door, spinning the noisy tumblers. "I forgot my glasses, and I...."

His nurse, Ricki. She took in the scene in one glance. "Oh, no," she said on a gasp, and turned to run.

Distracted, Travis whirled around and fired. Ricki fell against the safety glass window of the door with a pained scream.

Damon ran around the desk and picked up the chair Travis had used and threw it at him as he turned and ran, missing him completely, watching in dismay as his would-be murderer dashed out of the building and into the streets of Sycamore Springs.

##

"Ricki, are you all right?" Damon lifted her away from the door and began a frantic examination of his nurse. She was tall and stocky, and it took him almost a minute to find her pulse.

She opened one eye and regarded him arrogantly while he fumbled with his stethoscope. "Is he gone? Maybe we should pretend he got me for a few minutes longer, so he thinks he committed murder. Then he won't come back, and we'll be safe, and then the police can pick him up."

Damon held her, stunned. She wasn't hurt. She looked normal, constantly talking, making up her own scenario. "I heard you scream. I thought he shot you."

She struggled to get up. "No, I was trying to distract him, and it worked," she said arrogantly. "Comes from years of coddling and over-reacting to nervous patients. Often I must distract them to make them docile and accepting of medical protocols."

Damon immediately thought of Lisa. She wasn't like that. Must be an individual thing with nurses. Lisa was forthright and levelheaded. She'd never invent trouble.

"I saw him through the door before I came in. At first I figured you were just talking about hunting, but then I noticed how scared you looked and how strange he was acting, even if I couldn't hear much except the low murmur of your voices. Travis was always a violent man, all that hunting and killing," she said, standing up and brushing off her skirt.

Damon shivered. "No, he was never a violent man. As a matter of fact, he avoided confrontation with people. He hunted for sport, and although many believe that is morally wrong to kill defenseless animals for no reason, I've never seen him turn on a human until he turned on me. I didn't expect it."

"Well, it was no surprise to me," her voice shrill like a shrew. "I never liked him. Why did he want to shoot you? That's what he wanted, wasn't it, to kill you?"

Damon looked through the pharmaceutical samples in the top drawer of his desk and selected one package. He took out two pills and swallowed them without water. Anything to control the violent pounding of his heart. Darn it. That crazy Travis could have killed him.

"He says I'm responsible for Lyle's autism by giving him a shot on Injection Day."

Ricki broke out into a cackle. "That's crazy. Like Travis is an expert. He should know by now that you doctors rule along with the drug makers. Like he has any say in what happens to his grandson or anybody else in the family. We say what is going to happen with their health, and whatever you recommend, that is the course the parent's follow. What can they do to us? So, they'll sue. So what. For every attorney and expert they get, we can get a hundred who'll back us up with the full knowledge of the AMA and money provided by the drug manufacturers. We're untouchable, Doctor, completely untouchable."

Damon shuddered. He'd never had such a close brush with death. What good would the AMA have done him if Travis would have shot him?"

"Ricki, he made it sound like a shot for a shot, like an eye for an eye. I shot Lyle, and he was going to shoot me."

"He's crazy. He deserves to go to prison for interfering with us." Ricki picked up the phone. "Should I call the police for you, Doctor? Maybe they can arrest him before he gets out of town. They'll lock him up for the rest of his life. If they don't, he'll come after you. He won't stop until he kills you. That's how violent people are. They become obsessive. You know the studies."

Damon slowly took the phone out of her hand. "I need a minute. I never thought this would happen. I've always been loved by the people of Sycamore Springs. I've been their hero. This is the first time since Sam Perkins that someone wanted to kill me, and I couldn't get away. Some violent people are obsessive, but some are specific. It doesn't take a study to prove that. Travis is upset about his grandson, and he thinks I'm responsible. He nearly killed me over it, and we've been friends for years, or at least I thought we were."

She stared him down. "Friends don't hold a gun on friends. If you don't call the police, I will. I could have been killed, too."

Damon sat down and put one hand on his knee to try to stop the shaking racking his body. Adrenaline overload. He was almost in a state of minor shock. "I don't think anything will ever kill you, Ricki. You don't react inside. You'll live forever."

"That's what I intend to do. You call them now." She dialed for him. "I'll listen to be sure you get it right. I've always had your back."

He would have dismissed Ricki right there for addressing him in such a disrespectful manner if he wasn't so upset. She must have been waiting for the one time in his life he would feel weak. Now would be a most opportune moment. He was completely vulnerable. What if Ricki was right? What if Travis came back?

What if he made sure he finished what he started the next time?

Chapter 18

"Are you sure he'll be able to say something?" Damon asked Lisa and Millie across Dexter's hospital bed. "It would look ridiculous if we go to all this trouble to set up news cameras and Dexter won't know his lines."

Lisa looked at Millie. "Yes, we've coached him in what to say."

"Which is?"

"Dr. Damon Leviticus is a good doctor."

"A fine doctor. Make it a fine doctor. I like that better," he amended.

Damon nearly rubbed his hands together with glee. He still had nightmares over his attempted murder, but the thought of his being on television had carried him through the days that followed. Travis was no where to be found, despite a concentrated effort by the Sycamore Springs police department to locate him. Even the Sheriff had gotten involved, but Travis had disappeared. Pammi told them she didn't know where her father had gone, and she disavowed any knowledge of the murder attempt.

That bothered Damon, but not as much as the grapevine gossip that said that Pammi had taken Lyle to a specialist in Los Angeles. Now, that hurt. Who could know more than he did about his patients? What could some big time doctor know that he didn't? Hadn't he devoted his entire life to the practice of medicine? Hadn't he saved more lives than he lost? Did he have to make a pep tag out of that line for a slogan, or post a banner over his office door?

DR. DAMON LEVITICUS HAS SAVED MORE LIVES THAN HE'S LOST.

That had a successful ring to it.

Now was a good time to move forward. Dexter praising him for his efforts would revive his wounded spirit. Not that he could do much for Dexter. The paralysis with its onset in close proximity to the administration of the varicella live virus vaccine, had made him an invalid, and he would likely remain one for the rest of his life. At least he had had a active childhood. True, he wouldn't be able to have more children, but he couldn't support them anyway.

Of course, Damon had heard rumors that Aileen was going to sue him and the drug companies that made the vaccine, but he didn't care. He had malpractice insurance. Also, more importantly, the pharmaceutical manufacturer would pay for a top Los Angeles lawyer to defend him. They always took care of their own. He doubted if his malpractice insurance would pay a plugged nickel, as Travis used to say, when he could be found. Damon even doubted that Aileen would receive anywhere near the $250,000 maximum settlement from filing a claim with the National Vaccine Injury Compensation Program.

He'd given Aileen an arsenal of tranquilizers, but they didn't seem to be working. He heard that she said she wanted to kill him and then kill herself. Mothers were like that. Not his mother, an exceptionally strong woman given to few, if any emotional displays. His father believed in keeping private feelings private. Damon wondered if he had mistakenly supposed that all people, men and women of all ages past puberty, would be able to control their emotions as well as he had been able to do.

It didn't matter. He was the man of the hour and nothing was going to spoil it for him.

A tap on the outer door to Dexter's hospital room made Damon gasp. Damon must still be over-reacting to all stimuli from Travis' murder attempt. He whirled around, thinking it must be the camera crew.

"Damon?" It was Craig. "I came over to see if I could be of assistance to you during the show." He greeted Lisa with a handshake and Millie with a hug.

"Dad, I didn't know if you would be able to make it. Did you hear from the medical journal?"

"Yes. My article is being reviewed. I think they appreciate the methodology and analyses that I have presented."

Millie's eyes glowed with pride whenever she looked at her father.

Damon turned away. Why didn't Brandon ever look at him like that, with respect and admiration, instead of contempt and fear? Wasn't he as good a father? Didn't he make more money than Craig. They had a better house. They belonged to all the exclusive clubs.

Craig didn't believe in joining groups. He was all dedication with no time to enjoy anything except his research, which simultaneously served as his work and source of enjoyment. Yet, no matter how Damon compared himself to Craig, the irrefutable truth remained.

Craig's family loved him, and Damon's did not.

Millie gestured toward Craig, and they both stepped out of the room, leaving Damon with Lisa. She smiled a little too broadly, if he wanted to admit it or not. She probably didn't like Damon either, not that he cared. "Where's the crew," he asked.

Lisa looked over at Dexter asleep in the hospital bed. "They should be here soon. Do you want to examine Dexter? I'll step out of the room."

"No need." He dismissed her suggestion with the usual wave of his hand. "I've checked him over. No change."

Lisa looked out the vertical slats open over the window onto the parking lot across the street. Why did all hospital rooms look the same? Hopeless. Just like Dexter's future. She always thought he was a wild kid, but he had a right to live a normal life. He never killed anyone. He never paralyzed anyone. It didn't seem fair that the people and the industry responsible could walk around and their victims could not.

She'd said the same to Travis, and she wasn't surprised when she saw the light bulb of realization go on inside his hunting/fishing head. Suddenly, he and Lyle were the victims, the ones on the other end of the hunting rifle, the fishing rod. They had been caught by people far more powerful in a very dangerous game of who-gets-the-money-who-gets-the-pain.

Yet, she didn't expect him to attempt to murder Damon. She wondered how many victims would do the same if they had the opportunity. She assumed Travis didn't figure life was worth living for himself if his grandson was hurt. Family bonds went deep.

Millie backed through the door quietly. "The film crew is here. Do you want to wake up Dexter?"

Lisa shook her head and put her arm out to stop Damon from approaching the bed. "No, not yet. Let's wait." She patted Dexter's shoulder reassuringly, but he didn't move.

Craig nodded to her. "Lisa, why don't you and Millie go down the hall for a few minutes. I want to talk to Damon."

Lisa looked at him questioningly.

"It'll be okay," he said and turned to face Damon. From his peripheral vision, he saw both women leave the room. He had to ask for a private conversation. If he was going to get anywhere with Damon, he had to sidestep the ego issue.

"What is it, Craig?" Damon asked suspiciously. "I'm on the air in a few minutes." Damon didn't want to be alone with the man who was elected to the Phi Kappa Phi honor society and knew the answers automatically to important questions he himself had to look up first.

"I know. This is important. I've asked the crew to wait a minute."

Damon's face turned stormy. "You have no right to interfere with my crew."

Craig sighed. He probably shouldn't bother, but he wanted to help Aileen and Dexter. He worried about Aileen's deep depression and her outspoken desire to take her own life. She truly believed she had failed her son by not standing between him and the shot, the way Barbara had tried to do with Brandon. Craig tried to explain to Aileen that Brandon didn't listen anyway, went ahead and had the shot, but he didn't think she was listening. She stared into space while he was talking. He'd heard that Lisa had taken the bottle of tranquilizers that Damon had prescribed away from her and was doling them out a day's dosage at a time.

"First of all, Damon, this is not your crew. The crew belongs to the news channel. Second, I need a moment to appeal to you, because we're both persons with doctorate degrees. We meet on common ground."

Damon coughed exaggeratedly. "Really, Craig, we're hardly equals. I'm a practicing physician. You have a non-medical doctorate degree in computer science. Different training. Different skills."

"No, I disagree with you. We had very similar training, but our focus is different. I instigate the research, you selectively regurgitate it."

Damon jumped, his muscles tense. "If we're going to trade insults, then I'll tell you that you're non-medical doctorate degree is worthless, no matter what you say."

"You can tell me anything you want, it doesn't make it the truth. I'd venture to say that most of the utterances that miss the common sense filter that should be a part of the synaptic connections in your brain are not the truth. I want you to put your ill feelings toward me aside for a few minutes and help me consider the opportunity you have at this moment to help Dexter and all the other potential Dexter's in the world."

Damon crossed his arms in front of his chest. "And what opportunity would that be?"

Craig paused and then said firmly, "You could tell both sides of the story. You could be fair and honest. You could tell the news viewers the pros and cons of the universal varicella vaccination program."

Abruptly, Damon laughed, and then just as suddenly stopped. "There are no cons. There are only pros."

"That isn't true. There is going to be a major shingles epidemic in the United States and in other countries that may follow the lead of the U.S."

"That's absurd. Those children that are vaccinated have a lower incidence of shingles than those that contract the natural wild-type varicella virus."

"That is only half of the story. Unvaccinated children with a previous history of varicella currently experience shingles at the same rate as older adults. Also, within a decade, incidence of shingles will be significantly higher among adults as their cell-mediated immunity wanes due to the absence of boosting that naturally occurred in the community especially during yearly epidemics of chickenpox. For the first time in history, another booster varicella vaccination will have to be given to all adults to offset the effects of universal varicella vaccination. The number of shingles cases will remain higher than in the pre-licensure period for 30 or more years, essentially until a majority of the adult population dies out."

"But you must admit that if the incidence of shingles is less among vaccinees, the incidence of both chickenpox and shingles will eventually be lower."

"Yes, eventually, after 15 to 21 million more cases of shingles occur along with 5,000 deaths, over the next 50 years. All this suffering occurring among adults who did not receive the varicella vaccination, who had no warning of these deleterious effects, who were given no informed consent. This does not even consider the paralysis which has occurred in a few older vaccinees, as well as the potential problem that if the immune boost from the vaccine wanes, those vaccinated as children may become susceptible again to chickenpox at an older age when the disease has more morbidity. The full story concerning universal varicella vaccination, is that by administering the chickenpox vaccination to all healthy children at the age of 12 months, soon there will no longer be the immunologic boosting that occurred previously when natural varicella incidence was high in the community. There is also the issue of Thimerosal, and you probably used up the mercury-containing vaccine lots you had stocked for Injection Day. We know of several reported tragedies from your mass immunization program – Dexter, Lyle, Sylvia, and others whose names I don't even know. Don't you understand? You have an opportunity here to right the wrongs and present information on vaccines objectively. You have the chance to warn the medical consumer regarding the deleterious effects. You have to do it. It's your obligation as a fair and decent doctor and human being."

Damon regarded him coldly. "I don't have to do anything, and I understand only one thing."

"Which is?"

"You're standing in the way of my television appearance."

##

"Ready, Dr. Leviticus?" the nameless assistant director asked.

"Ready, Sir, whenever you are." Damon beamed his smile into the camera.

"That's fine, but don't look directly into the camera. Look at Millie when the TV correspondent asks you and Lisa the questions you all rehearsed, and then look at Dexter when I give you the cue. Are you sure that young man will be able to respond?"

Damon glanced at Dexter, seemingly asleep. "Of course, I'm sure. I'm his doctor."

The assistant stepped back, and Damon and Lisa moved closer for their staged "interview" with Millie. Damon checked the machines hooked up to Dexter. "Everything seems okay. Lisa, are you sure he knows his line, and why isn't he awake?"

She smiled and nodded. "Don't worry. He understands. He definitely knows his line, and he's conserving his energy."

Damon adjusted his stethoscope. "Good. Let's do this, before he forgets."

Lisa gave him a look she usually reserved for her more belligerent patients. "Yes, Doctor."

"Do you want a run-through?" the assistant asked.

Lisa broke in before Damon could answer. "No. The strain would be too much for Dexter. We'll do it on the first take."

The assistant shrugged. "Okay. Places." He paused and waited as Lisa and Millie stood on one side of Dexter's bed and Damon took an authoritative stance on the other. "And... action."

A man with a plastic smile suddenly appeared from the hallway, talking as he entered. "Tonight we are at the bedside of a young man stricken with paralysis last week. He is under the care of Dr. Damon Leviticus, renowned for his Injection Day, a mass inoculation program that took place in Sycamore Springs last month. If you recall, our news team covered it live. Good evening, Dr. Leviticus."

"Good evening," Damon answered in his most authoritative and intimidating manner.

Lisa knew she and Millie would not be introduced on camera. They were not important enough to warrant verbal mention. If they were lucky, the producer would add their names on screen in small type.

"What can you tell us about this young man, Doctor?"

Damon cleared his throat. "Dexter became paralyzed a few weeks ago. There is considerable controversy over this paralysis that has only rarely occurred following a varicella vaccination. We don't believe that his condition was vaccine-induced. It's merely a coincidence or chance happening that he received the vaccine in close proximity to the onset of the paralysis."

The anchorman looked confused. He pushed the microphone toward Lisa and now it was the TV correspondent's turn to cite what he had found. "There is considerable evidence, including a report from the CDC, reporting a 90% increase in shingles during a period of increasing use of the varicella vaccine. Other researchers have also suggested a major epidemic of shingles following the start of universal varicella vaccination."

Lisa nodded. "That's true. I have seen drastic increases in the number of both vaccinated and unvaccinated students that are experiencing shingles here in the Sycamore Springs School District. At first, some physicians were misdiagnosing the disease. One mother told me that her daughter, Sarah, has suffered from recurring childhood shingles. Sarah's last episode was resolved when the mother was finally able to get her on the right antiviral medication with the proper dosage. Sarah was seen by two pediatricians, one allergist and two dermatologists, including one of the top pediatric dermatologists in our nation. Perhaps because childhood shingles used to be so rare, her case was misdiagnosed as atopic dermatitis. The treatment for this condition, as you know, includes baths to keep the skin moist and topical agents to keep it lubricated. This only worsened Sarah's viral sores. Sarah was prescribed 23 different oral and topical medications, including many doses of cortisone and antihistamines in the past 20 months. The mother insisted that lab-work be done and Sarah's blood-work showed elevated levels of varicella zoster virus. By not receiving proper treatment early on, Sarah has suffered terribly and now has post-herpetic neuralgia. The mother was hoping that this case description would be aired on television to educate the audience on childhood shingles and make information more readily available to the general public." She gestured toward Millie, and he held the microphone across to her.

Millie looked toward her father for encouragement. He smiled, and she relaxed. "Lisa, who has been a school nurse for many years, has seen the number of students in special education classes increase dramatically over the past years. Interestingly, the Department of Education reports that the number of children aged 6 to 21 in the U.S. with autism spectrum disorders increased from 12,222 in 1992-1993 to 97,847 in 2001-2002, for an overall increase of 700% in the last decade. Many other deleterious affects go unreported since the physicians themselves along with their patients are not trained to even consider that onset of autism or other neurological problems might be connected with a previously administered vaccine. It is likely that two million children have previously been seriously affected by the Thimerosal in vaccines before the recommendation was made to eliminate it from the vaccine formulations. ADD and ADHD are very common today and these likely are the result of children having a mild sensitivity to Thimerosal-containing vaccines. Thimerosal is a 'preservative' which is 50% mercury by weight. Those children with highly sensitivity to Thimerosal, manifest autism or in some cases suffer death."

"Just a minute, young lady," Damon interrupted on a sputter that sent spittle across the bed. "This is not an open forum for speculation and lies."

Millie cleared her throat and said clearly. "I agree, that's why I reported only the documented evidence. Researchers Dr. Mark R. Geier and David A. Geier reported in the Journal of American Physicians and Surgeons a significant decrease in autism once the

Thimerosal had been removed.[60] If a national newscast isn't a forum for the truth, then what is?

Craig silently applauded.

Millie, encouraged, went on. "Since the sponsors of a local study would no longer permit my father to conduct objective research, my father resigned and sought to independently publish preliminary study results in a peer-reviewed medical journal. These results demonstrated unexpectedly high incidence of shingles among children who had a previous history of chickenpox. In the study community where vaccination coverage was already moderate to widespread, the incidence of shingles among children was similar to the same high rate found among older adults...[61] Personally, I don't see anything wrong with presenting a balanced view of vaccines on your news show."

So that there would be a measure of objectivity in this debate, the anchorman returned the microphone to Dr. Leviticus who replied, "We have seen dramatic declines in varicella, about a 70 to 80% decrease in cases during the six years since the Varivax® vaccine has been licensed.[62] The public health department reports a statistically significant decline in hospitalizations as well as deaths due to varicella disease."

The TV correspondent interrupted and asked Millie, "Can you explain why such documented success is subject to so much controversy and criticism?"

"According to Dr. Marc Brisson, Dr. W. John Edmunds, and others, this dramatic decline in the incidence of chickenpox observed by public health officials might lead to a significantly higher incidence of herpes zoster, commonly called shingles, over the next 50 years.[63] Thus, Dr. Leviticus is reporting only half the story. Trends in the annual incidence of shingles should be presented alongside the chickenpox data to show the full impact that the universal varicella vaccination program has on VZV disease."

Returning for a comment from Dr. Leviticus, the TV correspondent inquired, "What is this VZV disease that was just mentioned?"

Dr. Leviticus explained, "VZV is the varicella-zoster virus that is responsible for both chickenpox and shingles. After a person becomes infected with chickenpox, also called varicella or the primary infection, the varicella-zoster virus goes dormant for years and then for some reason, usually in adults 50 years and older, the virus can reactivate in a painful

---

[60] Early Downward Trends in Neurodevelopmental Disorders Following Removal of Thimerosal-Containing Vaccines. J. Am. Phys. and Surgeons 2006 Spring;11:8-13.

[61] Goldman GS. Incidence of herpes-zoster among children and adolescents in a community with moderate varicella vaccination coverage. Vaccine, 2003 Oct. 1; 21(27-30):4243-4249.

[62] Seward JF, Watson BM, Peterson CL, Mascola L, Pelosi JW, Zhang JX, Maupin TJ, Goldman GS, Tabony LJ, Brodovicz KG, Jumaan AO, Wharton M. Varicella disease after introduction of varicella vaccine in the United States, 1995-2000. JAMA 2002 Feb.;287(5):606-611.

[63] Brisson M, Edumunds WJ, Gay NJ Miller EM. Varicella Vaccine and Shingles. [Letter to Editor]. JAMA, 2002 May 1; 287(17):2211.

secondary infection called shingles or herpes zoster. It has been reported that overall medical costs due to shingles are four times more than those due to chickenpox."[64]

Pushing the microphone over to Millie, the TV correspondent commented, "So then it seems even a relatively small increase in shingles could offset the intended benefit of varicella vaccination."

Dr. Leviticus made a motion that he wanted to make the first response, so the microphone was quickly re-directed to him. "Trials of the varicella vaccine in Japan have demonstrated the vaccine to be safe and the duration of immunity has exceeded 20 years."

Now it was Millie's turn for a rebuttal response. "In Japan, only 1 in 5 children received the varicella vaccine so that the incidence of natural chickenpox remained high and this situation helped to boost the immune systems of these children. Similarly, many of the trials and post-licensing studies in the U.S. were conducted in communities where natural chickenpox was still high. This distorted estimates of the vaccine effectiveness, causing an overestimation of the duration of protection offered by the vaccine. In fact, a booster vaccine for children aged 12 months to 12 years has already been discussed and considered for approval by the Food and Drug Administration. The Universal Varicella Vaccination Program is largely a mass experiment on an uninformed public due to the fact that the U.S. is the first country to vaccinate every healthy child and this will nearly eradicate the boosting effect that had naturally existed during seasonal outbreaks of chickenpox in the U.S. communities."

Dr. Leviticus motioned for the microphone again. "The CDC has published a study that establishes varicella vaccine efficacy or efficiency at 84%, thus it provides a strong protection against chickenpox. This, in turn, helps parents since they no longer miss work to care for their ill children."

It was again Millie's turn. "That particular study presented an average of the vaccine's effectiveness over five years, 1997 to 2001.[65] During 1997 through 1999 when the incidence of natural chickenpox was still high, the vaccine efficacy was indeed very high—it peaked at 99% in 1999; however, it declined significantly in following years as exposures to natural chickenpox dramatically declined and vaccine efficacy dropped below 70% by 2002.[66] Another study by a Dr. K. Galil of the CDC reported a low 44% efficacy in a daycare setting."[67]

Millie had said enough and Dr. Leviticus was anxious for his rebuttal, citing the conclusion of a recent study: "There is a new tool, a high-potency VZV vaccine that has been

[64] Nowgesic E, Skowronski D, King A, Hockin J. Direct costs attributed to chickenpox and herpes zoster in British Columbia—1992 to 1996. Can. Commun. Dis. Rep. (CCDR), June 1, 1999; 25(11):100-104.

[65] Seward JF, Orenstein WA. Commentary: The Case for Universal Varicella Immunization. Pediatr. Infect. Dis. J., 2006 Jan.; 25(3):45-46.

[66] Goldman GS. Universal varicella vaccination: Efficacy trends and effect on herpes-zoster. Int. J. of Toxicol., 2005 Jul.-Aug.;24(4):205–213.

[67] Galil K, Lee B, Strine T, Carraher C, Baughman AL, Eaton M, Montero J, Seward J.Outbreak of varicella at a day-care center despite vaccination. N. Engl. J. Med. 2002 Dec. 12;347(24):1909-1915.

formulated. It has been shown by Dr. M. Oxman to reduce incidence of shingles in the elderly by 50%."

Millie was prepared for that argument. With the microphone passed back to her, "Offsetting this 50% reduction in shingles incidence mentioned by Dr. Leviticus, is the statistic given in a study by W. K. Yih and others, reporting that shingles incidence increased from 2.77 cases per 1,000 in 1998 to 5.25 cases per 1,000 in 2003.[68] Similar high percentage increases in shingles incidence using different methodology and in a different study population was reported by my father in the Varicella Active Surveillance Program (VASP), conducted in a community with a population of over 300,000."

The TV correspondent, having covered other medical issues, commented, "Millie, then what you are telling our viewers is that with all of this mass chickenpox vaccination thought to be responsible for increasing shingles incidence two-fold, followed by the shingles vaccine that reportedly reduces shingles by one-half, the U.S. population will essentially be back to about the same incidence of shingles that was occurring in our communities prior to the start of the universal varicella vaccination program. I know that historically, mass vaccination of adults has seldom been successful. Not only is there the issue of weak protective outcomes, but adults tend to experience a higher rate of adverse effects compared to children, including serious side effects." The correspondent noticed Millie was again ready to speak.

"Yes, Dexter, as an 18-year-old seems to have experienced a serious adverse effect. Another possible example of this type of serious event following immediately after a varicella booster, involved an adult female, 47-years-old, employed as a research coordinator in the infectious disease unit of a medical school. She and other employees were recruited for a manufacturer-sponsored study aimed at detecting the boosting effect of the vaccine. Following two doses of vaccine, she became quite ill with intestinal difficulties and was diagnosed with a rare collagenous colitis that was autoimmune in nature. She remains disabled and, because the change in her health was clearly associated with the second vaccine dosing, the event was reported to the Vaccine Adverse Events Reporting System (VAERS)."

Dr. Leviticus had heard enough. It was his turn to speak. "While this is suggestive of a serious side effect of the vaccine, causality was not proven in this case and it is erroneous to trust that every reaction reported in VAERS is vaccine related. A study authored by R. P. Wise and others from the CDC and FDA has reported on the safety of the varicella vaccine.[69] This was published September 13, 2000 in the *Journal of the American Association (JAMA)*, volume 284, issue 10 pages 1271 to 1279."

The TV correspondent interrupted, "Dr. Leviticus, I don't understand something here. Didn't you just say that the spontaneous reporting of adverse reactions in VAERS was

---

[68] Yih WK, Brooks DR, Lett SM, Jumaan AO, Zhang Z, Clements KM, Seward JF. The incidence of varicella and herpes zoster in Massachusetts as measured by the Behavioral Risk Factor Surveillance System (BRFSS) during a period of increasing varicella vaccine coverage, 1998-2003. BMC Public Health. 2005 Jun 16;5(1):68.
[69] Wise RP, Salive ME, Braun MM, Mootrey GT, Seward JF, Rider LG, Krause PR. Postlicensure safety surveillance for varicella vaccine. JAMA 2000 Sep. 13; 284(10):1271-1279.

unreliable, but then quoted a study by Wise and others from *JAMA* that reports vaccine safety based on the analysis of VAERS data? Also, you seemed to suggest that Millie's example of an adverse event resulting in disability did not prove causation when (1) the time of her illness closely followed vaccination and (2) there was lack of any other obvious cause. There appears to be a double standard here, when, for example, Millie cited a case that used these two criteria, while researcher Dr. S. Black and others can publish an entire study assuring safety based on a temporal relationship as the only criteria in the postmarketing evaluation.[70] It is illogical for our viewers to hear that the FDA or CDC acknowledge that reporting in VAERS does not prove causation and then state that VAERS serves to reassure the general public concerning the safety of a new vaccine."[71]

The microphone passed to Millie. "There is more to the study by Dr. M. Oxman and others that reported a 50% decrease in adults who were administered the shingles vaccine.[72] A substudy on adverse effects was conducted on one-sixth of the subjects during 42 days following vaccination. Based on that substudy, the cost to prevent one case of shingles was $5,900 at a conservative $100 per dose;[73] the vaccination cost was $100,000 to prevent one case of moderate to severe post herpetic neuralgia (PHN) among adults in their sixties."

Dr. Leviticus' turn to speak. "But we must all remember that chickenpox is much more serious than the public has been led to believe. There are 50 deaths per year in children out of the 4 million that contract chickenpox.[74] In other words, one child dies every week from chickenpox in the U.S."

Millie countered, "In perspective, a person has a greater chance of dying by being struck by lightning in the U.S. than of a child's dying from contracting chickenpox."[75]

The TV correspondent had to start wrapping up the shoot and said, "In summary, it appears there is at least some agreement that the initial assumptions used to justify the U.S. universal varicella vaccination program and its cost-benefit analysis are invalid. A single dose does not appear to provide lifelong immunity; there seems to be an immunologic-mediated

---

[70] Black S, Shinefield H, Ray P, Lewis E, Hansen J, Schwalbe J, Coplan P, Sharrar R, Guess H. Postmarketing evaluation of the safety and effective-ness of varicella vaccine. Pediatr. Infect. Dis. 1999 Dec; 18(12):1041-1046.

[71] Zhou W, Pool V, Iskander JK, English-Bullard R, Ball R, Wise RP, et al. Surveillance for safety after immunization: Vaccine Adverse Event Reporting System (VAERS)—United States, 1991-2001. *MMWR Surveill. Summ.* 3003;52:1-24.

[72] Oxman MN, Levin MJ, Johnson GR, Schmader KE, Straus SE, Gelb LD, *et al.* A vaccine to prevent herpes zoster and postherpetic neuralgia in older adults. N Engl J Med. 2005 Jun 2;352(22):2271-2284.

[73] Kauffman JM. New vaccine for shingles: is prevention really better than treatment? J. of Am. Physicians and Surgeons 2005;10:117.

[74] Seward JF, Orenstein WA. Commentary: The Case for Universal Varicella Immunization. Pediatr. Infect. Dis. J., 2006 Jan.; 25(3):45-46.

[75] Curran EB, Holle RL. Lightning fatalities, injuries, and damage reports in the United States from 1959-1994. U.S. Department of Commerce, October 1997, National Oceanic & Atmospheric Association (NOAA) Technical Memorandum NWS SR-193. Available online at http://www.nssl.noaa .gov/papers/techmemos/NWS-SR-193/techmemo-sr 193.html

link between chickenpox incidence and shingles incidence; and the vaccine is certainly not 100% safe."

The anchorman paused, obviously stunned by the deviation from the script.

In the silent moment, Damon took the floor. "Dexter, wake up, and tell the people watching all over the world what you believe in your heart."

The camera moved in for a close-up of Dexter's face. He opened his eyes. To Millie they were as clear and aware as the day he intimidated her in the boondocks.

"Yes, Dexter," she said with tears in her voice. "Tell the people what you feel."

The room because even quieter, and then over the hum of the machines that did for Dexter all the big and little things in life he could no longer do for himself, his voice rang out bold and strong.

"Dr. Leviticus," he said, "I hate you."

Chapter 19

Barbara ran her hand over the stained glass panels in the center of the heavy front door. She remembered the day she had bought it from the first antique store to open in Sycamore Springs at the beginning of the yuppie era. Quite a different California these days.

She had learned too much while married to Damon L. She thought it was amazing that people looked at the medical profession with trust, through rose-colored glass doors or through the haven of ignorance.

Was she doing the right thing, leaving her husband? Since Injection Day, his life had gone from good to bad to very bad. Many deleterious effects had been linked to the vaccines Damon had idealistically administered to the citizens of *his* town. Now what was he going to do?

She was being criticized for leaving him in his hour of need. That wasn't what bothered her. What she didn't like was that he hadn't told her the one thing that might have convinced her to stay with him.

He never said he needed her.

Instead, he steadfastly and belligerently defended the mass immunization campaign. Even Travis' murder attempt hadn't broken through his resolve to remain aloof in the presence of criticism.

Damon never needed anyone. He did his work, no matter the consequences, and then he came home. Nothing else filled his life. He had no contact with people except as patients and as audience members for his ego-building speeches.

She heard a sound behind her on the stairs and looked up. Damon was watching her from the landing. He had his glasses in one hand and a journal in the other.

"I didn't think you wanted to come back here, Barbara," he said quietly with no emotion in his voice.

She swallowed the tension in her throat, but it didn't make it go away. "I didn't. I had to be sure I wasn't leaving anything behind."

"You're leaving me behind."

"I don't think you'll even notice, Damon."

He walked slowly down the steps toward her, never taking his gaze from her face. "I would notice, every day and every night. I'd miss you. I have missed you these few months. I wish you'd reconsidered. If you're going to leave me, give it some more time and then go ahead, but not like this."

Would he say it now? Would he say he needed her? That he was sorry for all the hurt he had brought to her life?

"How much more time can I give it? It's been decades since we've been close. I don't think another few weeks or months will make any difference. We've slept on opposite sides of our bed for years. To say ours is a loveless marriage would be an understatement. I've asked for your understanding in the things that have meant so much to me, but you've ignored me and hurt me even more. I don't think you even know I'm in the same bed with you, let alone the same town. I really don't think you'll notice I've gone."

Damon put his report and glasses on the bottom step and moved closer. "If you leave me, I'll have to leave Sycamore Springs. It won't be the same without you."

"Of course it won't. When people leave, either by their own free will or through cosmic or medical interference, they don't come back. Things change. Lives change. Didn't you ever think about that? Action, reaction. When you do something, it has repercussions, and you should be held accountable for your actions and the inevitable reactions they cause."

"I mean it, Barbara. If you leave me, I'll move to another city, and good citizens of Sycamore Springs will be denied the doctor they need."

Anger welled up inside her tense stomach. "You're an arrogant nobody. The way I hear it around town, and I hear it all the time, people are blaming you for Lyle's autism and Sylvia's death. How about those unexpected cases of shingles coming to the attention of Lisa? And what of the major epidemic that looms a couple of years in the future? You're not a hero, you're a menace. Every word you've ever uttered to me or to this town has been a manipulation. Did you hear what I called you and I meant it? A menace."

"You're straying off the subject. Even now, I'm standing in front of you begging you to stay. I swear I'll be forced to leave town if you go."

She snorted with disgust. "You're manipulating me. You're forced to leave town because you know that Travis is going to come back for you, and you know he'll find you. You're a dead man if you stay. You're going to be on the run for the rest of your life, because you know he's not going to stop until he kills you.

Damon put his palms together as if he'd be in prayer. "I'm begging you. All the more reason for you to stay and help me, but if you don't think that all the material possessions my medical practice has been able to give you make up for the few problems we've had, then you may as well go."

She shook her head and sat down on the aged, expensive bench by the front door. "You're such a contradiction. You tell me to stay, then you tell me to go. You say you love Brandon, but you give him a shot despite the terrible reactions he had to most vaccines he'd previously received. It is likely you knew that Brandon already had antibodies to varicella and might not have needed the vaccine to begin with. You also knew Brandon would require a second varicella vaccine in 4 to 8 weeks, since this is specified for all those aged 13 years and older who receive the varicella vaccine."

"How did you know all of that?"

"Craig informed me. He also knew that you would support the ACIP recommendations and eagerly vaccinate pregnant women with the Thimerosal-containing flu vaccine. Also, that you would not hesitate to use your remaining supply of Thimerosal-containing vaccines on the children of Sycamore Springs. I know you honestly didn't think it mattered. But the inorganic mercury that derives from Thimerosal accumulates in the brain. This causes brain damage and sometimes death to those who for some reason are unable to excrete the toxin. More recent studies have implicated use of Thimerosal-containing vaccines in increases in childhood asthma, type 2 diabetes, obesity, certain cancers, food allergies, and other autoimmune disorders. These actions make you very dangerous."

"How can that make *me* dangerous?"

"Because ignorance is no excuse, especially for someone in medicine. People trust you not to hurt them anymore than they've already been hurt."

"I've never hurt you, Barbara."

"Yes, you have. You didn't let me have any more children, and you know how much I wanted them."

He huffed. "So, that's what this is really about. That old business. Haven't you gotten over that already?"

Tears stung her eyes. He'd never change. Arrogant and flawed to the end.

She stood quickly. "Goodbye, Damon. I never want to see you again, and believe me, it will take the end of the world for me to change my mind."

##

"Where are you going to go, Mom?"

Brandon watched her pack up the remainder of the possessions he knew meant the most to her. Strange, but they were things she had when she was very young. She bypassed everything expensive that his father had provided, either through personal gifts or access to credit cards. Barbara wasn't a material person. She valued people and life. Why had she married Damon? He was the opposite. People were a means to an end, and life was something he took for granted for himself and his family. He dismissed grief in other people as signs of weakness. Brandon always assumed his father had never lost anyone that mattered to him. Nothing had ever really happened to Dr. Damon Leviticus. He started at Point A, and was now at Point B. Whenever he had to do something different, for example Point C, he merely moved Point B farther down the path of his life. Nothing new ever happened to him that was bad or disturbing. He kept the control, and used up people like napkins at the diner whenever he needed someone to do his dirty work.

"I'm going to stay with an old acquaintance of mine. Janet and I were friends before I married Damon, and I need to be with someone I trust right now." Staying with Janet would give Barbara time to heal.

"Don't you trust me?" Brandon looked so vulnerable, like a young man with an immature past and no prospects for finding the security he needed within himself.

"Of course, but you have Millie, and I'll just be in the way. Besides, I feel betrayed that you didn't understand my grave concerns over your having another vaccination. You were too young to know the grief I went through with virtually every vaccine you were administered. The screaming, the high temperature, and febrile seizures. Your father, always concerned about building up his practice, didn't know the half of it because he was totally involved away from the home. I'm grateful you're still healthy, but I wish you would have listened to me. I honestly don't think you need me."

Brandon seemed genuinely confused to her. She didn't blame him. His had hardly been a normal life. She knew he also wasn't aware of how often she had spared him unnecessary medical treatments from his over-zealous father.

"I do need you. I have something to tell you."

About time.

"I've wanted to tell you for awhile, but I couldn't find the right time. It's one of the reasons I took the shot. I wanted to be sure I would be healthy and live to be very old. I have more at stake now than I've ever had. Millie and I are going to have a baby."

Tears formed in Barbara's eyes. How many times had she wanted to say the same words about herself? "That's wonderful news, Brandon."

"Will you stay now?"

"I can't. I have to make a new life for myself. Damon and I haven't had a real marriage for years. I'm only going to Los Angeles. It's an hour away. It will give you the space you need to become a husband and father, and the privacy I need to start all over again."

Brandon turned away.

Uh, oh. He was hiding something. Whenever he couldn't look her in the eye, she knew he didn't want her to know something.

"Is something wrong, Brandon?"

He nodded and turned back to her with an expression that was a mixture of worry and fear. "Millie wants to divorce me. She says I tricked her into the pregnancy."

What a strange thing for him to have done, if it were true. He was always an honest child. What could have made him do something deceptive? "Did you?"

"Maybe."

"There are no maybes when it comes to responsibility. A man becomes a man by his actions, not only his thoughts or intentions. You must accept responsibility for whatever happened between you and Millie and your unborn child, then I have a feeling she'll respect you. She probably figures I should finish bringing you up, so she doesn't have to. What she's too young to know is that sometimes a person reaches a level of maturity and stops. That person is content and has positive reinforcement for his actions, even if they are not quite up to standard. If you tricked, Millie, she doesn't trust you yet. Do something to earn her trust, and she'll respect you." So much for motherly advice to a grown man with a pregnant wife, but it was the best she could do under the circumstances, running from her husband, trying to save the last shred of her own life before Damon destroyed that too. Should she stay for Brandon's sake? No, he was an adult in every way. Besides, what good would she be to him if she couldn't salvage any of her identity?

Brandon watched her carefully, the way he always did when he was going to ask her something important. "Did you trust Dad when you met him?"

"Yes, but over the years, I witnessed events that made me believe that he did not embrace accountability for his actions. He used flawed and biased studies for validation. Studies conducted by pharmaceutical companies to promote their own products. He should have learned to think for himself. For example, he would read the research that Craig and others documented, yet he dismissed it. Anything outside the AMA and drug companies was considered as anti-vaccination propaganda. He was influenced by peer pressure and special interests in much the same way you were when you didn't want to refuse the shot. You thought your friends would laugh at you, but they would have admired you, and you might have even saved Dexter from his fate. If you would have left Injection Day, others might have had second thoughts wanting to first learn more themselves rather than relying on someone else to make healthcare decisions for them."

Brandon's eyes widened in disbelief. "Are you saying I'm responsible for what happened to Dexter because we all trusted the medical and pharmaceutical establishments?"

"Of course not. That's an illogical conclusion. That's blaming the victim, a tactic the doctors and drug makers love to use. They say the patient had a genetic defect or genetic predisposition, the patient shouldn't have consented, the patient was at fault. That is simply garbage. The patient is the victim. The doctors and the drug companies are the ones who are at fault."

Brandon exhaled with relief. "Would you go back to him if he learned to think for himself?"

She thought about that for only a minute. What was the use of pretending? Since she'd decided to leave Damon, she'd actually seen her reflection smile back at her from the mirror. "No, he's hurt too many people in the past, many more that will suffer in the future, and the harm he's done is irrevocable, causing continual disease and treatment cycles, requiring more and more vaccines. He can't make it right, no matter how hard he's going to try, and my guess is he'll hide behind the sanctions of the medical and pharmaceutical complex, and absolve himself of all blame."

"But if he were to try, why wouldn't you stay with him and help him? Wouldn't that be the right thing to do?

How easy was right and wrong for the people with little or no hurt in their past. "No, dear. Damon has hurt me too deeply for me to ever trust him again. I stayed with him for so many reasons, for you and also for me. I was too browbeaten to have left, but his Injection Day was one of the worst travesties Sycamore Springs has ever seen. I'm ashamed of him." She turned to finish packing, hiding the two tears that fell without a sound. She was also ashamed of herself for not leaving before.

"What did he do to you?" Brandon asked quietly, moving closer behind her. "I always wondered. Was it so bad? You never told me."

She had to wait a full minute to let the emotion and sorrow lessen so she could speak. "He made it impossible for you to have siblings, at least from me."

She heard him gasp. "I didn't know that," Brandon admitted softly. "I'm sorry."

"I'm sorry, too." She turned suddenly into his waiting embrace and hugged him fiercely.

##

"So, where are we going to live, Mil?"

She taped another box shut, pushing it carefully against the others to be shipped to the East coast once she got her dorm assignment. She wasn't leaving Sycamore Springs for a long time, but he knew it made her feel that soon her college degree would be a reality.

Brandon nudged her gently, but impatiently, out of the way. "Let me do the heavy stuff, okay?" What was the matter with her, taking chances like that with their child and her own health. Women, a constant source of worry for him. First, his mother was packing, and now the mother of his child.

"Sure, but I'm only pregnant. I'm not an invalid."

"You've got to be careful. Don't move anything. Don't take anything."

"Thanks for the advice." She smiled at him, and he felt better.

"You didn't take any catch-up vaccines on Injection Day, did you?" he asked, worried again. What if she had? What if it hurt the baby?

"No, not me," she replied. My father told me that I had all that were required when I was younger. I trust him."

Trust. Brandon felt a wave despair. How was he going to gain the trust and respect of the woman he loved?

"He and I recalled my case of chickenpox in first grade. He told me that likely this was sufficient to provide lifelong immunity. However he thought that immunity or protection against varicella was maintained somewhat by periodic exposures to other children with chickenpox and he was concerned that Injection Day would eliminate this vital boosting mechanism."

Brandon put his hand over the diminishing welt on his arm where his father had jabbed him, he thought extra hard for showmanship, with the injection. He'd seen a lot of kids walking around Sycamore with angry looking bumps and some bruises from the shots. Ricki was especially vicious in here technique and personality. He disliked her intensely, and he'd once asked his father why he'd hired her. He didn't answer him. So much for father and son loyalty.

"Do you think I'll have any bad side effects like Dexter did?" he asked, uneasy. She seemed to know so much.

Millie's heart turned over. Brandon was a frightened child, just like all people became once they crossed the line from citizens with free will to patients with ignored, so-called rights. What could she tell him? The truth would scare him, but a lie would hurt him even more. She couldn't undo what had been done to him.

"My father says that whoever took the chickenpox vaccine is not expected to experience any adverse reactions even though they may not have needed the injection due to having a previous undetected case of chickenpox. About 80% of adolescents who have an unknown history or no history of chickenpox, actually test positive for VZV antibodies and therefore do not require the vaccine. They may have had such a mild case, their parents simply did not recognize the symptoms of chickenpox, perhaps mistaking the appearance of the lesions for insect bites. However, for every varicella injection, there will be less naturally occurring varicella disease in the general population. Because of that, you and other adults will not receive the exposures to chickenpox that you would have naturally received in the community during the yearly epidemics of chickenpox in the community. The periodic exposures to chickenpox are what boosts your immunity to help suppress the reactivation of shingles. The pain from shingles can be excruciating and can continue even after the rash has disappeared. Chickenpox, on the other hand, is often a more mild disease than shingles with less hospitalizations, intense itching but not the incredible pain along the nerve pathways. Also, the scarring associated with chickenpox is of a different nature and in most cases is avoidable and minimal."

"In the near future, should the vaccination lose its effectiveness in protecting against chickenpox, mothers will not have natural immunity to varicella. Thus, their newborns may be more susceptible to disease. Also, should the mother contract varicella in the first trimester of her pregnancy, there is a small chance the disease can be transferred to the developing fetus resulting in deformities of the limbs in what is known as varicella syndrome.

Brandon stared at her. "All that – amazing! And I only thought I got a shot."

"We don't have time to go over the complete story. Nothing ever exists in a vacuum. Even if it appears to be in isolation, it is only in the laboratory. Out in the world, where real studies count the most, there are many factors. Consider that there exists the possibility that genetic variations might occur when the live Oka-strain varicella vaccine is transmitted to others[76] or mixes with the natural wild-type virus. Already, researchers have found both a vaccine strain and natural strain of varicella virus that is resistant to antiviral therapy.[77] A genetics researcher that my father knows has found single nucleotide polymorphisms, called SNPs, which are genetic changes from one varicella strain to the next. This is why he believes some children can manifest more than one case of chickenpox. The child is presented with a different or heterologous strain of chickenpox that is not recognized by the immune system as a result of exposure to the first case of chickenpox. Each person has their own unique set of circumstances and medical predispositions. Each unsuspecting person who is the subject, willing or not, of a study, is going to bring their own history, their own hereditary factors, their own undeniable past to the project. Robust conclusions can only be obtained when data are honestly collected and reported without prejudice."

Brandon turned away. "You're a smart woman, Millie. They say your father is a genius. It's really that when he finds a pattern that is unexpected or unexplained, he is not quick to dismiss it as erroneous, but is open-minded enough to consider that his previous understanding may need revision. He tries to objectively consider all options. In contrast, my father considers usually one and only one option that supports his thinking. There's a big difference. *You* didn't have to prove anything by taking the shot. *I* did."

---

[76] Grossberg R, Harpaz R, Rubtcova E, Loparev V, Seward JF, Schmid DS. Secondary transmission of varicella vaccine virus in a chronic care facility for children. J. Pediatr. 2006;148:842-844.

[77] Levin MJ, Dahl KM, Weinberg A, Giller R, Patel A, Krause PR. Development of resistance to acyclovir during chronic infection with the OKA vaccine strain of varicella-zoster virus, in an immunosuppressed child. J. Infect. Dis. 2003;188(7):945-947.

"No, you didn't," she said in strong disagreement. "What kind of a father are you going to be if you let people push you around? Just because people have a diploma, a piece of paper with their name on it stating that they sat in classrooms for a set number of years, doesn't mean they know what they're doing." She started working on packing another box.

Brandon sat down on the floor next to her and thought silently while he watched her sort through her childhood belongings. What a strange thing for her to say. Wasn't that exactly what she was going to do—sit in classrooms and listen to people who weren't as smart as she was, just so she could get a degree? "Then why are you doing it? Why are you going to sit in classrooms and waste those years dumbing yourself down for a degree while people are being hurt because you're not working writing investigative articles to expose them?"

Millie started to answer, but then stopped and stared at him. *Why was she going to college? To make herself a better journalist. Did that make sense? She would be sitting in classrooms with people who didn't know her father, people who hadn't had her advantages of an open-minded dialogue with intelligent people since birth.*

What was she doing?

"Gotcha, didn't I?" Brandon interrupted her thoughts with a smirk on his face. "Didn't think I could stop the Millie Train to Nowhere, did you?"

She sat down next to him and put her head on his shoulder. "Some people in college will be fair and dedicated like my father, won't they?"

Brandon shrugged. "Maybe, but I think most will be like my father—cookie cutter clones of the system."

Millie closed her eyes and pictured a roomful of Damon Leviticus'. She didn't like the narrow-minded, lemming-like view.

"What are my options, Brandon? Everyone goes to college, don't they?" All the kids in high school were going, if they could afford it or not. Loans were plentiful, roping teenagers into the credit system with grand promises of overly-inflated salaries, making it impossible for them to pay off their debt and live a credit-card free life at the same time. They were prisoners of the system, the company story of credit card debt, unfair bank charges, usury interest rates, and the necessity to take any job they could to pay their credit card bills and student loans.

"Do they? If they can get a loan and go in debt for the rest of their lives, they do so." At least they both agreed on that point. Brandon was really very levelheaded when it came to anything but the practice of medicine according to his father.

"My father has been saving ever since I was born so I could have everything," she said slowly, thinking about what she was about to do with her education for the first time, taking off the blinders, standing in the sun of reality—and not liking it.

"Nobody can have everything, Millie. Some people get a few things along the way, but most have to change with the times to make their lives unique and wonderful. You have everything you need right now to be an investigative journalist. What if you get a degree, and it turns out that it isn't the 'degree of the moment', or it happens that someone will have two degrees and outrank you. They won't. Nothing matters but intelligence and reason, and your parents have already given you these."

"But won't I need a degree to get a job?"

"Of course not. You don't want a common job that has the common prerequisite of a degree of any kind as long as you can say 'college graduate' on your resume. Big deal. It's just a racket to keep kids off the job market as long as possible. The same racket that forces people into early retirement with inviting termination packages."

Millie laughed. "Who's talking here? Is that you, Brandon? You've got a reputation of being only a jock, only showing up to class to stay on the team."

He nodded slowly. "I know. That's what's expected of me. I always do what's expected of me. That's why I took that shot, when my own mother warned me not to do it. It's because of that and the danger I'm now in because I moved blindly into an established practice—inoculations for a blind public. If I am not going to live the rest of my life as a puppet like my father, I have to take a stand now, and so do you."

That's why I love him. That's why I married him and wanted him to be the father of my baby. He has a mind, and he uses it.

"Is this a move to get me to stay in Sycamore?"

He moved closer and took both hands. He put one on her tummy and one on his heart. "Yes, Millie. Will you both stay here with me?"

##

Chapter 20

Sycamore Springs, California
2018

"At school, they were talking about your last play, Dad. How you ran thirty yards, and then you kicked that football to victory. I read the article about you in the paper. I wish I could have seen that."

Brandon put the newspaper down on the table and watched Mark over the rims of his glasses. Maybe Brandon needed new glasses. His eyes were more fatigued and sore than usual. He took off his glasses and rubbed his eyes—they seemed gritty. Any sort of reading, even for just a brief time, had become especially uncomfortable the past few days. Mark was watching him with that look of hero-worship that meant almost as much to him as his son's frequently expressed love.

Brandon replied to his son, "I wish you could have seen me play, too. I was really great," he said, proudly aware of his status in the sports community. "Who was talking about me? That was a long time ago when I was about your age."

Mark laughed and passed Brandon the football.

Brandon reached for it—and strangely he missed. He thought it was right where it was supposed to be, but instead it was somewhere else. That was it, he had to get his eyes examined. Not only was his vision becoming blurred, but his depth perception seemed very off as well.

"Don't give me that old man look. You can still beat me. I was just proud of you, that's all. The coach was talking about you. You're a legend. Your team always won because of you. You were the best player Sycamore ever had."

Brandon felt unsteady, getting progressively weaker over the past two weeks. He reflected on his experiences during the last couple of decades at the bad things that had happened. "No, I wasn't the best. Probably Dexter was better, before he got hurt. One time, just before Injection Day, he tackled me, and let me tell you, I thought he'd killed me for sure. He knocked the wind out of me, and I just lay there on the field, looking up at his grinning face, wondering if I'd have the strength to do the same to him that day. A few days after that, I punched him out for making a pass at your mother."

Brandon watched as Mark looked down at the floor, the same way he always did when memories and nostalgia overtook the conversation. They embarrassed him. Brandon understood. Mark was young and not much in the way of disappointment had happened to him yet.

Brandon, however, thought about Dexter every day, remembering how he saw Dexter confronting Millie in the boondocks years before, and how it could have been him instead of Dexter living out his life unable to enjoy a single, normal moment.

And Aileen. He thought about her, too. How she'd taken her own life when the tranquilizers Damon said she needed had turned her own mind against her one night when she was alone and under the influence of a pharmaceutical haze instead of in control of her own senses. Millie was sure it was a drug overdose that had induced a psychotic state. Aileen simply went to sleep and never woke again.

"You shouldn't think so much about the past, Dad. Mom said nothing was your fault. Damon does whatever he wants to do."

"Why don't you call him Grandfather the way you do to Craig?"

"Respect has gotta be earned, doesn't it? Craig's always helping people, writing about what's right and wrong, backing it up with facts and research, and building inventions that give us all better ways to live. He never backs down, no matter the pressure, no matter the odds. He is completely dedicated to his work."

"And Damon?"

"As far as I can tell, he's only caused pain and death. Nothing to respect there," Mark said frankly.

Brandon felt the sting of shame. Even his grandchild couldn't find anything good about Damon. Maybe he should stop hoping his father would do something not driven by greed and self-aggrandizement.

"I don't understand something, Mark. Maybe you can tell me. You're younger and smarter. Why is it that when someone is evil they survive, and when someone is good no one even remembers they were on the planet?" This question particularly plagued him. Evil people lived a long time.

Mark stared at him. "You think too much. Mom says you think more now than you used to. What difference does it make who's good and who's bad? Who's going to remember any of us years from now? Doesn't it matter whatever's going on at the moment? Just take care of yourself, right?"

"I used to think that way, but after years of living with your mother, I'm not so sure. Damon is always wrong about so many things, yet he only looked at what was in front of him. Craig is right about much more, because he looks at the who, what, why, when, where, and how of investigations. That's what research really is supposed to be, isn't it? Finding out the truth? What good is it to have all those opportunities, all those years of training, all those possibilities, and then promote half a story with only the positive propaganda or knowingly tell lies so that no one ever challenges incorrect assumptions or exposes unsafe practices?" What had turned him into a philosopher? He missed his ignorant jock days. Life was simpler then, divided between right and wrong, good and bad.

Mark put the football into his hands and held it there. "You know what I think, Dad? I think that if you died tomorrow, you wouldn't have really lived many of your years. That's the difference between you and Craig. He recognizes there are problems, but he tries to solve them. You just recognize there are problems."

Brandon smiled wryly. "I guess you respect Craig more than you respect me."

"Never. He's great, but you're my father, and I love you."

Brandon's eyes misted over and he felt an unfamiliar sting. "Isn't it strange, that you feel comfortable telling me you care about me, yet, if I died tomorrow, my own father would have never said he loved me? Isn't that sad?"

Mark looked at him unwaveringly. "Yeah, Dad, it is. But it isn't the end of the world. Why don't you forget about the past and live your life now?"

"I can't. My single act of cowardice, which was taking that shot, drove my mother away from my father, and made me sorry for the rest of my life, thinking I could have perhaps influenced persons on Injection Day to become more informed about their healthcare decisions and be wary of the continuous disease and treatment cycles that 'trusted' health officials and institutions promote for their own self-preservation and self-interests."

"That really disappoints me Dad—how you'll let some deranged old man ruin your life."

"It's just the luck of the draw." He rubbed a sore spot on his nose.

"Zits at your age, Dad? Gross, as your generation used to say."

"It's irritating. I'll have to ask your mother for something."

Mark stood up and hugged Brandon. "I'm going to find Hallie."

"Hallie? I thought you never went out with the same girl twice."

He grinned. "Maybe it's time I changed my ways."

##

"You can push now, Rochelle."

The lights in the delivery room glared against the sterile metal from the stirrups to the huge overhead lights. "I can't feel anything," she said.

"Well, that's because we've given you something to speed up labor, and then when that made it unbearable, we gave you a spinal. But I don't want you to miss the birth experience, so you can pretend to push anyway."

She looked puzzled, but it didn't matter. The hour was late, and he wanted to get home. He'd hurried her labor along as fast as medical science would allow without doing an emergency c-section. If she didn't deliver in a few minutes, he'd do that, too. God, he was tired.

"I want this baby so much, Dr. Leviticus. I came to you, even though you were no longer in Sycamore Springs, because I knew you'd help me be healthy, have a natural birth experience, and have a healthy baby. My husband and I have been trying for years."

"You'll have your baby, Rochelle, any minute now."

He signaled for forceps and used them. With a twist and a yank, the baby was born.

Silently.

Damon stared at it. It had stumps for both arms and one leg.

He looked up immediately at Rochelle, anticipating her screaming when he told her. "Now, Rochelle, I want you to be very calm," he began. "It was for a blessing."

##

"Later, an autopsy revealed the baby died from complications of classic Varicella Syndrome," Lisa whispered to Millie. "Because the wild-type, or natural, chickenpox had nearly been eradicated, Rochelle was never exposed to natural chickenpox and missed getting the vaccination. Rochelle contracted with chickenpox shortly after babysitting some children who she learned also contracted chickenpox. Unfortunately, Rochelle was in her first trimester of pregnancy. Chickenpox was passed on to the developing fetus. Really this scenario is also a possibility among those who are vaccinated if the protective effect wears off in adulthood."

Millie shuddered. The doctors and drug companies were responsible for yet another death from Injection Day. How far-reaching were the consequences going to be? She blessed her father every day for telling her all the facts, so she was not uninformed and left to the mercy of the self-promoting pharmaceuticals and health departments. Her father knew that the same company that manufactured the shingles vaccine, also manufactured Acyclovir, the antiviral used to treat shingles. How convenient it was to vaccinate children for chickenpox, cause a shingles epidemic, the same pharmaceutical company would further be enriched and supply the antiviral medication to treat shingles as well as a booster shingles vaccine to substitute for the natural exposure that adults previously received in the community when chickenpox incidence was high. A win-win-win situation promoting more greed.

"Will Rochelle have other children?" Millie asked.

"Lisa shook her head. "No, Damon talked her into signing a consent form for a hysterectomy, to spare her any more possibilities of the same thing happening. He had made a preliminary determination that attributed the deformities to a genetic defect and had not taken sufficient time to review Rochelle's medical history file to see that she had onset of varicella during her first trimester of pregnancy."

Millie slammed her fist down on Lisa's desk, startling them both. "Who is going to stop that man? He can't go on forever killing and destroying people, cutting out parts of their bodies they can use. He's a vicious murderer!"

Lisa shook from the strain. "I know they can't all be murderers, butchers. But those like Dr. L belong to the American Murder Association. Anyone who goes near them becomes sick, or sicker, and dies. They are the ultimate evil – sanctioned and mandated murder."

Millie put her head in her hands. "Barbara was butchered, too."

"I know. She told me once when we were at a class together. We need more control over the medical and pharmaceutical complex, more watchdog consumer groups that are independent and do not have the conflicts of interest. It's ignorance that keeps evil in power. Once we shine the bright light of truth on them, they'll be more careful."

Millie shuddered. "I'm not so sure. Maybe they'll only be more secretive; drawing people into treatments and drugs they don't need even more, so that the uninformed people won't know they've been butchered until it's too late."

"Like Dexter."

"Yes, but we did shine the bright light of television on him, and because of that, the station was flooded with calls and letters calling for improved vaccine safety testing and risk assessment of adverse vaccine reactions from the manufacturers. Then the national news picked it up, and it was all over the Internet."

"Damon hated that."

"Of course he did. He could not operate in secrecy anymore."

"Yes, he did, on Rochelle, even in another city after he ran out of Sycamore with Travis on his trail. Evil is mobile."

Millie smiled ruefully. "You're beginning to sound like me."

Lisa nodded and shuffled through some papers on her desk. She looked upset.

"Is there something you'd like to talk about?" Millie asked, perceptively.

Lisa looked up. There were tears in her eyes. "Paul left me."

Millie gasped. "After all these years? What happened?"

"He really loved another. I knew about that, but I didn't say anything. Everyone has a right to be happy, and he didn't love me anymore. I stay busy with my work and ignored the stares of his friends. But, after awhile, he lost interest in just about everything. He left Sycamore Springs last week. I don't think I'll see him again."

"What about Richard? Won't he come back to see his own son?"

"I doubt it. He was never one for family."

Millie leaned forward, concerned for her friend, a woman who gave unselfishly of herself and was so stepped on by everyone who could use her. "What are you going to do?"

"I'll keep on at school, but I'm also going to go to work for Craig. He's writing a book about his research, and he needs a research assistant."

Millie nodded approvingly. "Dad's going to help educate the public so that in the future, people will no longer be the willing experimental pawns of the health system.

"Amen."

##

"Can I talk to you, Dad?"

Millie touched the framed small poster on the wall. It read:

The heights by great men reached and kept
Were not attained by sudden flight,
But they, while their companions slept,
Were toiling upward in the night.

"You like Henry Wadsworth Longfellow?" Craig asked. "He's a favorite poet and philosopher of mine."

"I've seen this poem in your office since I was a little girl," she answered. "His words remind me of you."

Craig smiled. “I do stay up too late working.”

Millie turned toward him. “It’s not only the hours you keep, it’s about your work. Other men work far into the night, like Damon, yet they never reach any great heights.”

Craig shook his head. “Damon has problems, and they begin within himself. He’s power hungry, and he chose a personal way of life and a way of running his business life that feeds his ego. No one has to take advantage of people, no one has to hurt people. It’s all a choice. That’s why I left that epidemiological studies project after nearly 8 years of dedicated work. I had to bring my research to the public, so they would be informed in a balanced way—not only knowing the pros, but also identifying the cons of a universal varicella vaccination program. The health authorities focus on only one side of every issue—their side. For instance, did you know that an estimated two million children have been adversely affected by Thimerosal in vaccines, up until year 2000 when it was decided to finally have this preservative removed?”

“Yes, I had seen that figure before.”

“If you ask a doctor if vaccines are safe, most say, ‘yes’ without any hesitation.”

“Are they lying?”

“Most of them. Some refuse to believe otherwise, and that is a lie in itself.”

Millie stared out the window. So much had happened to her friends, so much more would happen to the world, and it would all be because of doctors and drugs. How could her father make a difference? He was only one man—a David against a Goliath. Even as a crusader for the truth, he was far out-numbered by those desiring to promote high vaccination rates and suppress the deleterious data despite the detriment to public health..

“Do you think people will listen to you?” she asked, worried.

“Yes, they will, and they’ll tell their friends, and they’ll tell more people, who’ll tell their relatives. That’s the beauty of truth. It is the fountain of life.”

Millie moved quietly to her father’s desk. It was covered with folders and papers, and it had a plaque at the front.

Beauty is truth, truth beauty.

“Is this new?” she asked.

“No, it’s very old. John Keats wrote that.”

She nodded. “No wonder the medical pharmaceutical complex is such an ugly industry.”

##

The phone rang twice in the dark room. Barbara pulled on her bathrobe and padded to the desk, careful not to wake Janet. “Hello?”

The voice on the other end was familiar in tone, but it had a frightened quality that made her skin crawl around her muscles. "Damon? Is that you? How did you get this number?"

"Faith gave it to me after I pleaded for it. You have to come back to Sycamore Springs right away. I'm leaving Denver tonight. I'm at the airport. For the love of God, get to the airport," he barely managed to say, his voice a stranglehold of emotion.

She drew herself up to her full height, straightening her back, shaking the remnants of sleep from her mind. Whatever he wanted, she was not going to be a part of it. He must be crazy, calling after all these years. How long had it been since she'd seen him last? The night on the stairs when he rubbed her face in the miserable past he had created for her.

"Forget it Damon. I told you I wouldn't want to see you again until the end of the world, and I meant it. I've moved on, and you must as well. Good-bye."

"Wait!"

Was that her ex-husband, shouting? He had never done that before. He was the epitome of calm. Cautiously, she put the phone back to her ear. Was he crying?

"Barbara, this isn't about you. It isn't about me. It's...."

He was beginning to scare her. "Tell me, Damon. What is it?"

"It's... Brandon."

Barbara's heart jumped into her throat. She could feel it pounding so loudly in her ears and feel it so strongly in her chest she thought she would die.

"Is he hurt?" Merciful heaven, was that her voice?

"He's... sick...." Damon managed on a sob.

"Explain that, right now," she yelled, her fear taking over. She was vaguely aware Janet was at her side, holding her by her shoulders, keeping her upright.

"Craig told me. Millie called him, because she recognized what was wrong based on articles she had found while conducting a literature search on shingles."

Barbara wanted to shriek into the phone. "You tell me right now, Damon, what's wrong with Brandon."

She heard silence, and then Damon said on a moan, "He has shingles."

Barbara exhaled with a sigh of relief. Shingles was very bad, but at least he had a good chance of recovery. He was young and strong. "How serious is it? The pain can be excruciating, but recovery can take from 4 to 8 weeks from what I've read. In a few cases it does recur, but...."

She stopped suddenly. Damon was barely able to control his emotions. He wasn't telling her something, and that scared her even more. He was never one to leave a detail out of a medical diagnosis, no matter who he frightened or hurt.

"What are you leaving out," she asked on a frightened whisper.

"The shingles aren't in the usual dermatome distribution on one side of the torso, but they have affected the ophthalmic branch of the trigeminal nerve affecting his eyes," Damon cried out. "In his eyes."

Barbara let the phone drop. It clattered to the floor. She stared at it as the strength ebbed out of her limbs, and she heard her own cry in the dark room.

"Have you blinded my baby? Will my child ever see me again?"

##

The drive from Los Angeles to Sycamore Springs usually took Barbara less than two hours depending on traffic. With the radio on, she was usually only two fast-food stops away from Brandon, Millie, and Mark.

This time the drive seemingly took forever. There were no fast-food stops on this trip. Janet looked worried, but she kept driving.

"What if I'm too late? What if...."

Janet patted her hand. "Don't do this to yourself. He's going to need you when you get there. You have to be strong for him. What do you know about shingles that have involvement of the eye and lens?"

She shuddered. "The classic symptoms start with a sore on the tip of the victim's nose, called Hutchinson's sign, which is the first indication that a branch of the trigeminal nerve is involved. Then the shingles virus can cause an irritation that scratches the cornea or tissue covering the lens...." How strange. She was never one not to finish her sentences. She must be more frightened than she thought she'd ever be. It was one thing when it was her that Damon had hurt, but now that it was her child, she couldn't think clearly, even though she knew that she had to stay calm for Brandon's sake.

By the time they approached the city limits of Sycamore Springs, she couldn't control her shaking. Yet, when Janet pulled in front of Brandon's house, she was only immobile long enough to realize that she had to be a pillar of strength, that she couldn't crumble. Brandon needed her.

Millie opened the door, and closed it quietly behind her, putting her finger to her lips. "He's finally sleeping," she whispered. "It's very bad, Barbara."

##

"I figured I'd see you again, Dr. L., in this world or the next."

Travis threw his weight against the motel room door, sending Damon backward into the room. The stench of unwashed previous guests filled Damon's nostrils along with the smell of a vengeful stalker.

"How many years has it been, Dr. Damon Leviticus, Pretender of the Faith?" Travis asked, a thick sneer covering his lips. "I'd heard you were back in town, and I figured you might need someone to take you around, show you the sights, the graves of the people you killed, the rooms where the 'impaired' have had to stay the last sixteen years, drooling over their canned food dinners, while you ate at the fanciest restaurants in Denver, at least that's the way I heard it."

What a time for his old nemesis to find him. Travis looked older and hadn't aged well. Damon figured it was the stupid factor along with Travis' hating him that had turned his hair to a shock of white and sunk his eyeballs deeply into his head. Some people took bad news too hard. If Travis had only accepted what had happened to Lyle as an unavoidable rare statistical event, then he might look better and have moved on, instead of harboring revenge all these years. Certainly, he couldn't still be carrying that gun, even though he was obviously still carrying that grudge.

"Get out of my way, Travis. Brandon is sick. He needs me." Damon tried to close the door to his motel room, but Travis stuck his foot onto the threshold. He had to stay in Travis' dump, because no one in Sycamore had room for him. Funny, he didn't expect to see Travis in town. Rumor had it that Travis had sold the motel and taken Pammi and Lyle to Mexico afterwards. He had apparently lost all his money trying to help Lyle. Why did he try? Hadn't Damon told Travis in no uncertain words that nothing more could be done for his grandson? Once again, Travis proved he was simply not listening to the people who knew more than he did.

"Don't have a minute for an old friend? That's not neighborly."

"We're not neighbors. We haven't been for years. I've been living in Denver. This is the first time I've set foot in Sycamore Springs since 2001. I'd moved on, and I've moved up."

Travis cackled with a hoarse laugh. "Denver? That's moving up? It's only a mile high. Heaven's the only really high place around. That's where Lyle's gonna go one day, when the good Lord puts him out of his misery. But you're never gonna see Heaven, Dr. L. They don't allow murderers in."

Damon snorted. "I've never murdered anyone."

"Let's see. Sarah Perkins, Aileen, Sylvia. And you gave a death in life to Dexter and Lyle. And what about Rochelle's baby? Doesn't look good for you. Nope, not good at all."

"How did you know about Rochelle? That was in the Denver paper last week, before I heard how sick Brandon was from Millie."

"News travels fast."

"Not that fast."

"It does if you've got friends. See, Michelle, that's my wife in case you don't remember, she took Rochelle and hid her in Denver during her first pregnancy, on account of nobody knowing who the father was. That baby was in good shape. Not like the one that only got a few breaths of life on this green earth."

Damon pushed Travis out of his way. "You are a raving lunatic. Go to you doctor. Tell him you need medication. You need something strong so you can cope with life as it happens to you. Everyone is a statistic. No one can control what happens to them and their family. That's why they trust doctors to fix things." He looked wildly around the room. How was he going to get out. Brandon needed him. He had the prescription drug famciclovir, call Famvir®, which supposedly has better absorption into the body than

Acyclovir, as the choice antiviral medication. As soon as he could see Brandon, he'd start him with a loaded dose." I can't talk to you now, don't you understand?"

"That's my grandson you destroyed, along with children and parents of folks who had been fooled to think you had the power to help them, the ability to heal them. Well, let me tell you something, Dr. L., you don't have any power at all. You're a murderer, a loser, and a fool, and the people you pimp for are the same. I'm going to have to make you pay for what you did. I'm going to hold you accountable for the lives you've ruined."

"Get out of my way," Damon shouted, pointing toward the door. "Those were not my children. They were not my grandchildren. Everyone is responsible for themselves. If they didn't want the shot, they shouldn't have come to me. I didn't put a gun to anyone's head. My own son needs me, and I'm going to help him."

Damon immediately recognized his ironic mistake, bringing up the gun episode. Travis had probably long forgotten the attempt on his life. What were the chances he'd carried around a weapon for nearly two decades waiting to see his imaginary foe again. Slim. Maybe six percent? That was statistically insignificant.

"Liar," Travis said menacingly and snarled with the look of a feral dog. "I've got something I've been meaning to give you for years, but every time I got close, you moved away or someone came between us."

"I don't know what you're talking about." He didn't. Maybe he could get to the cell phone in his pocket. He knew where the buttons were by touch. If he could turn it on without Travis hearing any signal, he could hit 911. Then he could figure out what to do from there."

He watched Travis' face for any sign of weakness. Everyone had signs of weakness. He relied on them with his patients. Then he knew how to make sure they did what he thought was best. When he approached a secure person, one who knew the options, well, then he had to try harder to find how to push their reluctant buttons. He could try fear, statistical references, fear, quoting drug company brochures, fear, quoting drug company testing, and when all else failed, fear. How else to make a believer out of a non-believer?

He must have hesitated too long and given the mad man in front of him time to think, because Travis reached into the waistband at the back of his jeans. It took Damon only a few seconds to recognize the gun from long ago. It gleamed evilly in the sparse room, catching the light from the cheap table lamp on the night stand.

Damon responded, "You're a sick man, Travis, a very sick man, to carry a grudge all these years. You need to be in a mental institution under the strictest supervision, medicated to the maximum allowable dose possible."

"Me?" He scratched his chin with the barrel of his gun. "Not me, Dr. L. I know I'm not the only person in the world. You're the one who should be locked up. You think people are pawns for some twisted game you play with your doctor friends. But they're not. People are humans, which is what you should have been, but you're not. You think you're the only one with a family, but you're wrong. Most people have someone they care about, someone who is their family."

Damon's blood pressure rose to the boiling point. "What has this got to do with me? Tell me right now. I'm not part of your family. If you care about them so much, go to them."

Travis stared at him. "You're even crazier than I thought. How did you ever get a job, let alone be in a position to have hurt so many people without any controls over your behavior? You have no grasp of reality at all. You think you're high and mighty, always talking down to me, and I let you, because then I can see your weakness. It's your pride, Dr. L., but you know what? You've got nothing to be proud about. You're a poor excuse for a human, taking the life's blood out of your patients to line your own pockets. Someone should have taken a shot at you long before I ever thought about it, but don't worry. I'm going to shoot you so full of holes, the cops won't be able to identify you without looking at your dental work, that is if you have any teeth left. I'm going to splatter you all over the walls of my motel. Fitting, don't you think? I had to sell this place to get enough money to take Lyle all over the country looking for a doctor who could help him. Know what? They were reluctant to get involved in a vaccine injury related case. They simply took my money and then after reviewing the charts told me they can't help Lyle."

Damon's temper flared higher. Every word Travis said, hit him like a lit match, building the conflagration of fury. How dare a moron like Travis think he could even speak to Damon? He's a medical doctor. He's above reproach. "Stop talking to me, or I'll call the police. You can't detain me against my will."

"Why not? You detain people against their will, but isn't that just like you, Dr. L., and all your doctor friends. I've heard from Sam Perkins that you called the police on him after you killed Sarah, because he was upset. You're not a good man, Dr. L. There's a special place and judgment reserved for butchers like you, and I'm going to send you there right now."

Panic hit Damon hard, strangely not for his own safety. He was reasonably sure, given enough time, he could talk his way out of the motel room, even if Travis were to try and shoot him. However, one thought froze his blood in his veins. What if Travis wounded him or killed him? Who would evaluate Brandon's condition and get him the needed antiviral drugs? Another physician might not be as familiar with this form of herpes zoster, called HZO or herpes zoster ophthalmicus, and might make some differential diagnosis that involves treatment of the rash symptoms only. Good thing he had friends in the drug companies, people who had taken him to dinner, people who cared for the well-being of his family. They had conveniently provided a box of free samples of Famvir® he had gathered together to take to Brandon. The pharmaceutical companies were his real, true friends. His friend had given him a box of the precious drugs because Damon had once testified in his friends favor on the witness stand regarding a pharmaceutical company involved in a drug-related death. This led to the pharmaceutical company being exonerated. They owed him one, and they knew it, he figured.

He wasn't going to let some gun-toting cowboy get in his way. He was an educated man, for God's sake, a righteous man. He'd served his community unselfishly since he was certified and took the Hippocratic oath to do so. No one had a right to stop him from helping the man who meant the most in the world to him.

He knew that he and Brandon had not had the closest of relationships since he had married Millie, the woman with no personality and no degree. She had turned his own son against him with unfounded speculation and lies, but that was all in the past. His son would love him again once Damon saved his life. After the situation was resolved, the newspapers and the media would report how Dr. Damon Leviticus had fought a meaningless ingrate for a gun, how he knew he might have to kill his would-be assassin, but he was willing to do it to reach Brandon in time. Who would blame him? A father running to his son with salvation in his hand?

He took a step forward. "I have to get to Brandon," Damon shouted. "I have antiviral drugs that can help him."

Travis stopped his further advancement with a vicious jerk of the gun. He looked interested. Damon saw the opening he had been waiting for, the show of vulnerability, the dropping of the guard for even an instant. Of course, why hadn't he seen it before? He could get to Travis. He loved Lyle. Damon loved Brandon. Of course. The love of family would get him out of the motel room alive.

Damon snickered. After he was safe in Brandon's house, he would call the police and have Travis arrested for attempted murder. What a great plan.

Travis eyed him suspiciously. "What's the matter with him?" he asked, a small amount of interest in his voice.

"Shingles. He's got shingles and they have affected his vision. That's what Millie said on the phone." Damon shuddered. He knew his daughter-in-law would be the harbinger of bad news. When he heard the sound of her voice telling him such unspeakable things, he hated her even more. It was all her fault. If she and her father wouldn't interfere all the time with the accepted standard of medical practice, Brandon wouldn't have gotten sick. She should have called him sooner, instead of waiting until his son's shingles had caused diminished sight.

Travis was watching him, distrustfully. "Are you lying to me, Dr. L? I remember that little talk you gave us all at the Spartacus Club, that hypocritical talk about how great you were, how you were going to save us all from having loss of income by our having to take time off from work to take care of our children with chickenpox. You're a lying murderer. You want me to believe that Brandon has shingles, but you said people who got the chickenpox vaccine were at a lower risk of shingles than those who got the natural disease. So that makes you a liar, right?"

"What are you babbling about? He has shingles. Let me out of here."

Travis rubbed his chin with his free hand. "How'd he get shingles? Was it from the chickenpox vaccine? If he had never had chickenpox and you hadn't given him the live virus by vaccinating him it would not be possible to have shingles. But I saw you give him a different shot than the one that turned my grandson into a vegetable on Injection Day. Brandon got the varicella shot, so why is his shingles case so serious?"

"I saved him from chickenpox by giving him the varicella vaccination," Damon confirmed. "But it is possible that he may have had a very mild case of natural chickenpox either before or after the administration of the vaccine that had gone undetected. Thus, he harbored both the attenuated vaccine strain of chickenpox and the natural strain of chickenpox. It is likely that the more dominant natural strain of chickenpox is what has reactivated as shingles affecting Brandon's eyes. Even though some children and adolescents get the chickenpox vaccine, they may still get a very mild case of chickenpox when exposed to either someone with shingles or a child with a natural case of chickenpox. It is called a breakthrough case."

"So, how did he...."

"People get shingles, you fool," Damon shouted, losing whatever control of whatever sanity he had left. "Get out of my way."

Taking advantage of Travis' bewilderment, he shoved him against the motel wall, yanked open the door and ran for his car. Would Travis follow him? Would he shoot him in the back of the head? Anything could happen when dealing with people who play God.

"Dr. L.," Travis called after him. "Don't leave. I've got something for you, something I've been saving for a long time. I want to give it to you."

Damon looked over his shoulder. Travis had raised the gun. It was pointed directly at him. They were only a few yards from each other. His car was parked outside the motel room door. Even if it wasn't, Travis was a crack shot. His life wasn't worth that plugged nickel his slow-witted friend was always talking about.

Desperate, Damon changed his tactics. "I'll make a deal with you. How about we make a deal, Travis, on the honor the Spartacus Club?" Damon shouted.

Travis almost smiled. A deal. What kind of a deal with a murderer like Damon did he think he'd make? *Look at the expression on Damon's face. He's scared. I've seen that expression before, on an animal I'm close enough to get to know before I kill it. It's good he's scared of me. I'm going to shoot him, sure as I'm standing here, Damon is going to die. Maybe the good Lord's helping me out here. There are all kinds of ways for a man to die. Guns and bullets don't make them suffer much. Makes their families suffer, though. Yes, there might be a better way for garbage like Dr. L to die.*

Like watching someone he loves suffer.

Like watching Brandon die.

A better plan would be for him to let Damon go and follow him. If Brandon suffers, it will be worse for Damon, because he'd know it. Yes, better to let Damon see Brandon suffering. He could kill him later. That would make it two deaths for Damon. He deserved both.

Damon looked triumphant, as if he'd won a prize in a fancy contest.

The good doctor said, "You can do anything you want to me later, if you stop interfering and let me hurry to save my boy."

Travis paused again. With any luck, Damon would get his due. He loved Brandon. What if something happened to the doctor's son?

##

"Barbara. What are you doing here?"

Damon stopped short at the sight of his wife in the driveway of Brandon's home. He hadn't seen her for over a decade. She looked very well, and very scared. She had aged, but she looked as if she took care of herself with expensive clothes and a young hairstyle. He would have been angry at her obvious prosperity if he wasn't scared himself.

She didn't back down or cower when she saw him, definitely not the same person who had left him defeated years ago. Maybe she hadn't been defeated after all. Maybe he hadn't gotten her the way he'd hoped he had and certainly he was humiliated by her disgraceful end to their marriage. If Brandon didn't need him so desperately, he would have turned on his educated heels and left her standing, agonizing, no doubt, about his contempt of her, but he was too scared.

"I came to see Hallie," she replied, with control in voice. "She's Janet's daughter, you know. Mark's in love with her."

"I haven't the time for women's gossip, my dear ex-wife," he said with a sputter, putting extra emphasis on the "ex".

She watched him with no emotion. "It doesn't work anymore, Damon. Save your hysterics for your patients. There are people and things in life far more important than you are, and right now we have one mountain of a problem." She better change the subject, if she was going to keep Damon under control. She, Millie, and Craig had debated long into the night if they should bring Damon into the mix. Finally, Craig, despite his intense worries about the consequences of such an idea, suggested that they should contact him. Millie had volunteered to be the one to make the call, having the least amount of years to have had to put up with Damon's dangerous pride.

"Have you heard about Brandon?" Damon blurted out. "He has shingles that has affected his vision."

Barbara watched him carefully, trying to judge how off-the-wall he was going to become if they gave him an opportunity to be of any real help. "Yes, I have heard. I saw for myself when I got here. Craig is helping us."

"Craig," Damon said, with a snarl. "Why are you asking him? I'm the doctor."

"But he knows how to keep his senses in working order when dealing with an emergency."

Damon smirked. "Big shot. Could he get these?" He reached into his pocket and pulled out the Famvir® he had to sell his soul to get. "I am the only one who is smart enough and successful enough to save the day and my child. I have spent my life doing and helping, and when I called in the favor, this is what I got in return." He waved the drugs over his head. "Salvation. Yes, do you hear me, Barbara, salvation. I am the only one who can help my boy."

He was going to be a big problem, she could see that. He hadn't changed in any way. He still thought the earth turned on its axis because of him.

"I don't want to deal with Craig or Millie. You tell me what happened," Damon said, ordering her to comply with a look on his face she had hoped to never see again. How had she stayed with him for all those years, seeing the hate and control in his eyes, being victimized by the tools of his murderous trade?

Brandon was the answer. She stayed with Damon to protect her child. What would have happened to a child of a doctor on Divorced Dad Weekends? How many more pills would he have been given instead of lunch?

She sighed and steeled herself for the questioning session. "He hadn't been feeling well, and then he developed a lesion on his nose and then the irritation seemed to spread to his eyes."

She waited.

"And?" he prompted with contempt.

"You're the doctor, Damon. You tell us."

He exploded in a shower of obscenities, which surprised her. He must be scared, that was the only explanation for him to resort to primitive expressions of frustration. He must fear his knowledge wouldn't be enough.

Of course, she knew something else would be eating at him at a level of his subconscious mind that even he wouldn't admit existed.

He was being consumed by guilt. Even a man as egocentric as Damon would see the cause and effect of the varicella vaccination and the increased incidence rate of shingles. Even a man as conceited as her ex-husband would have at least heard of Craig's highly published and publicized articles, including research of others that corroborated Craig's preliminary findings. Even a doctor unwilling to admit his mistakes, as Damon had always been, would have had to have been influenced by the turn-around by the medical profession to recognize the research once it had been made public, despite vicious attempts to suppress it.

"Maybe it isn't shingles. Did you ever think about that possibility, Barbara? Who gave any of you the right to make a medical diagnosis?"

Barbara felt the anger of revulsion rise in the bile creeping into her throat. "Craig had the local doctor send a sample scraping from the vesicle on his nose as well as a blood sample to the National VZV Laboratory in Atlanta, Georgia for analysis. The scraping came back positive for shingles, or herpes-zoster as you would diagnose it and the blood showed a three times increase in the VZV titer. We only called you because the local pharmacy in Sycamore Springs and those in the surrounding region were closed on Sunday and during the holidays that followed and we had hoped you would be able to start Brandon on some antiviral right away. We knew this medication would be most effective within 24 to 48 hours after the initial onset of the rash or even after up to four or five days."

The sound of her voice must have alerted the people in the house that something was wrong, that Damon was taking control. She had to keep her temper in check. She couldn't drive him away. He had a thread of hope in his hands.

The front door made a scraping sound as it opened into the foyer. Barbara had heard it countless times as she'd watched Mark dashing in and out with his friends. She remembered the times Brandon followed watching his son with pride, standing behind Millie, towering over her as they shared a worried look for their offspring. She herself glowed with proud family loyalty as she watched them, but Damon had never been part of their union, and he turned with a stare at the sound of the front door opening.

The first person to emerge was Millie, and her appearance further startled Damon. He jumped back and then moved cautiously forward. Barbara knew that Millie had seen Damon a few months before in her office, when she had made one last plea to him to at least consider her father's findings, and he'd refused with intense vehemence. Because of their near brawl, to hear how the gossip put it, Damon had left in his characteristic show of false pride without attending the dinner Millie and Brandon had planned in hopes of family unity.

"Is that you, Millie? I never would have recognized you. How could you have gotten so old in a few months?" She looked older than Barbara, a fact that startled and surprised him. At their last meeting, she said she would hold him accountable for what he did after he refused to publicly concede that Craig and other researchers that followed had been right. He remembered he'd been blinded by such hate for her and her father that he had dodged traffic getting back to his car instead of waiting his turn.

The women before him now looked haggard and sick from fear and worry. He'd seen that look countless times on the faces of his patients, but he had ignored them, every one. What difference did the emotional impact of illness make? He dealt only with the physical, and he dealt with it very well. Just to be sure he had the upper hand, he patted his pocket to confirm the medication was still there.

He turned his attention back to the people emerging from the house. Millie had one arm around Brandon to steady him. Brandon touched the door uncertainly as he tapped his foot on the planks of the front porch obviously hoping for a secure spot over the threshold to step without falling.

"I've got you," Millie said quietly, but Damon still heard her. Was she talking to a child? What nerve she had. Certainly Brandon didn't put up with this behavior all the time, did he? Once he was better, he'd make sure they had another father-son talk about not letting one's wife take the lead in matters.

Brandon wore sunglasses and a sweater even in the afternoon heat. He was thinner than he should have been, probably due to Millie's career keeping her out of the kitchen. His pants were baggy, and he wore loafers without any socks, as if he were using them for slippers, possibly for sure footing. The pain during the past week had been unbearable, no amount of prescription drugs even touched it. He was exhausted all the time and had almost completely lost his appetite.

He noticed one thing right away, based on his years of experience as a renowned doctor of medicine. His boy was quite ill. He could make that diagnosis from yards away.

Damon ran toward them, pulling the famciclovir drug of salvation from his pocket. "Brandon, you don't have anything to worry about. I'm here now, and I have these." He held the drugs out in front of him, but Brandon didn't seem to look in the right direction to see what his father had brought for him. Those fools. Had the antiviral arrived soon enough to be effective? Had they waited too long to diagnose the problem and call him? Now, he'd have to devise a full recovery plan, but he wasn't worried. Medical science could fix practically anything if the patient knew the right people, like him, for instance.

"This is all your fault," Damon yelled at Millie. "You interfered with me from the beginning. If you had stayed out of the art of medicine, your husband would not be in the predicament he's in. You've never been a good daughter-in-law."

"It is you who upset the natural balance of immunity in the community with your Injection Day mentality." Millie blanched. Was Damon insane? Couldn't he see that the present situation had everything to do with him? It was Brandon's tragedy. True, it may have been prevented by avoiding Injection Day and keeping chickenpox endemic in the community, but that was in the past, and now all attention had to be drawn to her husband to try to help him.

"Today, Damon, unbelievable as it may sound, is likely the first time in your life that even you will have to admit the subject is not Damon Leviticus, M.D. It is Brandon Leviticus, victim, son of a man with no conscience."

Damon paused and stared at her with an expression Millie could only describe as contempt.

"Is that how you see me, Mrs. Manchester-Leviticus?" he asked evenly.

"I can see through you for the liar and murderer you are. Did you think you could hide what you've done by running away? We all know why you had to rent a car to drive yourself to Travis' old motel. It's because there isn't a person in town who was willing to meet you at the airport. It's because there isn't a home in Sycamore Springs that would take you in. You're an outcast because of your actions and beliefs that hurt us all. How do you like it now, Doctor, when it's one of your very own that is stricken because of you."

Damon waved her out of his way. "Leave my boy alone. Leave him to me. I have the answer."

She didn't budge. "Don't you understand that this is not only about your son? What about the teacher's son, and the politician's child, and the construction worker's son? Aren't they valuable? Do you think you have the only child on the planet? Certainly even you have diagnosed more serious and a greater number of shingles cases in recent years than during your entire practice. Yes, one by one the shingles epidemic is having its toll on blinding some and crippling others in the community. Would you have moved heaven and earth to help any of them? Where is your social conscience?

Damon's explosive response to Barbara's accusations sent a shiver through the neighborhood, jarring Brandon out of his illness and pain.

"Is that you, Dad?" he asked, frantically. "I asked for them to call you. I wanted you to see how you've *impaired* my vision. They were all right. Look what you've done to me," he cried out.

Damon came closer. His heart thumped alarmingly, an unusual reaction for him in the face of patient distress, but he wasn't worried. This time the patient was his boy. It was natural for him to be upset. The first thing he had to do was reassure him. Then he could get close enough to administer a loading dose of Famvir® 500mg tablets. "Don't worry, Brandon," he said as calmly as possible. I've brought a miracle cure, an antiviral. I'm going to make you well."

Brandon shuddered. "No one can make me well. The local physician says I already have some damage to my cornea and if the antiviral does not keep the virus in check, I could lose all of my vision."

"He doesn't know what he's talking about," Damon said with a sputter. "He's not your father. I am. Trust me, only me."

Brandon stumbled down the front steps, pushing Millie away. She reached for him, but he eluded her grasp. "Mom, is that you? Are you here, too? Help me."

Damon shoved Barbara aside. "I'll go to him. I'm his doctor, I'm his father."

Brandon stopped and put his head in his hands, sobbing. "I can't see either of you very well. The virus is ravaging my eyes, but I can see you, Doctor, clearly with my heart. My mother was right. She warned me not to take the shot, but I had to. I wanted you to love me."

The words Damon had waited to hear ever since Brandon had run to Barbara instead of him for love. "I do love you, Brandon." Damon reached for him, to pull him into his arms for the hug he was always afraid to give him, because he knew it would not have been returned.

Brandon instantly stumbled to the side, knocking Damon's hands off him. "Don't touch me! I'm going blind, and it's because of you. You're an irresponsible murderer. You turn your family and your friends into statistics. We're nothing to you." He pushed hard against Damon's chest, forcing him backward. "You hate people." He shoved him again. "You want to hurt people because you are not human inside." Another push, holding onto his father's shirt as he forced him farther and farther away, keeping him close, pushing him away, knowing he was confused, wanting the comfort, fearing the pain. "You are my father. You should be my friend. I needed you and look what you did to me?" The final push knocked Damon over the curb, off his feet, onto the street, leaving him temporarily stunned with a superficial scrape on his elbow.

Barbara screamed.

Startled, Brandon squinted into the afternoon glare and saw a red pick-up truck barreling down the street, coming right for Damon. Nothing registered in his fogged mind for an instant, and then he saw his father holding him on his bike proudly in front of the neighborhood when he turned six years old, his father giving him one of the biggest presents he had ever seen, his father cheering him on at the fifty yard line— and suddenly he wanted Damon to live more than anything else in the world. He would have moved the mountains of Sycamore Springs stone by stone with his bare hands if that truck wouldn't hit his dad.

Brandon felt his anger replaced by the fear he felt for the safety of his parents when he was a little boy. He didn't want the car to hit his father. He didn't want Damon to die and leave him.

His father was in the path of a truck, and that was all he could see. They were part of a greater consciousness. Father and son. Both human. Above pettiness. Above all the hurt and pain that little bits of cells and souls called people could inflict on each other.

Why was the sun so hot? Why did it burn into him like a hot flame, searing his skin, burning into him the courage to see without his eyes, the bravery to act without his will. The late afternoon sun was taking the last of his vision, but the pickup truck was not going to take his father.

Brandon lunged toward Damon, pushing him out of the way, making sure he was out of the sure path of death.

He himself barely felt the impact of metal against himself. The last memory he had was the desperate touch of his father's skin on the palms of his hands, the aging fragility of his father's muscles and bones against the weight of his own body as he took his father's place in the scheme of life and death.

Damon was vaguely aware of a great commotion. He heard Barbara screaming and Craig shouting. Millie was sobbing. The pavement was hard under Damon's back, and he held his hands up to his face to see why they felt wet.

They were covered with blood.

He didn't think he'd been badly hurt. Whose blood could it be?

"Help you up, Dr. L?" a distant voice asked. It sounded like Travis. What was he doing in front of Brandon's house? Had he followed him? He felt himself hauled to his feet.

Dazed he blinked into the light. Brandon was lying in the middle of the street. He was bloody, and his neck was twisted at an unnatural angle. Damon felt the contents of his stomach lurch into his throat. That angle could only mean one thing.

Brandon was dead.

He stepped forward, his legs nearly frozen in fear. He had stepped on fragments of plastic. He looked down. The Famvir bottles with the drugs of salvation lay splintered on the asphalt.

Barbara advanced on him, battering his chest with her helpless fists. "He saved your worthless life," she barely managed to say, engulfed in shock. She crumpled to the sidewalk, inches from the shattered bottles. "It's the end of the world, Damon. The end of the world."

"No," he answered, galvanized into action. "He's got to be all right. He's young. He has everything to live for. I can get more medicine. I can revive him." He shook the lifeless body of his son. "Brandon, don't leave me. I'll help you. I'll find a way to save you. I love you."

Craig lifted Millie off Brandon, comforting her like the child she was at that moment. "He saved you, Damon. I don't know why. Men like you don't deserve salvation, especially from their victims. It's a vicious world, filled with greed and ambition, but you know what it comes down to, don't you? The sacrifice of the victim. It's always the martyrs that leave us too soon, and the villains that never know that the glory is gilded fool's gold."

Barbara moaned deep in her throat. "You killed my baby, as surely as if you had a gun. You killed my son."

“He’s my son, too. I did nothing to kill him. He was hit by a truck. It wasn’t me. It was fate.” Damon collapsed over Brandon, trying to protect him from death. “You’re telling lies, lies, lies.”

Epilogue

Dear Brandon,

It's me again, Millie. I just wanted to preserve some of my thoughts and memories of my life since you have fallen asleep in death. Had you still been alive, I would have told you that our younger son took his first steps today. I don't think he meant to do it on his own, but your mother and I were planning our move to Los Angeles, and he wanted something from across the living room. You know how impatient you've always been, and he takes after you, so he just got up, walked over and got it. Know what it was? Your picture, the one I keep by the sofa.

Your mother says he looks just like you. My parents say he's the smartest child they've ever seen, just as smart as his brother, even smarter than I am. I agree. He's just like you. Mark bought him a football, a very small football, and he loves it. He's going to play on his high school varsity team just like you did.

Mark will probably marry Hallie after they both graduate from college, but one never knows. Remember how you changed our plans that night? You were always a loving husband, which is why we have that second baby. Don't worry about him. I tell him about you every night. He knows you are asleep in the grave. When he's old enough, I'll tell him what happened, how you saved his grandfather's life, but I'll probably leave out some things, just for the sake of family pride.

No, I've never forgiven Damon. He went back to Denver, and I've heard he's gone on with his life with a new wife. Barbara was angry when she heard, saying things like he didn't deserve it. He doesn't. My father has a view of a larger consciousness, and he says that Damon will get his due.

Travis thinks he already did, watching you die, but he says it wasn't enough. I guess it's never enough.

I wanted to tell you that I got international publicity with my coverage of Craig's research. He's been published in several more medical journals. He's been interviewed as an expert on several radio shows and continues to write research articles and publish a medical journal. He was invited again to join the Spartacus Club, but he declined.

Negative trends, including violence and immorality seem to be escalating in Sycamore Springs. Students in public schools here are experiencing high stress and related physical problems—stomach aches, headaches, etc. When Billy is four, I am considering enrolling him in a nationally accredited distance learning program called Pearblossom Private School, Inc. (www.PearblossomSchool.com) which provides quality programs for kindergarten through 12th grade. The school will allow Billy to learn at his own pace and will grade tests the same day they are submitted through e-mail—thanks to my dad, Craig, who helped the school by writing this software. Craig highly recommends Pearblossom since they provides a high school diploma to those completing the requirements. I can tell already, Billy is going to be a fast learner and will probably graduate early.

Craig also enjoys teaching part time. He shared with me an illustration that will help me as I teach Billy. A certain man planted a rose and watered it faithfully and before it blossomed, he examined it. He saw the bud that would soon blossom, but noticed thorns upon the stem and he thought, "How can any beautiful flower come from a plant burdened with so many sharp thorns?" Saddened by this thought, he neglected to water the rose and it died before it could ever bloom. So it is with many people. Within each individual there is a rose. The wonderful qualities that were planted in us at birth which grow amid the thorns of our faults. Many of us look at ourselves and see only the thorns, the defects. We despair, thinking that nothing good can possibly come from us. We neglect to water the good within us, and eventually it dies. We never realize our potential. Craig went on to explain how some students do not see the rose within themselves; someone else must show it to them. One of the greatest gifts a teacher can possess is to be able to reach past the thorns and find the rose within others. If we show students the rose, they will conquer their thorns. Craig has been rewarded to see his students blossom many times over.

Life goes on in Sycamore Springs. The trees are green and the flowers bloom in profusion on the hillsides. Whenever I can, I take Billy out to the boondocks and let him run around with the freedom we once had together. He wants a puppy, and I told him he can have one as soon as he's old enough to help take care of it.

I also wanted to tell you that your life had great meaning, because you gave life to Mark and Billy, and because your sacrifice became a book. It was published along with my father's articles, and because of both of you, new vaccine-related legislation and vaccine injury compensation measures have been signed into law. Also, a regulatory commission is trying to ban the use of fluoride in water since studies have finally surfaced showing that water fluoridation did not prevent tooth decay, but instead, contributed to substantial illness. We are using a reverse osmosis water filter so that none of us receive the high toxic dose of fluoride that the water currently contains.

Billy is such a healthy child. I attribute this to my using natural birthing methods that use gravity to assist the process. Instead of using the often problematic birthing routine and practices that are disguised as standard medical practice, I found a doctor that allowed me to make my own birthing contract. Upon birth, usually within 30 seconds or so, the umbilical cord is clamped and subsequently cut. However, this procedure, called Instant Cord Clamping (ICC) or Early Cord Clamping (ECC), prevents as much as 60% of the newborn's blood volume from traveling from the placenta to the newborn (The Lippincott Manual of Nursing Practice, 7th edition, Chapter 38, J. B. Lippincott Company, Philadelphia-Toronto). This "standard" protocol, which "saves the attending physician's precious time", deprives the newborn of the volume of blood necessary to properly expand the newborn's heart and lungs. The newborn is also deprived of important enzymes, hormones, proteins, nutrients, stem cells, and iron reserves that would have otherwise transfused from the placenta to the newborn. (Reproduction, The Cycle of Life. K. Jensen. U.S. News Books. ISBN 0-89193-606-8, 1983, page 98) While the newborn appears alive and healthy, closer inspection often reveals brain damage that does not manifest itself until later years when the child starts to develop language and math skills. Further, the newborn must recover from an anemic condition (which takes up to two months to resolve) and may require resuscitation and/or blood transfusions that were all induced by the ICC/ECC procedure. The damage from ICC/ECC makes the newborn more vulnerable to infant diseases and probably predisposes ICC/ECC infants to asthma and other disorders. In this weakened state, the child may be more susceptible to serious adverse reactions to any vaccines and their adjuvants (consisting of heavy metals and other associated chemical/biological products mixed with the vaccine).

Another example of bad practice is the flat on-the-back or semi-sitting birthing position, which is the standard American protocol and certainly presents a convenient birthing position for the attending physician. Unfortunately, this position actually restricts the birth canal opening by as much as 30%, necessitating more episiotomies and C-section deliveries than a natural arched-back or squatting position that fully opens the birth canal and also takes advantage of gravity to aid delivery. (De Jonge A, Teunissen TA, Largo-Janssen AL. Supine position compared to other positions during the second stage of labor: a meta-analysis review. J. Psychosom. Obstet. Gynaelcol., 2004 Mar;25:35-45)

Well, I know how you start to get uninterested when I discuss too much science.

I think about you all the time. I remember all the amazing times we had together. One day, when we see each other again, I will tell you again about my deep love and respect for you.

Until my next letter —

Love,

Millie

THE END

Appendix I. Fifty Reasons to Oppose Fluoridation

Paul H. Connett, PhD
Professor of Chemistry
St. Lawrence University, NY 13617
Phone: +1 315 229 5853
Email: pconnett@stlawu.edu

Abstract

Water fluoridation is the practice of adding compounds containing fluoride to the water supply to produce a final concentration of fluoride of 1 part per million in an effort to prevent tooth decay. Trials first began in the U.S. in 1945, but before any of these trials were complete, the practice was endorsed by the U.S. Public Health Service in 1950. Since then fluoridation has been enthusiastically and universally promoted by U.S. health officials as being a "safe and effective" preventive for fighting tooth decay. However, even though most countries worldwide have not succumbed to America's enthusiasm for this practice, their teeth are just as good, if not better, than those countries that have. The "50 Reasons" offered in this article for opposing fluoridation are based on a thorough review of the scientific literature as regards both the risks and benefits of being exposed to the fluoride ion. Documentation is offered which indicates that the benefits of ingested fluoride have been exaggerated, while the numerous risks have been downplayed or ignored.

Keywords: water fluoridation, toxicity, criminal behavior

Introduction

This document, titled *50 Reasons to Oppose Fluoridation*, has an interesting history. In October 2000, Dr. Hardy Limeback and I were invited by Ireland's Ministry of Health and Children to present our concerns about water fluoridation to a panel called the "Fluoridation Forum." We accepted. Ireland is the only country in Europe which has mandatory fluoridation and currently over 70% of the Irish population is drinking fluoridated water.

When fluoridation opponents in Ireland heard that we had agreed to testify they were furious. They believed that this forum had been set up by the government merely to appear to deal with growing discontent about fluoridation. Opponents believed that most of the forum panel members had been hand picked to "whitewash" fluoridation, and by testifying, Dr. Limeback and I would give an illusion of legitimacy to an illegitimately established process and any product it produced.

We were in a dilemma. Although we also suspected that the opponents were correct in thinking the Forum was merely a rubber stamp for government policy, we both had a strong desire to bring the best science available to the panel. Had we chosen not to appear, proponents could have argued that there was no valid, scientific case to be made against fluoridation.

In the face of fierce opposition we proceeded to testify. In my testimony, however, I explained that many citizens felt the forum was "fixed." Then I offered the panel a challenge that could demonstrate to the Irish people and to us that the panel was truly going to perform an objective review of the issue. I presented the *50 Reasons to Oppose Fluoridation* and asked the panel to prepare a written, scientifically documented response and to make it publicly available.

Initially, the panel agreed and set up a sub-committee to do this. Forum minutes over the next year indicate several exchanges about how much progress was being made with the task. However, shortly before the forum report was completed, it was announced that the panel didn't have time to complete its answers. The cover excuse was that most of the 50 reasons were actually addressed in their 296 page report. This was blatantly untrue.

Subsequently, a group of 11 scientists, including Dr. Limeback and myself, issued a detailed critique of the forum's report which can be accessed at http://www.fluoridealert.org/ irish.forum-critique.htm

It now has been three and a half years since the *50 Reasons to Oppose Fluoridation* was presented to the Fluoridation Forum, and even though the Irish Minister of Health and Children, Mr. Michael Martin, has been questioned about this document in the Irish parliament, there still has been no formal answer to the questions. Meanwhile, citizens in other fluoridated countries (e.g.. Australia, Canada, New Zealand and United States) have asked their own local, state and federal health officials to respond to the "50 Reasons" document – also to no avail.

The 50 Reasons (updated April 12, 2004)

1) Fluoride is not an essential nutrient (NRC 1993 and IOM 1997). No disease has ever been linked to a fluoride deficiency. Humans can have perfectly good teeth without fluoride.

2) Fluoridation is not necessary. Most Western European countries are not fluoridated and have experienced the same decline in dental decay as the US (See data from World Health Organization in Table 1, and the time trends presented graphically at http://www.fluoridealert.org/who-dmft.htm). The reasons given by countries for not fluoridating are presented in Table 2.

3) Fluoridation's role in the decline of tooth decay is in serious doubt. The largest survey ever conducted in the US (over 39,000 children from 84 communities) by the National Institute of Dental Research (NIDR) showed little difference in tooth decay among children in fluoridated and non-fluoridated communities (Hileman 1989). According to NIDR researchers, the study found an average difference of only 0.6 decayed, missing and filled surfaces (DMFS) in the permanent teeth of children aged 5 to 17 years residing in either fluoridated or unfluoridated areas (Brunelle and Carlos 1990). This difference is less than one tooth surface! There are 128 tooth surfaces in a child's mouth. This result was not shown to be statistically significant. In a review commissioned by the Ontario government, Dr. David Locker concluded: "The magnitude of [fluoridation's] effect is not large in absolute terms, is often not statistically significant, and may not be of clinical significance" (Locker 1999).

4) Where fluoridation has been discontinued in communities from Canada, the former East Germany, Cuba and Finland, dental decay has not increased but has actually decreased (Maupome 2001; Kunzel and Fischer 1997, 2000; Kunzel 2000; and Seppa 2000).

5) There have been numerous recent reports of dental crises in U.S. cities (e.g., Boston, Cincinnati, New York City) which have been fluoridated for over 20 years. There appears to be a far greater (inverse) relationship between tooth decay and income level than with water fluoride levels.

6) Modern research (e.g., Diesendorf 1986; Colquhoun 1997; and De Liefde 1998) shows that decay rates were coming down before fluoridation was introduced and have continued to decline even after its benefits would have been maximized. Many other factors influence tooth decay. Some recent studies have found that tooth decay actually increases as the fluoride concentration in the water increases (Olsson 1979; Retief 1979; Mann 1987, 1990; Steelink 1992; Teotia 1994; Grobleri 2001; Awadia 2002; and Ekanayake 2002).

7) The Centers for Disease Control and Prevention (CDC 1999, 2001) has now acknowledged the findings of many leading dental researchers, that the mechanism of fluoride's benefits are mainly *topical* not *systemic*. Thus, you don't have to swallow fluoride to protect teeth. As the benefits of fluoride (if any exist) are topical, and the risks are systemic, it makes more sense, for those who want to take the risks, to deliver the fluoride directly to the tooth in the form of toothpaste. Since swallowing fluoride is unnecessary, there is no reason to force people (against their will) to drink fluoride in their water supply. This position was recently shared by Dr. Douglas Carnall, the associate editor of the British Medical Journal. His editorial appears in Table 3.

8) Despite being prescribed by doctors for over 50 years, the U.S. Food and Drug Administration (FDA) has never approved any fluoride supplement designed for ingestion as safe or effective. Fluoride supplements are designed to deliver the same amount of fluoride as ingested daily from fluoridated water (Kelly 2000).

9) The U.S. fluoridation program has massively failed to achieve one of its key objectives, i.e. to

lower dental decay rates while holding down dental fluorosis (mottled and discolored enamel), a condition known to be caused by fluoride. The goal of the early promoters of fluoridation was to limit dental fluorosis (in its mildest form) to 10% of children (NRC 1993, pp. 6-7). A major U.S. survey has found 30% of children in optimally fluoridated areas had dental fluorosis on at least two teeth (Heller 1997), while smaller studies have found up to 80% of children impacted (Williams 1990; Lalumandier 1995 and Morgan 1998). The York Review estimates that up to 48% of children in optimally fluoridated areas worldwide have dental fluorosis in all forms and 12.5% with symptoms of aesthetic concern (McDonagh, 2000).

10) Dental fluorosis means that a child has been overdosed on fluoride. While the mechanism by which the enamel is damaged is not definitively known, it appears fluorosis may be a result of either inhibited enzymes in the growing teeth (Dan Besten 1999), or through fluoride's interference with G-protein signaling mechanisms (Matsuo 1996). In a study in Mexico, Alarcon-Herrera (2001) has shown a linear correlation between the severity of dental fluorosis and the frequency of bone fractures in children.

11) The level of fluoride put into water (1 ppm) is up to 200 times higher than normally found in mothers' milk (0.005 – 0.01 ppm) (Ekstrand 1981; Institute of Medicine 1997). There are no benefits, only risks, for infants ingesting this heightened level of fluoride at such an early age (this is an age where susceptibility to environmental toxins is particularly high).

12) Fluoride is a cumulative poison. On average, only 50% of the fluoride we ingest each day is excreted through the kidneys. The remainder accumulates in our bones, pineal gland, and other tissues. If the kidney is damaged, fluoride accumulation will increase, and with it, the likelihood of harm.

13) Fluoride is very biologically active even at low concentrations. It interferes with hydrogen bonding (Emsley 1981) and inhibits numerous enzymes (Waldbott 1978).

14) When complexed with aluminum, fluoride interferes with G-proteins (Bigay 1985, 1987). Such interactions give aluminum-fluoride complexes the potential to interfere with many hormonal and some neurochemical signals (Strunecka and Patocka 1999; Li 2003).

15) Fluoride has been shown to be mutagenic, cause chromosome damage and interfere with the enzymes involved with DNA repair in a variety of cell and tissue studies (Tsutsui 1984; Caspary 1987; Kishi 1993; and Mihashi 1996). Recent studies have also found a correlation between fluoride exposure and chromosome damage in humans (Sheth 1994; Wu 1995; Meng 1997; and Joseph 2000).

16) Fluoride forms complexes with a large number of metal ions that include metals which are needed in the body (like calcium and magnesium) and metals (like lead and aluminum) which are toxic to the body. This can cause a variety of problems. For example, fluoride interferes with enzymes where magnesium is an important co-factor and fluoride can help facilitate the uptake of aluminum and lead into tissues where these metals would not otherwise go (Mahaffey 1976; Allain 1996; Varner 1998).

17) Rats fed for one year with 1 ppm fluoride in their water, using either sodium fluoride or aluminum fluoride, had morphological changes to their kidneys and brains, an increased uptake of aluminum in the brain, and the formation of beta amyloid deposits which are characteristic of Alzheimer's disease (Varner 1998).

18) Aluminum fluoride was recently nominated by the Environmental Protection Agency (EPA) and National Institute of Environmental Health Sciences (NIEHS) for testing by the National Toxicology Program. According to EPA and NIEHS, aluminum fluoride currently has a "high health research priority" due to its "known neurotoxicity" (BNA 2000). If fluoride is added to water which contains aluminum, then aluminum fluoride complexes will form.

19) Animal experiments show that fluoride accumulates in the brain and exposure alters mental behavior in a manner consistent with a neurotoxic agent (Mullenix 1995). Rats dosed prenatally demonstrated hyperactive behavior. Those dosed postnatally demonstrated hypoactivity (i.e., under activity or "couch potato" syndrome). More recent animal experiments have reported that fluoride can damage the brain (Wang 1997; Guan 1998; Varner 1998; Zhao 1998; Zhang 1999; Lu 2000; Shao 2000; Sun 2000; Bhatnagar 2002; Chen 2002, 2003; Long 2002; Shivarajashankara 2002a, b; Shashi 2003; and Zhai 2003) and impact learning and behavior (Paul

1998; Zhang 1999, 2001; Sun 2000; Ekambaram 2001; Bhatnagar 2002).

20) Five studies from China show a lowering of IQ in children associated with fluoride exposure (Lin Fa-Fu 1991; Li 1995; Zhao 1996; Lu 2000; and Xiang 2003a, b). One of these studies (Lin Fa-Fu 1991) indicates that even just moderate levels of fluoride exposure (e.g., 0.9 ppm in the water) can exacerbate the neurological defects of iodine deficiency.

21) Studies by Jennifer Luke (2001) showed that fluoride accumulates in the human pineal gland to very high levels. In her Ph.D. thesis Luke has also shown in animal studies that fluoride reduces melatonin production and leads to an earlier onset of puberty (Luke 1997).

22) In the first half of the 20th century, fluoride was prescribed by a number of European doctors to reduce the activity of the thyroid gland for those suffering from hyperthyroidism (over active thyroid) (Stecher 1960; Waldbott 1978). With water fluoridation, we are forcing people to drink a thyroid-depressing medication which could, in turn, serve to promote higher levels of hypothyroidism (underactive thyroid) in the population, and all the subsequent problems related to this disorder. Such problems include depression, fatigue, weight gain, muscle and joint pains, increased cholesterol levels, and heart disease.

It bears noting that according to the Department of Health and Human Services (1991) fluoride exposure in fluoridated communities is estimated to range from 1.6 to 6.6 mg/day, which is a range that actually overlaps the dose (2.3 to 4.5 mg/day) shown to decrease the functioning of the human thyroid (Galletti and Joyet 1958). This is a remarkable fact, particularly considering the rampant and increasing problem of hypothyroidism in the United States (in 1999, the second most prescribed drug of the year was Synthroid, which is a hormone replacement drug used to treat an underactive thyroid). In Russia, Bachinskii (1985) found a lowering of thyroid function, among otherwise healthy people, at 2.3 ppm fluoride in water.

23) Some of the early symptoms of skeletal fluorosis, a fluoride-induced bone and joint disease that impacts millions of people in India, China, and Africa, mimic the symptoms of arthritis (Singh 1963; Franke 1975; Teotia 1976; Carnow 1981; Czerwinski 1988; DHHS 1991). According to a review on fluoridation by *Chemical & Engineering News*, "Because some of the clinical symptoms mimic arthritis, the first two clinical phases of skeletal fluorosis could be easily misdiagnosed" (Hileman 1988). Few if any studies have been done to determine the extent of this misdiagnosis, and whether the high prevalence of arthritis in America (1 in 3 Americans have some form of arthritis - CDC, 2002) is related to our growing fluoride exposure, which is highly plausible. The causes of most forms of arthritis (e.g., osteoarthritis) are unknown.

24) In some studies, when high doses of fluoride (average 26 mg per day) were used in trials to treat patients with osteoporosis in an effort to harden their bones and reduce fracture rates, it actually led to a *higher* number of fractures, particularly hip fractures (Inkovaara 1975; Gerster 1983; Dambacher 1986; O'Duffy 1986; Hedlund 1989; Bayley 1990; Gutteridge 1990. 2002; Orcel 1990; Riggs 1990; and Schnitzler 1990). The cumulative doses used in these trials are exceeded by the lifetime cumulative doses being experienced by many people living in fluoridated communities.

25) Nineteen studies (three unpublished, including one abstract) since 1990 have examined the possible relationship of fluoride in water and hip fracture among the elderly. Eleven of these studies found an association, eight did not. One study found a dose-related increase in hip fracture as the concentration of fluoride rose from 1 ppm to 8 ppm (Li 2001). Hip fracture is a very serious issue for the elderly, as a quarter of those who have a hip fracture die within a year of the operation, while 50 percent never regain an independent existence All 19 of these studies are given at the end of the reference section).

26) The only government-sanctioned animal study to investigate whether or not fluoride causes cancer, found a dose-dependent increase in cancer in the target organ (bone) of the fluoride-treated (male) rats (NTP 1990). The initial review of this study also reported an increase in liver and oral cancers, however, all non-bone cancers were later downgraded–with a questionable rationale–by a government-review panel (Marcus 1990). In light of the importance of this study, EPA Professional Headquarters Union has requested that Congress establish an independent review to examine the study's results (Hirzy 2000).

27) A review of national cancer data in the U.S. by the National Cancer Institute (NCI) revealed a significantly higher rate of bone cancer in young men in fluoridated versus unfluoridated areas (Hoover 1991). While the NCI concluded that fluoridation was not the cause, no explanation was provided to explain the higher rates in the fluoridated areas. A smaller study from New Jersey (Cohn 1992) found bone cancer rates to be up to 6 times higher in young men living in fluoridated versus unfluoridated areas. Other epidemiological studies have failed to find this relationship (Mahoney 1991; Freni 1992).

28) Fluoride administered to animals at high doses wreaks havoc on the male reproductive system - it damages sperm and increases the rate of infertility in a number of different species (Kour 1980; Chinoy 1989; Chinoy 1991; Susheela 1991; Chinoy 1994; Kumar 1994; Narayana 1994a, b; Zhao 1995; Elbetieha 2000; Ghosh 2002; and Zakrzewska 2002). While studies conducted at the FDA have failed to find reproductive effects in rats (Sprando 1996, 1997, 1998), an epidemiological study from the U.S. has found increased rates of infertility among couples living in areas with 3 or more ppm fluoride in the water (Freni 1994), and 2 studies have found a reduced level of circulating testosterone in males living in high fluoride areas (Susheela 1996 and Barot 1998).

29) The fluoridation program has been very poorly monitored. There has never been a comprehensive analysis of the fluoride levels in the bones, blood, or urine of the American people or the citizens of other fluoridated countries. Based on the sparse data that has become available, however, it is increasingly evident that some people in the population—particularly people with kidney disease—are accumulating fluoride levels that have been associated with harm to both animals and humans, particularly harm to bone (Connett 2004).

30) Once fluoride is put in the water it is impossible to control the dose each individual receives. This is because 1) some people (e.g., manual laborers, athletes, diabetics, and people with kidney disease) drink more water than others, and 2) we receive fluoride from sources other than the water supply. Other sources of fluoride include food and beverages processed with fluoridated water (Kiritsy 1996 and Heilman 1999), fluoridated dental products (Bentley 1999 and Levy 1999), mechanically deboned meat (Fein 2001), teas (Levy 1999), and pesticide residues on food (Stannard 1991 and Burgstahler 1997).

31) Fluoridation is unethical because individuals are not being asked for their informed consent prior to medication. This is standard practice for all medication, and one of the key reasons why most of western Europe has ruled against fluoridation (see Table 2).

As one doctor aptly stated, "No physician in his right senses would prescribe for a person he has never met, whose medical history he does not know, a substance which is intended to create bodily change, with the advice: 'Take as much as you like, but you will take it for the rest of your life because some children suffer from tooth decay.' It is a preposterous notion."

32) While referenda are preferential to imposed policies from central government, it still leaves the problem of individual rights versus majority rule. Put another way – does a voter have the right to require that their neighbor ingest a certain medication (even if it's against that neighbor's will)?

33) Some individuals appear to be highly sensitive to fluoride as shown by case studies and double blind studies (Shea 1967; Waldbott 1978; and Moolenburg 1987). In one study, which lasted 13 years, Feltman and Kosel (1961) showed that about 1% of patients given 1 mg of fluoride each day developed negative reactions. Can we as a society force these people to ingest fluoride?

34) According to the Agency for Toxic Substances and Disease Registry (ATSDR 1993), and other researchers (Juncos and Donadio 1972; Marier and Rose 1977; Johnson 1979), certain subsets of the population may be particularly vulnerable to fluoride's toxic effects; these include: the elderly, diabetics and people with poor kidney function. Again, can we in good conscience force these people to ingest fluoride on a daily basis for their entire lives?

35) Also vulnerable are those who suffer from malnutrition (e.g., calcium, magnesium, vitamin C, vitamin D and iodide deficiencies and protein poor diets) (Massler and Schour 1952; Marier and Rose 1977; Lin Fa-Fu 1991; Chen 1997; Teotia 1998). Those most likely to suffer from poor nutrition are the poor, who are precisely the people being targeted by new fluoridation programs. While being at heightened risk, poor families are less able to afford

avoidance measures (e.g., bottled water or removal equipment).

36) Since dental decay is most concentrated in poor communities, we should be spending our efforts trying to increase the access to dental care for poor families. The real "Oral Health Crisis" that exists today in the United States, is not a lack of fluoride but poverty and lack of dental insurance. The Surgeon General has estimated that 80% of dentists in the U.S. do not treat children on Medicaid.

37) Fluoridation has been found to be ineffective at preventing one of the most serious oral health problems facing poor children, namely, baby bottle tooth decay, otherwise known as early childhood caries (Barnes 1992 and Shiboski 2003).

38) The early studies conducted in 1945–1955 in the U.S. that helped to launch fluoridation, have been heavily criticized for their poor methodology and poor choice of control communities (De Stefano 1954; Sutton 1959, 1960 and 1996; Ziegelbecker 1970). According to Dr. Hubert Arnold, a statistician from the University of California at Davis, the early fluoridation trials "are especially rich in fallacies, improper design, invalid use of statistical methods, omissions of contrary data, and just plain muddleheadedness and hebetude." In 2000, the British Government's "York Review" could give no fluoridation trial a grade A classification – despite 50 years of research (McDonagh 2000; see Table 3 for commentary).

39) The U.S. Public Health Service first endorsed fluoridation in 1950, prior to the completion of one single trial (McClure 1970)!

40) Since 1950, it has been found that fluorides do little to prevent pit and fissure tooth decay, a fact that even the dental community has acknowledged (Seholle 1984; Gray 1987; PHS 1993; and Pinkham 1999). This is significant because pit and fissure tooth decay represents up to 85% of the tooth decay experienced by children today (Seholle 1984 and Gray 1987).

41) Despite the fact that we are exposed to far more fluoride today than we were in 1945 (when fluoridation began), the "optimal" fluoridation level is still 1 part per million, the same level deemed optimal in 1945 (Marier and Rose 1977; Levy 1999; Rozier 1999; and Fomon 2000)!

42) The chemicals used to fluoridate water in the U.S. are not pharmaceutical grade. Instead, they come from the wet scrubbing systems of the superphosphate fertilizer industry. These chemicals (90% of which are sodium fluorosilicate and fluorosilicic acid), are classified hazardous wastes contaminated with various impurities. Recent testing by the National Sanitation Foundation suggest that the levels of arsenic in these chemicals are relatively high (up to 1.6 ppb after dilution into public water) and of potential concern (NSF 2000 and Wang 2000).

43) These hazardous wastes have not been tested comprehensively. The chemical usually tested in animal studies is pharmaceutical grade sodium fluoride, not industrial grade fluorosilicic acid. The assumption being made is that by the time this waste product has been diluted, all the fluorosilicic acid will have been converted into free fluoride ion, and the other toxics and radioactive isotopes will be so dilute that they will not cause any harm, even with lifetime exposure. These assumptions have not been examined carefully by scientists, independent of the fluoridation program.

44) Studies by Masters and Coplan (1999, 2000) show an association between the use of fluorosilicic acid (and its sodium salt) to fluoridate water and an increased uptake of lead into children's blood. Because of lead's acknowledged ability to damage the child's developing brain, this is a very serious finding yet it is being largely ignored by fluoridating countries.

45) Sodium fluoride is an extremely toxic substance – just 200 mg of fluoride ion is enough to kill a young child, and just 3-5 grams (e.g., a teaspoon) is enough to kill an adult. Both children (swallowing tablets/gels) and adults (accidents involving fluoridation equipment and filters on dialysis machines) have died from excess exposure.

46) Some of the earliest opponents of fluoridation were biochemists and at least 14 Nobel Prize winners are among numerous scientists who have expressed their reservations about the practice of fluoridation (see Table 4).

47) The recent Nobel Laureate in Medicine and Physiology, Dr. Arvid Carlsson (2000), was one of the leading opponents of fluoridation in Sweden, and part of the panel that recommended that the Swedish government reject the practice, which they did in 1971. According to Carlsson: "I am quite convinced that water fluoridation, in a not-too-distant future, will be consigned to medical history...Water fluoridation goes against leading principles of

pharmacotherapy, which is progressing from a stereotyped medication – of the type 1 tablet 3 times a day – to a much more individualized therapy as regards both dosage and selection of drugs. The addition of drugs to the drinking water means exactly the opposite of an individualized therapy" (Carlsson 1978).

48) While pro-fluoridation officials continue to promote fluoridation with undiminished fervor, they cannot defend the practice in open public debate – even when challenged to do so by organizations such as the Association for Science in the Public Interest, the American College of Toxicology, or the U.S. Environmental Protection Agency (Bryson 2004). According to Dr. Michael Easley, a prominent lobbyist for fluoridation in the U.S., "Debates give the illusion that a scientific controversy exists when no credible people support the fluorophobics' view" (see Table 5).

In light of proponents' refusal to debate this issue, Dr. Edward Groth, a Senior Scientist at Consumers Union, observed that "the political profluoridation stance has evolved into a dogmatic, authoritarian, essentially antiscientific posture, one that discourages open debate of scientific issues" (Martin 1991).

49) Many scientists, doctors and dentists who have spoken out publicly on this issue have been subjected to censorship and intimidation (Martin 1991). Most recently, Dr. Phyllis Mullenix was fired from her position as Chair of Toxicology at Forsyth Dental Center for publishing her findings on fluoride and the brain; and Dr. William Marcus was fired from the EPA for questioning the government's handling of the NTP's fluoride-cancer study (Bryson 2004). Tactics like this would not be necessary if those promoting fluoridation were on secure scientific ground.

50) The Union representing the scientists at U.S. EPA headquarters in Washington DC is now on record as opposing water fluoridation (Hirzy 1999). According to the Union's Senior Vice President, Dr. William Hirzy: "In summary, we hold that fluoridation is an unreasonable risk. That is, the toxicity of fluoride is so great and the purported benefits associated with it are so small – if there are any at all – that requiring every man, woman and child in America to ingest it borders on criminal behavior on the part of governments."

Conclusion

When it comes to controversies surrounding toxic chemicals, invested interests traditionally do their very best to discount animal studies and quibble with epidemiological findings. In the past, political pressures have led government agencies to drag their feet on regulating asbestos, benzene, DDT, PCBs, tetraethyl lead, tobacco and dioxins. With fluoridation we have had a fifty year delay. Unfortunately, because government officials have put so much of their credibility on the line defending fluoridation, and because of the huge liabilities waiting in the wings if they admit that fluoridation has caused an increase in hip fracture, arthritis, bone cancer, brain disorders or thyroid problems, it will be very difficult for them to speak honestly and openly about the issue. But they must, not only to protect millions of people from unnecessary harm, but to protect the notion that, at its core, public health policy must be based on sound science, not political expediency. They have a tool with which to do this: it's called the Precautionary Principle. Simply put, this says: if in doubt leave it out. This is what most European countries have done and their children's teeth have not suffered, while their public's trust has been strengthened.

It is like a question from a Kafka play. Just how much doubt is needed on just one of the health concerns identified above, to override a benefit, which when quantified in the largest survey ever conducted in the U.S., amounts to less than one tooth surface (out of 128) in a child's mouth?

For those who would call for further studies, I say fine. Take the fluoride out of the water first and then conduct all the studies you want. This folly must end without further delay.

Postscript

Further arguments against fluoridation, can be viewed at http://www.fluoridealert.org. Arguments for fluoridation can be found at http://www.ada.org and a more systematic presentation of fluoride's toxic effects can be found at http://www.Slweb .org/bibliography.html

Acknowledgements

I would like to acknowledge the help given to

me in the research for this statement to my son Michael Connett and to Naomi Flack for the proofreading of the text. Any remaining mistakes are my own.

Table 1. World Health Organization Data: DMFT (Decayed, Missing and Filled Teeth status for 12-year-olds by country.

Country	DMFTs	Year	Water/Salt Fluoridation Status*
Australia	0.8	1998	More than 50% of water is fluoridated
Zurich, Switzerland	0.84	1998	Water is unfluoridated, but salt is fluoridated
Netherlands	0.9	1992-93	No water fluoridation or salt fluoridation
Sweden	0.9	1999	No water fluoridation or salt fluoridation
Denmark	0.9	2001	No water fluoridation or salt fluoridation
UK *(England and Wales)*	0.9	1996-97	11% of water supplies are fluoridated
Ireland	1.1	1997	More than 50% of water is fluoridated
Finland	1.1	1997	No water fluoridation or salt fluoridation
Germany	1.2	2000	No water fluoridation, but salt fluoridation is common
U.S.	1.4	1988-91	More than 50% of water is fluoridated
Norway	1.5	1998	No water fluoridation or salt fluoridation
Iceland	1.5	1996	No water fluoridation or salt fluoridation
New Zealand	1.5	1993	More than 50% of water is fluoridated
Belgium	1.6	1998	No water fluoridation, but salt fluoridation is common
Austria	1.7	1997	No water fluoridation, but salt fluoridation is common
France	1.9	1998	No water fluoridation, but salt fluoridation is common

Data from *WHO Oral Health Country/Area Profile Programme*
Department of Noncommunicable Diseases Surveillance/Oral Health WHO Collaborating Centre, Malmö University, Sweden
http://wwwWhocollab.od.mah.se/euro.html

Table 2. Statements on fluoridation by governmental officials from several countries.

Germany: "Generally, in Germany fluoridation of drinking water is forbidden. The relevant German law allows exceptions to the fluoridation ban on application. The argumentation of the Federal Ministry of Health against a general permission of fluoridation of drinking water is the problematic nature of compuls[ory] medication." (Gerda Hankel-Khan, Embassy of Federal Republic of Germany, September 16, 1999) www. fluoridealert.org/germany.jpeg

France: "Fluoride chemicals are not included in the list [of 'chemicals for drinking water treatment']. This is due to ethical as well as medical considerations." (Louis Sanchez, Directeur de la Protection de l'Environment, August 25, 2000) www. fluoridealert.org/france.jpeg

Belgium: "This water treatment has never been of use in Belgium and will never be (we hope so) into the future. The main reason for that is the fundamental position of the drinking water sector that it is not its task to deliver medicinal treatment to people. This is the sole responsibility of health services." (Chr. Legros, Directeur, Belgaqua, Brussels, Belgium, February 28, 2000) www.fluoridation.com/c-belgium.htm

Luxembourg: "Fluoride has never been added to the public water supplies in Luxembourg. In our views, the drinking water isn't the suitable way for medicinal treatment and that people needing an addition of fluoride can decide by their own to use the most appropriate way, like the intake of fluoride tablets, to cover their [daily] needs." (Jean-Marie RIES, Head, Water Department, Administration De L'Environment, May 3, 2000) www.fluoridealert.org/luxembourg.jpeg

Finland: "We do not favor or recommend fluoridation of drinking water. There are better ways of providing the fluoride our teeth need." (Paavo Poteri, Acting Managing Director, Helsinki Water, Finland, February 7, 2000) www.fluoridation.com /c-finland.htm

"Artificial fluoridation of drinking water supplies has been practiced in Finland only in one town, Kuopio, situated in eastern Finland and with a population of about 80,000 people (1.6% of the Finnish population). Fluoridation started in 1959 and finished in 1992 as a result of the resistance of local population. The most usual grounds for the resistance presented in this context were an individual's right to drinking water without additional chemicals used for the medication of limited population groups. A concept of "force-feeding" was also mentioned.

Drinking water fluoridation is not prohibited in Finland but no municipalities have turned out to be willing to practice it. Water suppliers, naturally, have always been against dosing of fluoride chemicals into water." (Leena Hiisvirta, M.Sc., Chief Engineer, Ministry of Social Affairs and Health, Finland, January 12, 1996) www.fluoridealert.org/finland .jpeg

Denmark: "We are pleased to inform you that according to the Danish Ministry of Environment and Energy, toxic fluorides have never been added to the public water supplies. Consequently, no Danish city has ever been fluoridated." (Klaus Werner, Royal Danish Embassy, Washington DC, December 22, 1999) www.fluoridation.com/c-denmark.htm

Norway: "In Norway we had a rather intense discussion on this subject some 20 years ago, and the conclusion was that drinking water should not be fluoridated." (Truls Krogh & Toril Hofshagen, Folkehelsa Statens institutt for folkeheise (National Institute of Public Health) Oslo, Norway, March 1, 2000) www.fluoridation.com/c-norway.htm

Sweden: "Drinking water fluoridation is not allowed in Sweden...New scientific documentation or changes in dental health situation that could alter the conclusions of the Commission have not been shown." (Gunnar Guzikowski, Chief Government Inspector, Livsmedels Verket – National Food Administration Drinking Water Division, Sweden, February 28, 2000) www.fluoridation.com/c-sweden.htm

Netherlands: "From the end of the 1960s until the beginning of the 1970s drinking water in various places in the Netherlands was fluoridated to prevent caries. However, in its judgment of June 22, 1973 in case No. 10683 (Budding and co. versus the City of Amsterdam) the Supreme Court (Hoge Road) ruled there was no legal basis for fluoridation. After that judgment, amendment to the Water Supply Act was prepared to provide a legal basis for fluoridation. During the process it became clear that there was not enough support from Parliament [sic] for this amendment and the proposal was withdrawn." (Wilfred Reinhold, Legal Advisor, Directorate Drinking Water, Netherlands, January 15, 2000) www.fluoridation.com/c-netherlands.htm

Northern Ireland: "The water supply in Northern Ireland has never been artificially fluoridated except in 2 small localities where fluoride was added to the water for about 30 years up to last year. Fluoridation ceased at these locations for operational reasons. At this time, there are no plans to commence fluoridation of water supplies in Northern Ireland." (C.J. Grimes, Department for Regional Development, Belfast, November 6, 2000) www.fluoridealert.org/Northern-Ireland.jpeg

Austria: "Toxic fluorides have never been added to the public water supplies in Austria." (M. Eisenhut, Head of Water Department, Osterreichische Yereinigung fur das Gas-und Wasserfach Schubertring 14, A-1015 Wien, Austria, February 17, 2000) www.fluoridation.com/c-austria.htm

Czech Republic: "Since 1993, drinking water has not been treated with fluoride in public water supplies throughout the Czech Republic. Although fluoridation of drinking water has not actually been proscribed it is not under consideration because this form of supplementation is considered as follows:

(a) uneconomical (only 0.54% of water suitable for drinking is used as such; the remainder is employed for hygiene etc. Furthermore, an increasing amount of consumers (particularly children) are using bottled water for drinking (underground water usually with fluoride)

(b) unecological (environmental load by a foreign substance)

(c) unethical ("forced medication")

(d) toxicologically and phyiologically debateable (fluoridation represents an untargeted form of supplementation which disregards actual individual intake and requirements and may lead to excessive health-threatening intake in certain population groups; [and] complexation of fluor in water into non biological active forms of fluor." (Dr. B. Havlik, Ministerstvo Zdravotnictvi Ceske Republiky, October 14, 1999) www.fluoridealert .org/czech.jpeg

Table 3. Statement of Douglas Carnall, Associate Editor of the British Medical Journal, published on the BMJ website (http://www.bmj.com) on the day that the York Review on Fluoridation was published.

British Medical Journal, October 7, 2000, Reviews, Website of the week: Water fluoridation.

Fluoridation was a controversial topic even before Kubrick's Base Commander Ripper railed against "the international communist conspiracy to sap and impurify all of our precious bodily fluids" in the 1964 film Dr Strangelove. This week's BMJ shouldn't precipitate a global holocaust, but it does seem that Base Commander Ripper may have had a point. The systematic review published this week (p 855) shows that much of the evidence for fluoridation was derived from low quality studies, that its benefits may have been overstated, and that the risk to benefit ratio for the development of the commonest side effect (dental fluorosis, or mottling of the teeth) is rather high.

Supplementary materials are available on the BMJ's website and on that of the review's authors, enhancing the validity of the conclusions through transparency of process. For example, the "frequently asked questions" page of the site explains who comprised the advisory panel and how they were chosen ("balanced to include those for and against, as well as those who are neutral"), and the site includes the minutes of their meetings. You can also pick up all 279 references in Word97 format, and tables of data in PDF. Such transparency is admirable and can only encourage rationality of debate.

Professionals who propose compulsory preventive measures for a whole population have a different weight of responsibility on their shoulders than those who respond to the requests of individuals for help. Previously neutral on the issue, I am now persuaded by the arguments that those who wish to take fluoride (like me) had better get it from toothpaste rather than the water supply (see www.derweb .co.uk/bfs/index.html and www.npwa.freeserve.co.uk/index.html for the two viewpoints).

Douglas Carnall, Associate Editor
British Medical Journal

Table 4. List of 14 Noble Prize winners who have opposed or expressed reservations about fluoridation.

1) Adolf Butenandt (Chemistry, 1939)
2) Arvid Carlsson (Medicine, 2000)
3) Hans von Euler-Chelpin (Chemistry, 1929).
4) Walter Rudolf Hess (Medicine, 1949)
5) Corneille Jean-François Heymans (Medicine, 1938)
6) Sir Cyril Norman Hinshelwood (Chemistry, 1956)
7) Joshua Lederberg (Medicine, 1958)
8) William P. Murphy (Medicine, 1934)
8) Giulio Natta (1963 Nobel Prize in Chemistry)
10) Sir Robert Robinson (Chemistry, 1947)
11) Nikolai Semenov (Chemistry, 1956)
12) James B. Sumner (Chemistry, 1946)
13) Hugo Theorell (Medicine, 1955)
14) Artturi Virtanen (Chemistry, 1945)

Table 5. Quotes on debating fluoridation from Dr. Michael Easley, Director of the National Center for Fluoridation Policy and Research, and one of the most active proponents of fluoridation in the U.S. (Easley 1999).

Easley's quotes typify the historic contempt that proponents have had to scientific debate.

"A favorite tactic of the fluorophobics is to argue for a debate so that 'the people can decide who is right.' Proponents of fluoride are often trapped into consenting to public debates."

"Debates give the illusion that a scientific controversy exists when no credible people support the fluorophobics' view."

"Like parasites, opponents steal undeserved credibility just by sharing the stage with respected scientists who are there to defend fluoridation;" and,

"Unfortunately, a most flagrant abuse of the public trust occasionally occurs when a physician or a dentist, for whatever personal reason, uses their professional standing in the community to argue against fluoridation, a clear violation of professional ethics, the principles of science and community standards of practice."

References

Agency for Toxic Substances and Disease Registry (ATSDR) (1993). Toxicological Profile for Fluorides, Hydrogen Fluoride, and Fluorine (F). U.S. Department of Health & Human Services, Public Health Service. ATSDR/TP-91/17.

Allain P, et al. (1996). Enhancement of aluminum digestive absorption by fluoride in rats. *Research Communications in Molecular Pathology and Pharmacology* 91: 225-31.

Arnold HA. (1980). Letter to Dr. Ernest Newbrun. May 28, 1980. http://www.fluoridealert.org/uc-davis.htm

Awadia AK, et al. (2002). Caries experience and caries predictors - a study of Tanzanian children consuming drinking water with different fluoride concentrations. *Clinical Oral Investigations* (2002) 6:98-103.

Bachinskii PP, et al. (1985) Action of the body fluorine of healthy persons and thyroidopathy patients on the function of hypophyseal-thyroid the system. *Probl Endokrinol* (Mosk) 31: 25-9. http://www.fluoridealert.org/epa-sf/appendix-e.pdf

Barnes GP, et al. (1992). Ethnicity, location, age, and fluoridation factors in baby bottle tooth decay and caries prevalence of Head Start children. *Public Health Reports* 107: 167-73.

Barot VV. (1998). Occurrence of endemic fluorosis in human population of North Gujarat, India: human health risk. *Bulletin of Environmental Contamination and Toxicology* 61: 303-10.

Bayley TA, et al. (1990). Fluoride-induced fractures: relation to osteogenic effect. *Journal of Bone and Mineral Research* 5(Suppl 1):S217-22.

Bentley EM, et al. (1999). Fluoride ingestion from toothpaste by young children. *British Dental Journal* 186: 460-2.

Bhatnagar M, et al. (2002). Neurotoxicity of fluoride: neurodegeneration in hippocampus of female mice. *Indian Journal of Experimental Biology* 40: 546-54.

Bigay J, et al. (1987). Fluoride complexes of aluminium or beryllium act on G-proteins as reversibly bound analogues of the gamma phosphate of GTP. *EMBO Journal* 6:2907-2913.

Bigay J, et al. (1985). Fluoroaluminates activate transducin-GDP by mimicking the gamma-phosphate of GTP in its binding site. *FEBS Letters* 191:181-185.

Brunelle JA, Carlos JP. (1990). Recent trends in dental caries in U.S. children and the effect of water fluoridation. *Journal of Dental Research* 69(Special edition): 723-727.

Bryson C. (2004). The Fluoride Deception. Seven Stories Press, New York.

Burgstahler AW, et al. (1997). Fluoride in California wines and raisins. *Fluoride* 30: 142-146.

Carlsson A. (1978). Current problems relating to the pharmacology and toxicology of fluorides. *Journal of the Swedish Medical Association* 14: 1388-1392.

Carnow BW, Conibear SA. (1981). Industrial fluorosis. *Fluoride* 14: 172-181.

Caspary WJ, et al (1987). Mutagenic activity of fluorides in mouse lymphoma cells. *Mutation Research* 187:165-80.

Centers for Disease Control and Prevention (CDC). (2002). Prevalence of Self-Reported Arthritis or Chronic Joint Symptoms Among Adults – United States, 2001. *Mortality and Morbidity Weekly Review* 51: 948-950.

Centers for Disease Control and Prevention (CDC). (2001). Recommendations for Using Fluoride to Prevent and Control Dental Caries in the United States. *Morbidity and Mortality Weekly Report* 50(RR14): 1-42.

Centers for Disease Control and Prevention (CDC). (1999). Achievements in Public Health, 1900-1999: Fluoridation of Drinking Water to Prevent Dental Caries. *Mortality and Morbidity Weekly Review* 48: 933-940.

Chen J, et al. (2003). Selective decreases of nicotinic acetylcholine receptors in PC12 cells exposed to fluoride. *Toxicology* 183: 235-42.

Chen J, et al. (2002). [Studies on DNA damage and apoptosis in rat brain induced by fluoride] *Zhonghua Yu Fang Yi Xue Za Zhi* 36(4):222-224.

Chen YC, et al. (1997). Nutrition survey in dental fluorosis-afflicted areas. *Fluoride* 30(2):77-80.

Chinoy NJ, Narayana MV. (1994). In vitro fluoride toxicity in human spermatozoa. *Reproductive Toxicology* 8:155-9.

Chinoy NJ, et al. (1991). Microdose vasal injection of sodium fluoride in the rat. *Reproductive Toxicology* 5: 505-12.

Chinoy NJ, Sequeira E. (1989). Effects of fluoride on the histoarchitecture of reproductive organs of the male mouse. *Reproductive Toxicology* 3: 261-7.

Cohn PD. (1992). A Brief Report On The Association Of Drinking Water Fluoridation And The Incidence of Osteosarcoma Among Young Males. New Jersey Department of Health Environ. Health Service: 1- 17.

Colquhoun J. (1997) Why I changed my mind about Fluoridation. *Perspectives in Biology and Medicine* 41: 29-44. http://www.fluoride-journal.com/98-31-2/312103 .htm

Connett M. (2004). Fluoride & Bone Damage: Published Data. Submission to National Research Council (NRC). http://www.fluoridealert.org/bone-data.pdf

Connett, P. (2000). Fluoride: A Statement of Concern. Waste Not #459. January 2000. Waste Not, 82 Judson Street, Canton, NY 13617. http://www.fluoridealert.org/fluoride-statement .htm

Czerwinski E, et al. (1988). Bone and joint pathology in fluoride-exposed workers. *Archives of Environmental Health* 43: 340-343.

Dambacher MA, et al. (1986). Long-term fluoride therapy of postmenopausal osteoporosis. *Bone* 7: 199-205.

De Liefde B. (1998). The decline of caries in New Zealand over the past 40 Years. *New Zealand Dental Journal* 94: 109-113.

Department of Health & Human Services. (U.S. DHHS) (1991). Review of Fluoride: Benefits and Risks. Report of the Ad Hoc Committee on Fluoride, Committee to Coordinate Environmental Health and Related Programs. Department of Health and Human Services, USA.

DenBesten, P (1999). Biological mechanism of dental fluorosis relevant to the use of fluoride supplements. *Community Dentistry and Oral Epidemiology* 27: 41-7.

De Stefano TM. (1954). The fluoridation research studies and the general practitioner. *Bulletin of Hudson County Dental Society*. February.

Diesendorf M.(1986). The mystery of declining tooth decay. *Nature.* 322: 125-129. http://www.fluoridealert.org/diesendorf .htm

Ditkoff BA, Lo Gerfo P. (2000). The Thyroid Guide. Harper-Collins. New York.

Easley, M. (1999). Community fluoridation in America: the unprincipled opposition. Unpublished.

Ekambaram P, Paul V. (2001). Calcium preventing locomotor behavioral and dental toxicities of fluoride by decreasing serum fluoride level in rats. *Environmental Toxicology and Pharmacology* 9(4):141-146.

Ekanayake L, Van Der Hoek W. (2002). Dental caries and developmental defects of enamel in relation to fluoride levels in drinking water in an arid area of sri lanka. *Caries Research* 36: 398-404.

Ekstrand J, et al. (1981). No evidence of transfer of fluoride from plasma to breast milk. *British Medical Journal* (Clin Res Ed). 283: 761-2.

Elbetieha A, et al. (2000). Fertility effects of sodium fluoride in male mice. *Fluoride* 33: 128-134.

Emsley J, et al (1981). An unexpectedly strong hydrogen bond: ab initio calculations and spectroscopic studies of amide-fluoride systems. *Journal of the American Chemical Society* 103: 24-28.

Fein NJ, Cerklewski FL. (2001). Fluoride content of foods made with mechanically separated chicken. *Journal of Agricultural Food Chemistry* 49(9):4284-6.

Feltman R, Kosel G. (1961). Prenatal and postnatal ingestion of fluorides - Fourteen years of investigation - Final report. *Journal of Dental Medicine* 16: 190-99.

Fomon SJ, et al. (2000). Fluoride intake and prevalence of dental fluorosis: trends in fluoride intake with special attention to infants. *Journal of Public Health Dentistry* 60: 131-9.

Franke J, et al. (1975). Industrial fluorosis. *Fluoride* 8: 61-83.

Freni SC. (1994). Exposure to high fluoride concentrations in drinking water is associated with decreased birth rates. *Journal of Toxicology and Environmental Health* 42: 109-121.

Freni SC, Gaylor DW. (1992). International trends in the incidence of bone cancer are not related to drinking water fluoridation. *Cancer* 70: 611-8.

Galletti P, Joyet G. (1958). Effect of fluorine on thyroidal iodine metabolism in hyperthyroidism. *Journal of Clinical Endocrinology* 18: 1102-1110. http://www.fluoridealert.org/galletti.htm

Gerster JC, et al. (1983). Bilateral fractures of femoral neck in patients with moderate renal failure receiving fluoride for spinal osteoporosis. *British Medical Journal* (Clin Res Ed) 287(6394):723-5.

Ghosh D, et al. (2002). Testicular toxicity in sodium fluoride treated rats: association with oxidative stress. *Reproductive Toxicolology* 16(4):385.

Gotzsche A. (1975). The Fluoride Question: Panacea or Poison? Stein and Day Publishers, New York.

Gray, AS. (1987). Fluoridation: time for a new base line? *Journal of the Canadian Dental Association* 53: 763-5.

Grobleri SR, et al. (2001). Dental fluorosis and caries experience in relation to three different drinking water fluoride levels in South Africa. *International Journal of Paediatric Dentistry* 11(5):372-9.

Guan ZZ, et al (1998). Influence of chronic fluorosis on membrane lipids in rat brain. *Neurotoxicology and Teratology* 20: 537-542.

Gutteridge DH, et al. (2002). A randomized trial of sodium fluoride (60 mg) +/- estrogen in postmenopausal osteoporotic vertebral fractures: increased vertebral fractures and peripheral bone loss with sodium fluoride; concurrent estrogen prevents peripheral loss, but not vertebral fractures. *Osteoporosis International* 13(2):158-70.

Gutteridge DH, et al. (1990). Spontaneous hip fractures in fluoride-treated patients: potential causative factors. *Journal of Bone and Mineral Research* 5 Suppl 1:S205-15.

Hanmer R. (1983). Letter to Leslie A. Russell, D.M.D, from Rebecca Hanmer, Deputy Assistant Administrator for Water, US EPA. March 30, 1983.

Hedlund LR, Gallagher JC. (1989). Increased incidence of hip fracture in osteoporotic women treated with sodium fluoride. *Journal of Bone and Mineral Research* 4: 223-5.

Heller KE, et al (1997). Dental caries and dental fluorosis at varying water fluoride concentrations. *Journal of Public Health Dentistry* 57: 136-143.

Hileman B. (1989). New studies cast doubt on fluoridation benefits. *Chemical and Engineering News* May 8. http://www .fluoridealert .org/NIDR.htm

Hileman B. (1988). Fluoridation of water: Questions about health risks and benefits remain after more than 40 years. *Chemical and Engineering News*. August 1: 26-42. http://www .fluoridealert.org/hileman.htm

Hirzy JW. (1999). Why the EPA's Headquarters Union of Scientists Opposes Fluoridation. Press release from National Treasury Employees Union. May 1. http://www .fluoridealert.org/HP-Epa.htm

Hoover RN, et al. (1991). Time trends for bone and joint cancers and osteosarcomas in the Surveillance, Epidemiology and End Results (SEER) Program. National Cancer Institute In: Review of Fluoride: Benefits and Risks Report of the Ad Hoc Committee on Fluoride of the Committee to Coordinate Environmental Health and Related Programs US Public Health Service. pp F1 -F7.

Inkovaara J, et al. (1975). Prophylactic fluoride treatment and aged bones. *British Medical Journal* 3: 73-4.

Institute of Medicine. (1997). Dietary Reference Intakes for Calcium, Phosphorus, Magnesium, Vitamin D, and Fluoride. Standing Committee on the Scientific Evaluation of Dietary Reference Intakes, Food and Nutrition Board. National Academy Press.

Johnson W, et al. (1979). Fluoridation and bone disease in renal patients. In: Johansen E, Taves DR, Olsen TO, Eds. Continuing Evaluation of the Use of Fluorides. AAAS Selected Symposium. Westview Press, Boulder, Colorado. pp. 275-293.

Joseph S, Gadhia PK. (2000). Sister chromatid exchange frequency and chromosome aberrations in residents of fluoride endemic regions of South Gujarat. *Fluoride* 33: 154-158.

Juncos LI, Donadio JV. (1972). Renal failure and fluorosis. *Journal of the American Medical Association* 222: 783-5.

Kelly JV. (2000). Letter to Senator Robert Smith, Chairman of Environment and Public Works Committee, U.S. Senate, August 14, 2000. http://www.fluoridealert.org/fda.htm

Kilborn LG, et al. (1950). Fluorosis with report of an advanced case. *Canadian Medical Association Journal* 62: 135-141.

Kiritsy MC, et al. (1996). Assessing fluoride concentrations of juices and juice-flavored drinks. *Journal of the American Dental Association* 127: 895-902.

Kishi K, Ishida T. (1993). Clastogenic activity of sodium fluoride in great ape cells. *Mutation Research* 301:183-8.

Kour K, Singh J. (1980). Histological finding of mice testes following fluoride ingestion. *Fluoride* 13: 160-162.

Kumar A, Susheela AK. (1994). Ultrastructural studies of spermiogenesis in rabbit exposed to chronic fluoride toxicity. *International Journal of Fertility and Menopausal Studies* 39:164-71.

Kumar JV, Green EL. (1998). Recommendations for fluoride use in children. *NY State Dental Journal* 64: 40-7.

Kunzel W, Fischer T. (2000). Caries prevalence after cessation of water fluoridation in La Salud, Cuba. *Caries Research* 34: 20-5.

Kunzel W, et al. (2000). Decline in caries prevalence after the cessation of water fluoridation in former East Germany. *Community Dentistry and Oral Epidemiology* 28: 382-389.

Kunzel W, Fischer T. (1997). Rise and fall of caries prevalence in German towns with different F concentrations in drinking water. *Caries Research* 31: 166-73.

Lalumandier JA, et al. (1995). The prevalence and risk factors of fluorosis among patients in a pediatric dental practice. *Pediatric Dentistry* 17: 19-25.

Levy SM, Guha-Chowdhury N. (1999). Total fluoride intake and implications for dietary fluoride supplementation. *Journal of Public Health Dentistry* 59: 211-23.

Li L. (2003). The biochemistry and physiology of metallic fluoride: action, mechanism, and implications. *Critical Reviews of Oral Biology and Medicine* 14: 100-14.

Li XS. (1995). Effect of fluoride exposure on intelligence in children. *Fluoride* 28: 189-192.

Lin FF, et al. (1991). The relationship of a low-iodine and high-fluoride environment to subclinical cretinism in Xinjiang. *Iodine Deficiency Disorder Newsletter.* Vol. 7. No. 3. http://www.fluoridealert.org/IDD.htm

Locker D. (1999). Benefits and Risks of Water Fluoridation. An Update of the 1996 Federal-Provincial Sub-committee Report. Prepared for Ontario Ministry of Health and Long Term Care.

Long YG, et al. (2002). Chronic fluoride toxicity decreases the number of nicotinic acetylcholine receptors in rat brain. *Neurotoxicology and Teratology* 24: 751-7.

Lu XH, et al. (2000). Study of the mechanism of neurone apoptosis in rats from the chronic fluorosis. *Chinese Journal of Epidemiology* 19: 96-98.

Luke J. (2001). Fluoride deposition in the aged human pineal gland. *Caries Research* 35: 125-128.

Luke J. (1997). The Effect of Fluoride on the Physiology of the Pineal Gland. Ph.D. Thesis. University of Surrey, Guildord.

Mahaffey KR, Stone CL. (1976).. Effect of High Fluorine (F) Intake on Tissue Lead (Pb) Concentrations. *Federation Proceedings* 35: 256.

Mahoney MC, et al. (1991). Bone cancer incidence rates in New York State: time trends and fluoridated drinking water. *American Journal of Public Health* 81: 475-9.

Mann J,et al. (1990). Fluorosis and dental caries in 6-8-year-old children in a 5 ppm fluoride area. *Community Dentistry and Oral Epidemiology* 18: 77-9.

Mann J, et al. (1987). Fluorosis and caries prevalence in a community drinking above-optimal fluoridated water. *Community Dentistry and Oral Epidemiology* 15: 293-5.

Marcus W. (1990). Memorandum from Dr. William Marcus, to Alan B. Hais, Acting Director Criteria & Standards Division ODW, US EPA. May 1, 1990. http://www.fluoridealert .org/marcus.htm

Martin B. (1991). Scientific Knowledge in Controversy: The Social Dynamics of the Fluoridation Debate. SUNY Press, Albany NY.

Massler M, Schour I. (1952). Relation of endemic dental fluorosis to malnutrition. *Journal of the American Dental Association* 44: 156-165.

Masters R, et al. (2000). Association of silicofluoride treated water with elevated blood lead. *Neurotoxicology* 21: 1091-1099.

Masters RD, Coplan M. (1999). Water treatment with silicofluorides and lead toxicity. *International Journal of Environmental Studies* 56: 435-449.

Matsuo S, et al. (1998). Mechanism of toxic action of fluoride in dental fluorosis: whether trimeric G proteins participate in the disturbance of intracellular transport of secretory ameloblast exposed to fluoride. *Archives of Toxicology* 72: 798-806.

Maupome G, et al. (2001). Patterns of dental caries following the cessation of water fluoridation. *Community Dentistry and Oral Epidemiology* 29: 37-47.

McClure F. (1970). Water fluoridation, the search and the victory. US Department of Health, Education, and Welfare, Washington DC.

McDonagh M, et al. (2000). A Systematic Review of Public Water Fluoridation. NHS Center for Reviews and Dissemination,. University of York, September 2000. http://www .fluoridealert.org/york.htm

Meng Z, Zhang B. (1997). Chromosomal aberrations and micronuclei in lymphocytes of workers at a phosphate fertilizer factory. *Mutation Research* 393: 283-288.

Mihashi,M. and Tsutsui,T.(1996). Clastogenic activity of sodium fluoride to rat vertebral body-derived cells in culture. *Mutation Research* 368: 7-13.

Moolenburgh H. (1987). Fluoride: The Freedom Fight. Mainstream Publishing, Edinburgh.

Morgan L, et al. (1998). Investigation of the possible associations between fluorosis, fluoride exposure, and childhood behavior problems. *Pediatric Dentistry* 20: 244-252.

Mullenix P, et al. (1995). Neurotoxicity of sodium fluoride in rats. *Neurotoxicology and Teratology* 17: 169-177.

Narayana MV, et al. (1994). Reversible effects of sodium fluoride ingestion on spermatozoa of the rat. *International Journal of Fertility and Menopausal Studies* 39: 337-46.

Narayana MV, Chinoy NJ. (1994). Effect of fluoride on rat testicular steroidogenesis. *Fluoride* 27: 7-12.

National Research Council. (1993). Health Effects of Ingested Fluoride. National Academy Press, Washington DC.

National Sanitation Foundation International (NSF). (2000) Letter from Stan Hazan, General Manager, NSF Drinking Water Additives Certification Program, to Ken Calvert, Chairman, Subcommittee on Energy and the Environment, Committee on Science, US House of Representatives. July 7. http://www.keepersofthewell.org/product_pdfs/NSF_respons e.pdf

National Toxicology Program [NTP] (1990). Toxicology and Carcinogenesis Studies of Sodium Fluoride in F344/N Rats and B6C3f1 Mice. Technical report Series No. 393. NIH Publ. No 91-2848. National Institute of Environmental Health Sciences, Research Triangle Park, N.C. The results of this study are summarized in the Department of Health and Human Services report (DHHS,1991) op cit.

O'Duffy JD, et al. (1986). Mechanism of acute lower extremity pain syndrome in fluoride-treated osteoporotic patients. *American Journal of Medicine* 80: 561-6.

Olsson B. (1979). Dental findings in high-fluoride areas in Ethiopia. *Community Dentistry and Oral Epidemiology* 7: 51-6.

Orcel P, et al. (1990). Stress fractures of the lower limbs in osteoporotic patients treated with fluoride. *Journal of Bone and Mineral Research* 5(Suppl 1): S191-4.

Paul V, et al. (1998). Effects of sodium fluoride on locomotor behavior and a few biochemical parameters in rats. *Environmental Toxicology and Pharmacology* 6: 187–191.

Pinkham, JR, ed. (1999). Pediatric Dentistry Infancy Through Adolescence. 3rd Edition. WB Saunders Co, Philadelphia.

Public Health Service (PHS). (1993). Toward improving the oral health of Americans: an overview of oral health status, resources, and care delivery. *Public Health Reports* 108: 657-72.

Retief DH, et al. (1979). Relationships among fluoride concentration in enamel, degree of fluorosis and caries

incidence in a community residing in a high fluoride area. *Journal of Oral Pathology* 8: 224-36.
Riggs BL, et al. (1990). Effect of Fluoride treatment on the Fracture Rates in Postmenopausal Women with Osteoporosis. *New England Journal of Medicine* 322: 802-809.
Rozier RG. (1999). The prevalence and severity of enamel fluorosis in North American children. *Journal of Public Health Dentistry* 59: 239-46.
Schnitzler CM, et al. (1990). Bone fragility of the peripheral skeleton during fluoride therapy for osteoporosis. *Clinical Orthopaedics* (261): 268-75.
Seholle RH. (1984). Preserving the perfect tooth (editorial). *Journal of the American Dental Association* 108: 448.
Seppa L, et al. (2000). Caries trends 1992-98 in two low-fluoride Finnish towns formerly with and without fluoride. *Caries Research* 34: 462-8.
Shao Q, et al. (2000). [Influence of free radical inducer on the level of oxidative stress in brain of rats with fluorosis*]. Zhonghua Yu Fang Yi Xue Za Zhi* 34(6):330-2.
Shashi A. (2003). Histopathological investigation of fluoride-induced neurotoxicity in rabbits. *Fluoride* 36: 95-105.
Shea JJ, et al. (1967). Allergy to fluoride. *Annals of Allergy* 25:388-91.
Sheth FJ, et al. (1994). Sister chromatid exchanges: A study in fluorotic individuals of North Gujurat. *Fluoride* 27: 215-219.
Shiboski CH, et al. (2003). The association of early childhood caries and race/ethnicity among California preschool children. *Journal of Public Health Dentistry* 63:38-46.
Shivarajashankara YM , et al. (2002). Brain lipid peroxidation and antioxidant systems of young rats in chronic fluoride intoxication. *Fluoride* 35: 197-203.
Shivarajashankara YM , et al. (2002). Histological changes in the brain of young fluoride-intoxicated rats. *Fluoride* 35: 12-21.
Singh A, Jolly SS. (1970). Fluorides and Human Health. World Health Organization. pp 239-240.
Singh A, et al. (1963). Endemic fluorosis: epidemiological, clinical and biochemical study of chronic fluoride intoxication in Punjab. *Medicine* 42: 229-246.
Sprando RL, et al. (1998). Testing the potential of sodium fluoride to affect spermatogenesis: a morphometric study. *Food and Chemical Toxicology* 36: 1117-24.
Sprando RL, et al. (1997). Testing the potential of sodium fluoride to affect spermatogenesis in the rat. *Food and Chemical Toxicology* 35: 881-90.
Sprando RL, et al. (1996). Effect of intratesticular injection of sodium fluoride on spermatogenesis. *Food and Chemical Toxicology* 34: 377-84.
Stannard JG, et al. (1991). Fluoride Levels and Fluoride Contamination of Fruit Juices. *Journal of Clinical Pediatric Dentistry* 16: 38-40.
Stecher P, et al. (1960). The Merck Index of Chemicals and Drugs. Merck & Co., Inc, Rathway NJ. p. 952
Steelink C. (1992). Fluoridation controversy. *Chemical & Engineering News* (Letter). July 27: 2-3.
Strunecka A, Patocka J. (1999). Pharmacological and toxicological effects of aluminofluoride complexes. *Fluoride* 32: 230-242.
Sun ZR, et al. (2000). Effects of high fluoride drinking water on the cerebral functions of mice. *Chinese Journal of Epidemiology* 19: 262-263.
Susheela AK. (1993). Prevalence of endemic fluorosis with gastrointestinal manifestations in people living in some North-Indian villages. *Fluoride* 26: 97-104.
Susheela AK, Kumar A. (1991). A study of the effect of high concentrations of fluoride on the reproductive organs of male rabbits, using light and scanning electron microscopy. *Journal of Reproductive Fertility* 92: 353-60.
Sutton P. (1996). The Greatest Fraud: Fluoridation. Lorne, Australia: Kurunda Pty, Ltd.
Sutton P. (1960) Fluoridation: Errors and Omissions in Experimental Trials. Melbourne University Press. Second Edition.
Sutton, P. (1959). Fluoridation: Errors and Omissions in Experimental Trials. Melbourne University Press. First Edition.
Teotia M, et al. (1998). Endemic chronic fluoride toxicity and dietary calcium deficiency interaction syndromes of metabolic bone disease and deformities in India: year 2000. *Indian Journal of Pediatrics* 65: 371-81.
Teotia SPS, Teotia M. (1994). Dental caries: a disorder of high fluoride and low dietary calcium interactions (30 years of personal research). *Fluoride* 27: 59-66.
Teotia SPS, et al. (1976). Symposium on the non-skeletal phase of chronic fluorosis: The Joints. *Fluoride* 9: 19-24.
Tsutsui T, Suzuki N, Ohmori M, Maizumi H. (1984). Cytotoxicity, chromosome aberrations and unscheduled DNA synthesis in cultured human diploid fibroblasts induced by sodium fluoride. *Mutation Research* 139:193-8.
Waldbott GL, et al. (1978). Fluoridation: The Great Dilemma. Coronado Press, Inc., Lawrence, Kansas.
Waldbott GL. (1965). A Battle with Titans. Carlton Press, NY.
Wang C, et al. (2000). Treatment Chemicals contribute to Arsenic Levels. Opflow (a journal of the American Water Works Association). October 2000.
Wang Y, et al. (1997). [Changes of coenzyme Q content in brain tissues of rats with fluorosis]. *Zhonghua Yu Fang Yi Xue Za Zhi* 31: 330-3.
WHO (Online). WHO Oral Health Country/Area Profile Programme. Department of Noncommunicable Diseases Surveillance/Oral Health. WHO Collaborating Centre, Malmö University, Sweden. http://www.whocollab.od.mah.se/euro .html
Williams JE, et al. (1990). Community water fluoride levels, preschool dietary patterns, and the occurrence of fluoride enamel opacities. *Journal of Public Health Dentistry* 50: 276-81.
Wu DQ, Wu Y. (1995). Micronucleus and sister chromatid exchange frequency in endemic fluorosis. *Fluoride* 28: 125-127.
Xiang Q, et al. (2003a). Effect of fluoride in drinking water on children's intelligence. *Fluoride* 36: 84-94.
Xiang Q. (2003b). Blood lead of children in Wamiao-Xinhuai intelligence study. *Fluoride* 36: 138.
Zakrzewska H, et al. (2002). In vitro influence of sodium fluoride on ram semen quality and enzyme activities. *Fluoride* 35: 153-160.
Zhang Z, et al. (2001). [Effects of selenium on the damage of learning-memory ability of mice induced by fluoride]. *Wei Sheng Yan Jiu* 30: 144-6.
Zhang Z, et al. (1999). [Effect of fluoride exposure on synaptic structure of brain areas related to learning-memory in mice] [Article in Chinese]. *Wei Sheng Yan Jiu* 28:210-2.

Zhao ZL, et al. (1995). The influence of fluoride on the content of testosterone and cholesterol in rat. *Fluoride* 28: 128-130.

Ziegelbecker R. (1970). A critical review on the fluorine caries problem. *Fluoride* 3: 71-79.

Zhai JX, et al. (2003). [Studies on fluoride concentration and cholinesterase activity in rat hippocampus]. *Zhonghua Lao Dong Wei Sheng Zhi Ye Bing Za Zhi* 21: 102-4.

Zhao XL, Wu JH. (1998). Actions of sodium fluoride on acetylcholinesterase activities in rats. *Biomedical and Environmental Sciences* 11: 1-6

Zhao LB, et al (1996). Effect of high-fluoride water supply on children's intelligence. *Fluoride* 29: 190-192.

References to 19 studies that consider possible association of hip fracture and fluoridated-water

Studies reporting an association between fluoridated water (1 ppm fluoride) and hip fracture

[1a] Cooper C, et al. (1990). Water fluoride concentration and fracture of the proximal femur. *Journal of Epidemiology and Community Health;* 44:17–9.

[1b] Cooper C, et al. (1991). Water fluoridation and hip fracture. *JAMA;* 266:513–4 (letter, a reanalysis of data presented in 1990 paper).

[2] Danielson C, et al. (1992). Hip fractures and fluoridation in Utah's elderly population. *Journal of the American Medical Association;* 268:746–8.

[3] Hegmann KT, et al. (2000). The Effects of Fluoridation on Degenerative Joint Disease (DJD) and Hip Fractures. Abstract #71, of the 33rd Annual Meeting of the Society For Epidemiological research, June 15-17, 2000. Published in a Supplement of *American Journal of Epidemiology;* P. S18.

[4] Jacobsen SJ, et al. (1992). The association between water fluoridation and hip fracture among white women and men aged 65 years and older; a national ecologic study. *Annals of Epidemiology;* 2:617–26.

[5] Jacobsen SJ, et al. (1990). Regional variation in the incidence of hip fracture: US white women aged 65 years and olders. *JAMA;* 264(4):500-2.

[6a] Jacqmin-Gadda H, et al. (1995). Fluorine concentration in drinking water and fractures in the elderly. *JAMA;* 273:775–6 (letter).

[6b] Jacqmin-Gadda H, et al. (1998). Risk factors for fractures in the elderly. *Epidemiology;* 9(4):417–23. (An elaboration of the 1995 study referred to in the JAMA letter).

[7] Keller C. (1991) Fluorides in drinking water. Unpublished results. Discussed in Gordon, S.L. and Corbin, S.B,(1992) Summary of Workshop on Drinking Water Fluoride Influence on Hip Fracture on Bone Health. *Osteoporosis International;* 2:109–17.

[8] Kurttio PN, et al. (1999). Exposure to natural fluoride in well water and hip fracture: A cohort analysis in Finland. *American Journal of Epidemiology;* 150(8):817–24.

[9] May DS, Wilson MG. (1992). Hip fractures in relation to water fluoridation: an ecologic analysis. Unpublished data, discussed in Gordon SL, and Corbin SB. (1992). Summary of Workshop on Drinking Water Fluoride Influence on Hip Fracture on Bone Health. *Osteoporosis International;* 2:109–17.

Studies reporting an association between water-fluoride levels higher than fluoridated water (4 ppm+) and hip fracture

[10] Li Y, et al. (2001). Effect of long-term exposure to fluoride in drinking water on risks of bone fractures. *Journal of Bone and Mineral Research;* 16: 932–9.

[11] Sowers M, et al. (1991). A prospective study of bone mineral content and fracture in communities with differential fluoride exposure. *American Journal of Epidemiology;* 133: 649–60.

Studies reporting no association between water fluoride and hip fracture

(Note: An association was actually found between fluoride and some form of fracture – e.g., wrist and hip – in 4 out of 8 of these studies.)

[12] Cauley J, et al. (1995). Effects of fluoridated drinking water on bone mass and fractures: the study of osteoporotic fractures. *Journal of Bone and Mineral Research;* 10:1076–86.

[13] Feskanich D, et al. (1998). Use of toenail fluoride levels as an indicator for the risk of hip and forearm fractures in women. *Epidemiology;* 9:412–6. Note: While this study didn't find an association between water fluoride and hip fracture, it did find an association – albeit non-significant 1.6 (0.8-3.1) – between fluoride exposure and elevated rates of forearm fracture.

[14] Hillier S, et al. (2000). Fluoride in drinking water and risk of hip fracture in the UK: a case control study. *The Lancet*; 335:265–9.

[15] Jacobsen SJ, et al. (1993). Hip Fracture Incidence Before and After the Fluoridation of the Public Water Supply, Rochester, Minnesota. *American Journal of Public Health;* 83:743–5.

[16] Karagas MR, et al. (1996). Patterns of Fracture among the United States Elderly: Geographic and Fluoride Effects. *Annals of Epidemiology;* 6:209–16. Note: As with Feskanich (1998) this study didn't find an association between fluoridation and hip fracture, but it did find an association between

fluoridation and distal forearm fracture, as well as proximal humerus fracture. "Independent of geographic effects, men in fluoridated areas had modestly higher rates of fractures of the distal forearm and proximal humerus than did men in nonfluoridated areas."

[17] Lehmann R, et al. (1998). Drinking Water Fluoridation: Bone Mineral Density and Hip Fracture Incidence. *Bone;* 22:273–8.

[18] Phipps KR, et al. (2000). Community water fluoridation, bone mineral density and fractures: prospective study of effects in older women. *British Medical Journal;* 321:860–4. Note: As with Feskanich (1998) and Karagas (1996), this study didn't find an association between water fluoride and hip fracture, but it did find an association between water fluoride and other types of fracture - in this case, wrist fracture. "There was a non-significant trend toward an increased risk of wrist fracture."

[19] Suarez-Almazor M, et al. (1993). The fluoridation of drinking water and hip fracture hospitalization rates in two Canadian communities. *American Journal of Public Health;* 83:689–93. Note: While the authors of this study conclude there is no association between fluoridation and hip fracture, their own data reveals a statistically significant increase in hip fracture for men living in the fluoridated area. According to the authors, "although a statistically significant increase in the risk of hip fracture was observed among Edmonton men, this increase was relatively small (RR=1.12)."

Appendix II. Summary of Highlights of the Simpsonwood Meeting

June 7-8, 2000
Simpsonwood Retreat Center
Norcross, Georgia

Abstract

A meeting was convened by the Centers for Disease Control and Prevention (CDC) to discuss the findings of Dr. Thomas Verstraeten relating to the positive statistical association between Thimerosal-containing vaccines and neurodevelopmental disorders. There were 51 scientists and physicians in attendance, including Dr. Howe of Smith-Kline Beecham, Dr. Guess of Merck, Dr. Blum of Wyeth, and Dr. White of North American Vaccine.

One of the concluding speakers, Dr. Clements on Page 247 concludes: "I am really concerned that we have taken off like a boat going down one arm of the mangrove swamp at high speed, when in fact there was not enough discussion really early on about which way the boat should go at all. ... I know how we handle it from here is extremely problematic. The ACIP (Advisory Committee on Immunization Practices) is going to depend on comments from this group in order to move forward into policy, and I have been advised that whatever I say should not move into the policy area because that is not the point of this meeting. ... But that pure science has resulted in splitting the atom or some other process which is completely beyond the power of the scientists who did the research to control it. And what we have here is people who have, for every best reason in the world, pursued a direction of research. But there is now the point at which the research results have to be handled, and even if this committee decides that there is no association and that information gets out, the work that has been done and through the freedom of information that will be taken by others, will be used in ways beyond the control of this group. And I am very concerned about that as I suspect it is already too late to do anything regardless of any professional body and what they say...."

The transcript of this meeting was finally obtained through the Freedom of Information Act, despite the fact that each page of the transcript was stamped "DO NOT COPY OR RELEASE" and "CONFIDENTIAL."

Keywords: Thimerosal, neurodevelopmental disorders, vaccines

Attendees: 51 scientists and physicians
Of special interest:
Dr. Howe: Smith-Kline Beecham;
Dr. Guess: Merck;
Dr. Blum: Wyeth;
Dr. White: North American Vaccine.

A meeting was convened by the Centers for Disease Control and Prevention (CDC) to discuss the findings of Dr. Thomas Verstraeten relating to the positive statistical association between Thimerosal-containing vaccines and neurodevelopmental disorders.

Dr. Bernier: Page 12 "In the United States there was a growing recognition that cumulative exposure [to Thimerosal in vaccines] may exceed some of the guildlines [established by regulatory agencies including the Agency for Toxic Substances and Disease Registry (ATSDR), the FDA, and the Environmental Protection Agency]."

Dr. Johnston: Page 20 "...there is absolutely no data including animal data, about the potential for synergy, additivity or antagonism, all of which can occur in binary metal mixtures that relate and allow us to draw any conclusions from the simultaneous exposure to these two salts in vaccines."

Dr. Clarkson: Page 21: "There is an issue that pharmacokinetics might be different too. Again this is all animal work, but the animal studies suggested, for example, a suckling animal does not eliminate methylmercury until the end of the suckling period, and there is a mechanism on the study for that. So there could be an age difference in the excretion rates."

Dr. Rapin: Page 22: "I don't know if anyone has looked at the literature of old Pinks disease which was present in the twenties or thirties when mothers wore shields that contained mercury." (Editorial comment: it was a teething powder that was rubbed on the baby's gums)

Dr. Weil: Page 24: "One, up until this last discussion we have been talking about chronic exposure. I think it's clear to me anyway that we are talking about a problem that is probably more related to bolus acute exposures, and we also need to know that the migration problems and some of the other developmental problems in the central nervous system go on for quite a period after birth. But from all of the other studies of toxic substances, the earlier you work with the central nervous system, the more likely you are to run into a sensitive period for one of these effects, so that moving from one month or one day of birth to six months of birth changes enormously the potential for toxicity. There are just a host of neurodevelopmental data that would suggest that we've got a serious problem. The earlier we go, the more serious the problem.

The second point I could make is that in relationship to aluminum, being a nephrologist for a long time, the potential for aluminum and central nervous system toxicity was established by dialysis data. To think there isn't some possible problem here is unreal."

Dr. Verstraeten: Page 31: " It is sort of interesting that when I first came to the CDC as a NIS officer a year ago only, I didn't really know what I wanted to do, but one of the things I knew I didn't want to do was studies that had to do with toxicology or environmental health. Because I thought it was too much confounding and it's very hard to prove anything in those studies. Now it turns out that other people also thought that this study was not the right thing to do, so what I will present to you is the study that nobody thought we should do."

Dr. Verstraeten: Page 40: "..we have found statistically significant relationships between the exposures and outcomes for these different exposures and outcomes. First, for two months of age, an unspecified developmental delay, which has its own specific ICD9 code. Exposure at three months of age, Tics. Exposure at six months of age, an attention deficit disorder. Exposure at one, three and six months of age, language and speech delays which are two separate ICD9 codes. Exposure at one, three and six months of age, the entire category of neurodevelopmental delays, which includes all of these plus a number of other disorders."

Dr. Verstraeten: Page 42: "But one thing that is for sure, there is certainly an under-ascertainment of all of these because some of the children are just not old enough to be diagnosed. So the crude incidence rates are probably much lower that what you would expect because the cohort is still very young."

Dr. Verstraten: Page 44: "Now for speech delays, which is the largest single disorder in this category of neurologic delays. The results are a suggestion of a trend with a small dip. The overall test for trend is highly statistically significant above one."

Dr. Verstraten: Page 45: "What this represents is the overall category of developmental delays, of which I have excluded speech delays because of the impression we had was some of the calculations were driven by this speech group, which was making up about half of this category. After excluding this speech group, the trend is also apparent in this group and the test for trend is also significant for this category excluding speech."

Dr. Weil: Page 75: "I think that what you are saying is in term of chronic exposure. I think that the alternative scenario is that this is repeated acute exposures, and like many repeated acute exposures, if you consider a dose of 25 micrograms on one day, then you are above threshold. At least we think you are, and then you do that over and over to a series of neurons where the toxic effect may be the same set of neurons or the same set of neurologic processes, it is conceivable that the more mercury you get, the more effect you are going to get."

Dr. Verstraeten: Page 76: "What I have done here, I am putting into the model instead of mercury, a number of antigens that the children received, and what do we get? Not surprisingly, we get very similar estimates as what we got for Thimerosal because every vaccine put in the equation has Thimerosal. So for speech and the other ones maybe it's not so significant, but for the overall group it is also significant....Here we have the same thing, but instead of number of antigens, number of shots. Just the number of vaccinations given to a child, which is also for nearly all of them significantly related."

Dr. Guess: Page 77: So this essentially is a 7% risk per antigen, in a vaccine like DPT you've got three antigens."

Dr. Verstraten: Page 77: "Correct."

Dr. Egan: Page 77: "Could you do this calculation for aluminum?"

Dr. Verstraeten: Page 77: "I did it for aluminum...Actually the results were almost identical to ethylmercury because the amount of aluminum goes along almost exactly with the mercury one."

Dr. Verstraeten: Page 78: "Then the last slide I wanted to show, there was a question concerning if there was any way from this data that we could estimate what would happen in the future if there is Thimerosal-free HepB and Thimerosal-free haemophilus influenza vaccine and only DTP has Thimerosal." Page 79 "The second column would be the same scenario but now at six months. Assuming they have received two additional DTPs, so between three and six months of age they have increased their ethylmercury amounts by 50 micrograms. If I do in this current cohort with all its limitations, because there is also the Hep B that exists in this cohort*, I can't really take it out. It is significant for this one disorder which is language delay and it is quite high. Together with that, speech or language delay which is a combination of these two disorders, also becomes significant." *Dr. Verstraeten could not determine which children got Hep B at birth in some cases so it was difficult to back the birth dose of Hep B out of the data.

Dr. Davis: Page 85: "Now in terms of a search for pre-disposing factors, this is actually going to be important in what I will talk about tomorrow, but I will mention it today and put a little seed in your mind. Which is that serious and chronic otitis media, by history being mentioned by the pediatrician or the specialist, was present 38% of the time."

Dr. Bernier: Page 113: "We have asked you to keep this information confidential. We do have a plan for discussing these data at the upcoming meeting of the Advisory Committee on Immunization Practices on June 21 and June 22. At that time CDC plans to make a public release of this information, so I think it would serve all of our interests best if we could continue to consider these data. The ACIP work group will be considering also. If we could consider these data in a certain protected environment. So we are asking people who have a great job protecting this information up until now, to continue to do that until the time of the ACIP meeting. So to basically consider this embargoed information. That would help all of us to use the machinery that we have in place for considering these data and for arriving at policy recommendations."

Dr. Brent: Page 130: "Dr. Jones brought up a suggestion when we were talking in the coffee break. The collaborative perinatal project had 50,000 parents. The registered them right from the beginning of pregnancy and then they followed them very closely. It was subsidized. Probably all of these children had DTP. Was mercury in the DTP in the fifties and sixties? Well, that is still on the computer and available to you. One of the things I have been taught about Epidemiology is repetition. In other words, if you could get another body of patients and demonstrate the same thing, it makes it more convincing."

Dr. Verstraeten: Page 131: "I would be the first person to try and analyze that. I have been asking all over if there is another data set I could look at and try to replicate it in a very oriented manner without doing another, analysis."

Dr. Brent: Page 131: "Well, it's on the eleventh floor of the Archives Building in Washington, D.C. and certainly any government employee would have access to that data"

Dr. Verstraeten: Page 131: "So what we want to avoid is multiple comparisons just for the specific outcomes that we are interested in. That's one and then at the same time at the U.K., there is another data set of General Practitioners, where we have asked them if they can replicate our findings there. So we are waiting for those results."

Dr. Verstraeten: Page 142: "But if I can have the next slide, here instead of the proportional hazard model, we did a logistic regression model. I didn't use person time here and it's a bit tough to define exactly the control group. However, if I do it for all ages and not looking at different years, and this is for speech, the outcome is almost identical to the proportional hazard model, which suggests to me that it is not a question of bringing the diagnosis forward, but it is really the overall number that drives this estimate."

Dr. Rapin: Page 143: "I would like to make a comment. We have been focusing on all these acquired causes including mercury and prematurity, and you had a list of confounding variables that should be considered in future studies. What we know today about all of the developmental disorders is that environmental factors are in fact rather unimportant in the case of these deficits and the major cause is genetic…I find it a little difficult knowing this and putting in autism. The major cause is not environmental, it is genetic and that we are focusing just on these environmental events or adventitious events when we haven't considered, and you told us that you don't have data for example on siblings, your study does not lend itself to considering the major variable."

Dr. Johnson: Page 144: "Well, I think the assumption is that those genetic predispositions would be randomly distributed".

Dr. Rapin: Page 144: "But you don't know that."

Dr. Johnson: Page 144: "No, that's an interlining assumption".

Dr. Rapin: Page 144: "I understand that, but you don't know that".

Dr. Johnson: Page 144: "Just on principle, Dr. Rapin, it seems to me that the more we learn about genetics or the more we learn about let's say autism, the more we shift towards focusing on genetic causes, but would you rule out the possibility, and let's move away from autism, that some of these are genetic predisposition and then the second hit?"

Dr. Rapin: Page 144: "Not at all. I think that it is in fact an attractive hypothesis".

Dr. Johnson: Page 145: "Right, thank you."

Dr. Chen: Page 151: "One of the reasons that led me personally to not be so quick to dismiss the findings was that on his own Tom independently picked three different outcomes that he did not could be associated with mercury and three out of three had a different pattern across different exposure levels as compared to the ones that again on a priority basis we picked as biologically plausible to be due to mercury exposure."

Dr Brent: Page 161: "Wasn't true that if you looked at the population that had 25 micrograms you had a certain risk and when you got to 75 micrograms you had a higher risk."

Dr. Verstraeten: Page 161: "Yes, absolutely, but these are all at the same time. Measured at the same age at least."

Dr. Brent: Page 161: "I understand that, but they are different exposures."

Dr. Verstraeten: Page 161: "Yes".

Dr. Brent: Page 161: "What is your explanation? What explanations would you give for that?"

Dr. Verstraeten: Page 161: "Personally, I have three hypotheses. My first hypotheses is it parental bias. The children that are more likely to be vaccinated are more likely to be picked up and diagnosed. Second hypothesis, I don't know. There is a bias that I have not recognized, and nobody has yet told me about it. Third hypothesis. It's true, it's Thimerosal. Those are my hypotheses."

Dr. Brent: Page 161: "If its true, which or what mechanisms would explain the finding with?"

Dr. Verstraeten: Page 162: "You are asking for biological plausibility?"

Dr. Brent: Page 162: "Well, yes"

Dr. Verstraeten: Page 162: "When I saw this, and I went back through the literature, I was actually stunned by what I saw because I thought it is plausible. First of all there is the Faeroe study, which I think people have dismissed too easily, and there is a new article in the same Journal that was presented here, the Journal of Pediatrics, where they have looked at PCB. They have looked at other contaminants in seafood and they have adjusted for that, and still mercury comes out. That is one point. Another point is that in many of the studies with animals, it turned out that there is quite a different result depending on the dose of mercury. Depending on the route of exposure and depending on the age at which the animals were exposed. Now, I don't know how much you can extrapolate that from animals to humans, but that tells me mercury at one month of age is not the same as mercury at three months, at 12 months, prenatal mercury, later mercury. There is a whole range of plausible outcomes from mercury. On top of that, I think that we cannot so easily compare the U.S. population to Faeroe or Seychelles populations. We have different mean levels of exposure. We are comparing high to high in the Seychelles, high to high in the Faeroe and low to low in the U.S., so I am not sure how easily you can transpose one finding to another one. So basically to me that leaves all the options open, and that means I can not exclude such a possible effect."

Dr. Brent: Page 191: "Finally, the thing that concerns me most, those who know me, I have been a pin stick in the litigation community because of the nonsense of our litigious society. This will be a resource to our very busy plaintiff attorneys in this country when this information becomes available. They don't want valid data. At that is my biased opinion.. They want business and this could potentially be a lot of business."

Dr. Koller: Page 192. "..As you increase the vaccination, you increase effects, but you don't know. You have modified live viruses. You have different antigens. There is a lot of things in those vaccinations other than mercury, and we don't know whether this is a vaccination effect or a mercury effect. But I am almost sure it is not a mercury effect. Positive as a matter of fact, and there are several experts particularly that have reviewed this, the methylmercury aspect who would agree with that due to dose response."

Dr. Johnson: Page 193: "Are you really comfortable with the way neurologic function was tested in the Seychelles?"

Dr. Koller: Page 193: "I have to admit that there were many other tests that could have been conducted.... We are talking about very subjective, very sensitive assays and yes, there could have been others done and there should be more done..."

Dr. Roger Bernier: Page 198: "...the negative findings need to be pinned down and published...other less responsible parties will treat this as a signal." In other words, Dr. Bernier is suggesting that a manuscript should be written that demonstrates no association between Thimerosal-containing vaccines and nuerodevelopmental disorders.

Dr. Johnson: Page 198: "This association leads me to favor a recommendation that infants up to two years old not be immunized with Thimerosal-containing vaccines if suitable alternative preparations are available. I do not believe the diagnosis justifies compensation in the Vaccine Compensation Program at this point. I deal with causality, it seems pretty clear to be that the data are not sufficient one way or the other. My gut feeling? It worries me enough. Forgive this personal comment, but I got called out at eight o'clock for an emergency call and my daughter-in-law delivered a son by C-Section. Our first male in the line of the next generation, and I do not want that grandson to get a Thimerosal-containing vaccine until we know better what is going on. It will probably take a long time. In the meantime, and I know there are probably implications for this internationally, but in the meantime I think I want that grandson to only be given Thimerosal-free vaccines.".

Dr. Dick Johnson: Page 199: "This association leads me to favor a recommendation that infants up to two years old not be immunized with Thimerosal-containing vaccines if suitable alternative preparations are available."

Dr. Brent: Page 205: "I personally want to congratulate Dr. Johnson on his grandson. I have a small series of 11 children all who received the Thimerosal vaccine and they are all geniuses of course. But as Dr. Rapin points out, the genetics was probably most important."

Dr. Rapin: Page 205: "My grandchildren are geniuses too, I have two."

Dr. Weil: Page 207: "The number of dose related relationships are linear and statistically significant. You can play with this all you want. They are linear. They are statistically significant. The positive relationships are those that one might expect from the Faroe Islands studies. They are also related to those data we do have on experimental animal data and similar to the neurodevelopmental tox data on other substances, so that I think you can't accept that this is out of the ordinary. It isn't out of the ordinary."

Dr. Weil: Page 208: "The rise in the frequency of neurobehavioral disorders whether it is ascertainment or real, is not too bad. It is much too graphic. We don't see that kind of genetic change in 30 years."

Dr. Brent: Page 229: "The medical/legal findings in this study, causal or not, are horrendous and therefore, it is important that the suggested epidemiological, pharmokinetic, and animal studies be performed. If an allegation was made that a child's neurobehavioral findings were caused by Thimerosal containing vaccines, you could readily find a junk scientist who would support the claim with "a reasonable degree of certainty". But you will not find a scientist with any integrity who would say the reverse with the data that is available. And that is true. So we are in a bad position from the standpoint of defending any lawsuits if they were initiated and I am concerned."

Dr. Meyers: Page 231: "Can I go back to the core issue about the research? My own concern, and a couple of your said it, there is an association between vaccines and outcome that worries both parents and pediatricians. We don't really know what that outcome is, but it is one that worries us and there is an association with vaccines. We keep jumping back to Thimerosal, but a number of us are concerned that Thimerosal may be less likely than some of the potential associations that have been made. Some of the potential associations are number of injections, number of antigens, and other additives. We mentioned aluminum and I mentioned yesterday aluminum and mercury. Antipyretics and analgesics are better utilized when vaccines are given. And then everybody mentioned all of the ones that we can't think about in this quick time period that are a part of this association, and yet all of the questions I hear we are asking have to do with Thimerosal. My concern is we need to ask the questions about the other potential associations, because we are going to the Thimerosal-free vaccine. If many of us don't think that is a plausible association because of the levels and so on, then we are missing looking for the association that may be the important one."

Dr. Caserta: Page 234: "One of the things I learned at the Aluminum Conference in Puerto Rico that was tied into the metal lines in biology and medicine that I never really understood before, is the interactive effect of different ions and different metals when they are together in the same organism. It is not the same as when they are alone, and I think it would be foolish for us not to include aluminum as part of our thinking with this."

Dr. Clements: Page 247: "I am really concerned that we have taken off like a boat going down one arm of the mangrove swamp at high speed, when in fact there was not enough discussion really early on about which way the boat should go at all. And I really want to risk offending everyone in the room by saying that perhaps this study should not have been done at all, because the outcome of it could have, to some extent, been predicted, and we have all reached this point now where we are left hanging, even though I hear the majority of consultants say to the Board that they are not convinced there is a causality direct link between Thimerosal and various neurological outcomes. I know how we handle it from here is extremely problematic. The ACIP is going to depend on comments from this group in order to move forward into policy, and I have been advised that whatever I say should not move into the policy area because that is not the point of this meeting. But nonetheless, we know from many experiences in history that the pure scientist has done research because of pure science. But that pure science has resulted in splitting the atom or some other process which is completely beyond the power of the scientists who did the research to control it. And what we have here is people who have, for every best reason in the world, pursued a direction of research. But there is now the point at which the research results have to be handled, and even if this committee decides that there is no association and that information gets out, the work that has been done and through the freedom of information that will be taken by others, will be used in ways beyond the control of this group. And I am very concerned about that as I suspect it is already too late to do anything regardless of any professional body and what they say…."

Appendix III. Mercury Toxicity: Genetic Susceptibility and Synergistic Effects

Boyd E. Haley, PhD
Professor and Chair, Department of Chemistry, University of Kentucky

Abstract

Mercury toxicity and intoxication (poisoning) are realities that every American needs to face. Both the Environmental Protection Agency and National Academy of Science state that between 8 to 10% of American women have mercury levels that would render any child they gave birth to neurological disorders. One of six children in the USA have a neurodevelopmental disorder according to the Centers for Disease Control and Prevention. Yet our dentistry and medicine continue to expose all patients to mercury. This article discusses the obvious sources of mercury exposures that can be easily prevented. It also points out that genetic susceptibility and exposures to other materials that synergistically enhance mercury and ethylmercury toxicity need to be evaluated, and that by their existence prevent the actual determination of a "safe level" of mercury exposure for all. The mercury sources we consider are from dentistry and from drugs, mainly vaccines, that, in today's world are not only unnecessary sources, but also sources that are being increasingly recognized as being significantly deleterious to the health of many.

Keywords: mercury toxicity, ethylmercury toxicity, Thimerosal toxicity, amalgams, antibiotic susceptibility to neurotoxicity, hormone susceptibility to neurotoxicity

1. Introduction

Mercury toxicity and intoxication (poisoning) are realities that every American needs to face. This article discusses mercury intoxication and several normally appearing factors that increase the susceptibility to mercury toxicity. The sources considered are dentistry and mercury from drugs, mainly vaccines, that, in today's world are not only unnecessary sources, but also sources that are being increasingly recognized as being significantly deleterious to the health of many who are so exposed.

2. Mercury from dentistry

Let us begin by discussing mercury exposure from dental amalgams. Figure 1 is a segment from a movie showing the emission of mercury vapors from a 50 year old amalgam; it is still releasing mercury at the temperature of a cup of coffee. The point of this figure is to provide visual evidence that mercury is indeed released by dental amalgams. It has been reported in a World Health Organization review of mercury that 80% of the mercury vapors inhaled are retained by the human body [1]. This is why dental amalgams have been found to be the major contributor to human body mercury burden. The visualization of mercury emitting from amalgams presents irrefutable evidence that spokespersons for the American Dental Association (ADA) are exceptionally deceptive when they state there is no danger of mercury exposure from dental amalgams.

Figure 1. Visualization of mercury emitting from a dental amalgam. The filling is 50 years old. The tooth was extracted 15 years ago. (Credits: www.uninformedcosent.com)

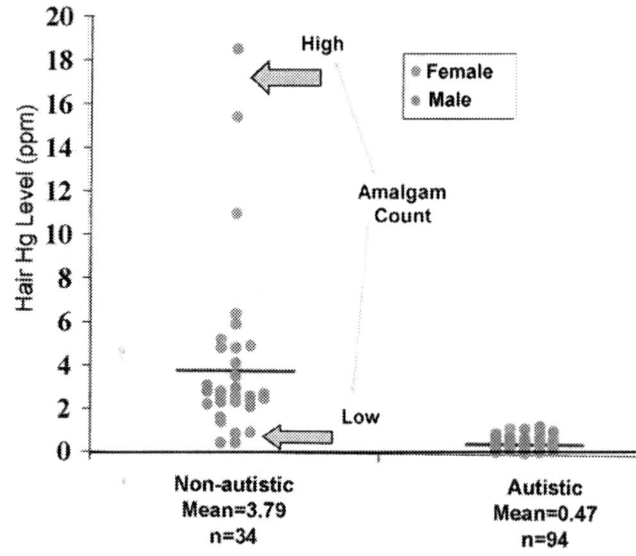

Figure 2. Birth-hair mercury of autistic vs. control groups [2]

This data in Figure 2 show that normal children have birth hair levels of mercury that correlate with the number of amalgam fillings in the birth mother; whereas, in sharp contrast, the autistic children have exceptionally low levels of birth hair mercury, no matter what the number of amalgam fillings are found in the birth mother. This data strongly implies that autistic children represent a subset of the population that does not effectively excrete mercury from their cells.

Mercury vapor, when it enters the body spends a very short time in the blood. Mercury vapor (Hg^o) is a hydrophobic entity and is rapidly absorbed through cell membranes into cells where certain enzymes, such as catalyase, rapidly converts it to Hg^{2+}, the reactive and toxic form of mercury called inorganic mercury. It would be nearly impossible for the body to substantially excrete either Hg^o or Hg^{2+} from the body in their original form. To rid the body of Hg^{2+} it must first be taken intracellular where it can be complexed with glutathione. It is primarily the mercury-glutathione complex that is excreted from the cells into the blood to be cleared by the bilary transport system in the liver. Therefore, it is primarily the mercury-glutathione complex that is measured in the blood, urine, feces and hair as elevated after mercury exposures. It is not the original Hg^o as it would prefer partioning into the more hydrophobic cells of the body.

Therefore, the lack of mercury in the birth hair of autistics strongly implies that they cannot effectively excrete mercury most likely by not being able to effectively couple Hg^{2+} with glutathione. Research by Dr. Jill James of the University of Arkansas has partially explained this phenomenon by demonstrating that autistics are quite low in glutathione, the sequester of mercury that exists intracellular and used by the body in the normal excretion process [3].

Figure 3 demonstrates that considering the mercury exposures from dietary fish, vaccines and amalgams versus the predicted birth hair mercury levels that again the normal children have the predicted birth hair mercury levels; whereas, the autistic children show no significant increase. Considering the data from birth mothers with 8 to 15 amalgams the mercury hair ratio was 12 to 1 in normals versus autistics. There can be little doubt that in this cohort group, the autistics do not biochemically excrete mercury in a similar fashion as do normal children.

Also, as expected, amalgams are the major contributor to mercury body burden, not the mother's fish diet. In considering different exposures as contributing to mercury body burden one should consider the reactive potential of the mercury. Mercury in fish has already reacted with proteins and other protective molecules or atoms in fish (e.g., glutathione, selenium, and other proteins); this is why the fish does not die of mercury toxicity. This bound mercury, or methylmercury, is not as toxic as an equal amount of the pure equivalent. Therefore, while there may be an equal exposure to mercury from a tuna fish sandwich as from an amalgam or vaccine, the mercury from the amalgam or vaccine has much more toxic potential. The Thimerosal-containing vaccine given in the past to infants on the day of birth would be safe by EPA standards, based on adolescents eating fish, if the infant weighed 275 pounds.

Figure 3. Actual versus predicted birth hair mercury levels [2]

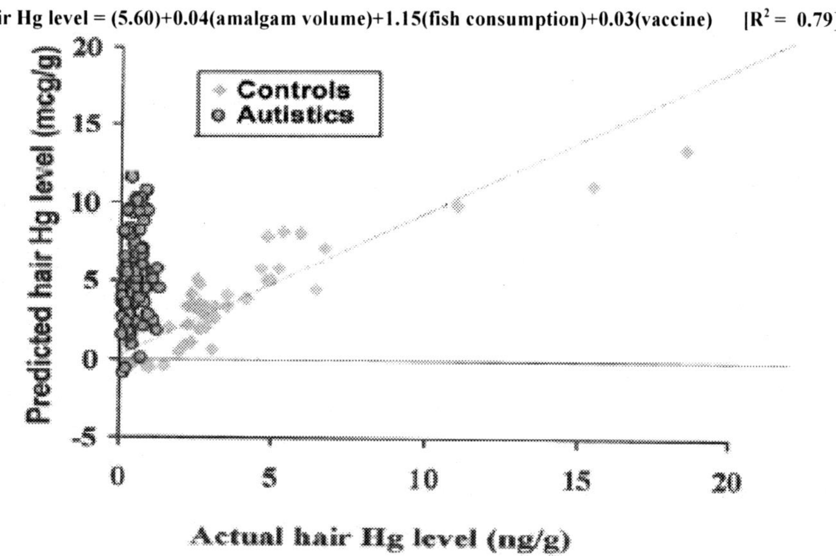

Figure 4. Mercury birth hair levels vs. amalgam in autistics and control groups [2]

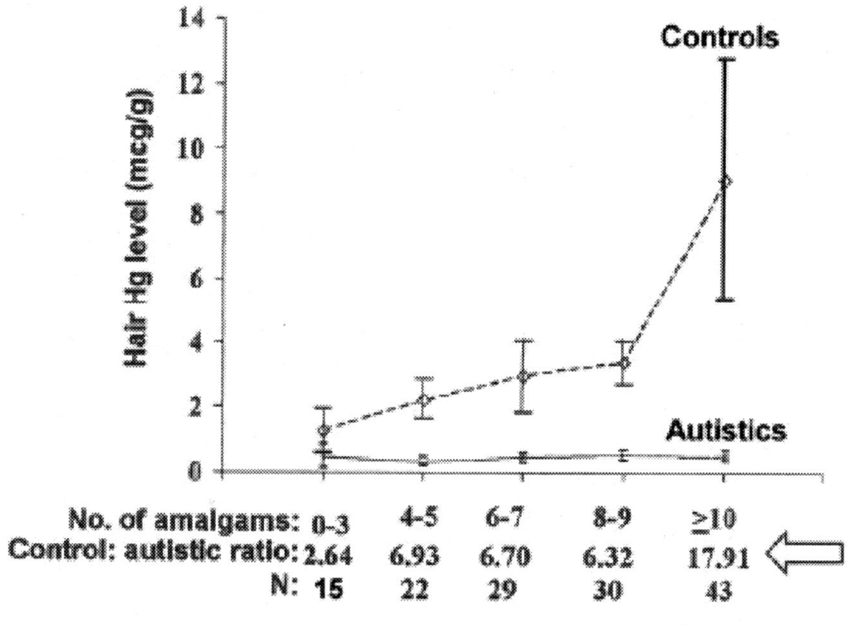

Figure 4 shows that, as expected, the birth hair mercury levels in normal children are determined more by their birth mother's number of amalgams than by any other exposure, such as fish in the mother's diet. In contrast, autistic children born of mothers with greater than 10 amalgam fillings still do not have significant levels of mercury in their birth hair. This confirms that autistic children do not handle mercury biochemically like normal children. The most likely explanation is they are poor excretors. Work from Dr. Jeff Bradstreet [4] and others have shown that autistics do have higher body burdens of mercury than normals. This supports the hypothesis that autistics are in reality poor mercury excretors who retain mercury and are thusly more severely affected by low dose exposures.

Figure 5. Birth-hair mercury by severity of autism [2]

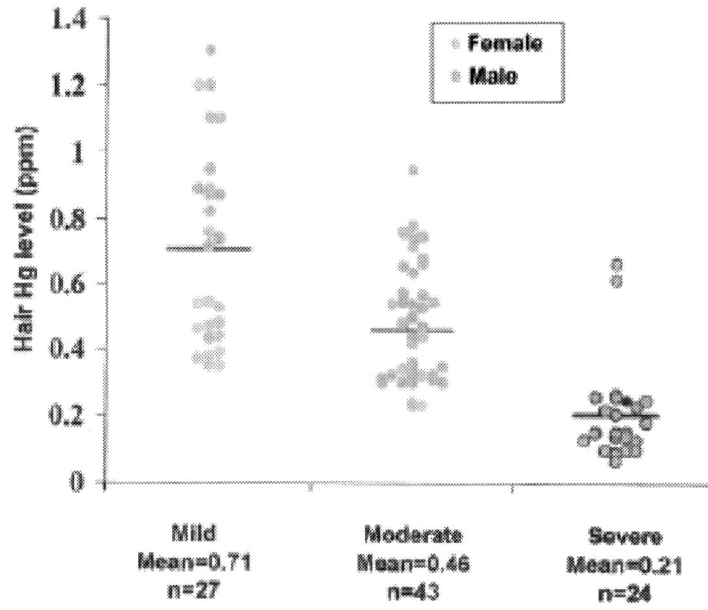

The major observation of this data is that the lower the birth hair mercury level the more likely the severity of the autism. This fits into the hypothesis as follows: the lower the ability to excrete mercury the more mercury that is retained by the cells of the body and the more toxic the exposure to the infant (Fig. 5).

Another observation is that of comparing boys to girls. Note that the females mostly fall below the average line in each level of severity and that the "severe category" has only one female (Fig. 5). This indicates that a female must be a much poorer mercury excretor than the males to become autistic at that level. Bottom line, it takes more retention of mercury to make a female autistic than it does for a male. We feel the male/female ratio of about four gives us a hint as to the causal element in autism. We also think that the differential effects of estrogen versus testosterone on mercury toxicity to neurons may explain the increased susceptibility of males to autism.

3. Synergistic effects: Thimerosal, aluminum hydroxide and Neomycin

It is well documented in the literature that mercury toxicity is synergistic with other heavy metals such as cadmium and lead. It is also known that certain antibiotics greatly enhance the toxicity of Thimerosal in ocular solutions and that antibiotics prevent test animals from effectively excreting mercury. The major known difference between males and females is their hormones. We therefore investigated the possible involvement of aluminum cation (found in vaccines), antibiotics (neomycin) and male versus female (estrogen versus testosterone) on the toxic effects of 50 nanomolar (nM) Thimerosal on neurons in culture. Neurons can be cultured for 24 hours without much death (Fig. 6). Fifty nanomolar Thimerosal alone (solid circles [•]) will cause the death of about 70% of the neurons within 24 hours. The synergistic effects of aluminum, neomycin and testosterone are shown (Fig. 6) and are as follows:

Aluminum: Aluminum hydroxide alone (solid triangles [▲]) at 500 nM showed no significant death of cells at 6 hours, and only slight toxicity over the 24-hour period. Thimerosal at 50 nM effected only a slight increase in neuron death at 6 hours. However, in the presence of 50 nM Thimerosal plus 500 nM aluminum hydroxide (open triangles [Δ]), the neuronal death increases to roughly 60%, an amazing increase and clearly demonstrates the synergistic effects of other metals on mercury toxicity and certainly Thimerosal toxicity.

Neomycin: At 1.75 mcg neomycin alone (solid squares [■]) did not cause a significant increase in neuronal death after 12 hours. In the presence of 50 nM Thimerosal (open squares [□]) the rate of death at same point increased from about 40% to 60%, a 20% increase in rate of death.

A report on infants treated topologically with Thimerosal for umbilical cord infections resulted in the deaths of 10 of 13 exposed with corresponding increased mercury levels in their internal organs [5]. This lead to the withdrawal of Thimerosal as a topical antiseptic available across the counter, but did not prevent the CDC and FDA from approving injection into day old infants on the day of birth.

4. Hormonal effects: Testosterone and Estrogen

Figure 6. Synergistic toxicities. (Dr. Mark Lovell, collaborator)

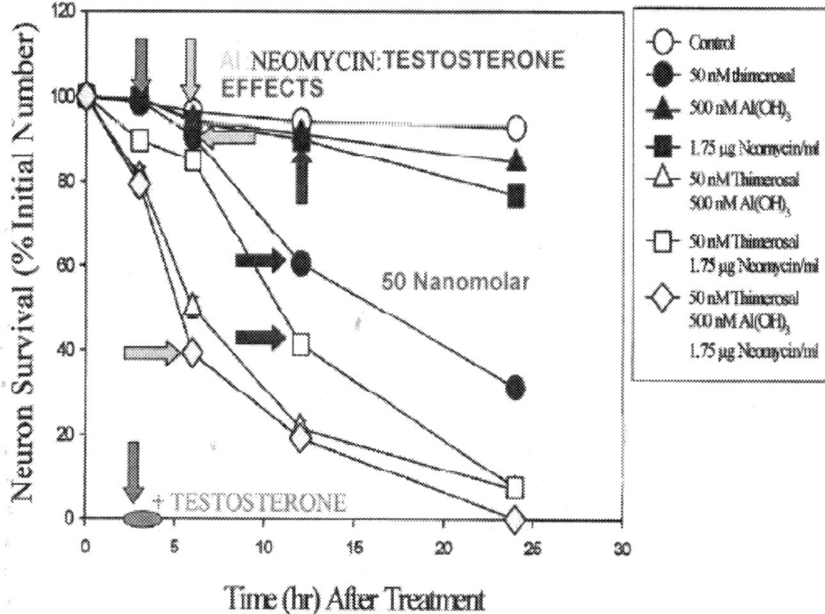

Testosterone and estrogen-like compounds give vastly different results. Using female hormones we found them not toxic to the neurons alone and to be consistently protective against Thimerosal toxicity. In fact, at high levels they could afford total protection for 24 hours against neuronal death in this test system (data not plotted). However, testosterone which appeared protective at very low levels (0.01 to 0.1 micromolar), dramatically increased neuron death at higher levels (0.5 to 1.0 micromolar). In fact, 1.0 micromolar levels of testosterone that by itself did not significantly increase neuron death (red flattened oval), within 3 hours when added with 50 nanomolar Thimerosal (solid circles) caused 100% neuron death. Fifty nanomolar Thimerosal at this time point did not significantly cause any cell death.

These testosterone results, while not conclusive because of the in vitro neuron culture type of testing, clearly demonstrated that male versus female hormones may play a major role in autism risk and may explain the high ratio of boys to girls in autism (4 to 1) and autism related disorders.

5. Thimerosal and ionic mercury: Additive effects

Infants are obviously exposed to mercury from the amalgams of the birth mother and, shortly after birth, from the Hepatitis B vaccines that contained Thimerosal. An experiment was done to compare the combined toxicity of Thimerosal and inorganic mercury. In this neuron culture system both Thimerosal and inorganic mercury were toxic to cells at the low nanomolar levels. Inorganic mercury at 25 nanomolars caused more neuron death at the early exposure times but after 12 hours the toxicity of Thimerosal was greater. It probably took some time for the ethylmercurihydroxide, the initial Thimerosal metabolite that forms rapidly, to be released and it is therefore not as initially as toxic. However, as the Thimerosal releases the "ethylmercury" it becomes effectively lethal to the neurons (Fig. 7).

We combined the levels of inorganic mercury and Thimerosal at levels which alone gave about 50% neuron death at 24 hours to determine their combined effects (Fig. 7). They appeared to be additive instead of synergistic. This implies that both inorganic mercury(II) ions and the ethylmercurihydroxide from Thimerosal cause neuronal death by similar mechanisms.

6. Inorganic mercury poisoning: Acrodynia and Pink Disease

The valid argument against any data obtained using neurons in culture is that the body has protection mechanisms against the toxic exposure that prevents the toxin from getting near the neurons and causing any biochemical abnormalities. However, we have a historical fact that proves a low exposure to mercury can cause a severe neurological disease in infants. Acrodynia, or Pink Disease, was known to affect 1 in 500 children in the late 1800s into the early 1940s. A practicing physician noted that most of the children who suffered from this illness came from the more affluent families, as the disease was much less prevalent in the poorer populations in his area. He also noted that the use of teething powders containing calomel (mercurous chloride, Hg_2Cl_2, 84.98% mercury by weight) was closely associated with the illness and recommended that these teething powders no longer be used. His patients recovered, he reported this and these teething powders were removed from the market and the disease disappeared into history.

Figure 7. Hg and Thimerosal display additive toxicities

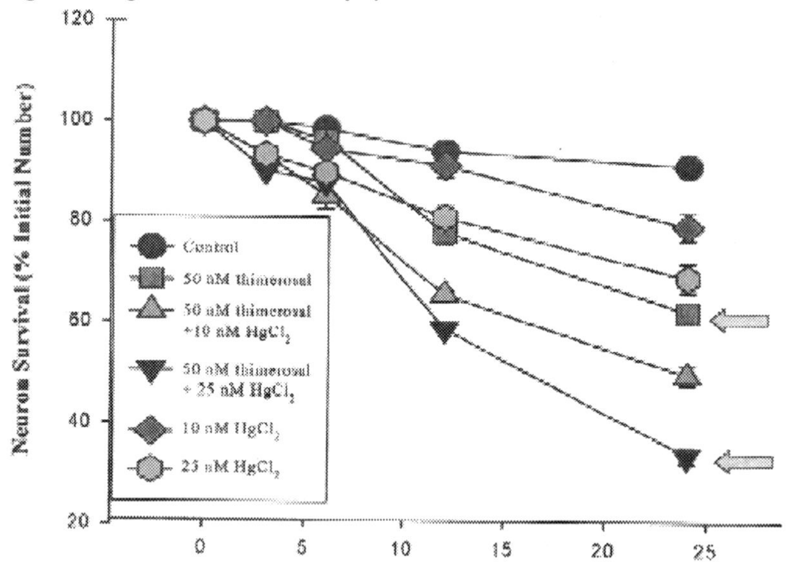

Calomel is still used today in many diaper rash treatments and other ointments used to treat skin irritations, though the use of organic mercury compounds, like Thimerosal and phenyl mercuric acetate, was banned in 1998 in such products. Calomel is one of the least toxic forms of mercury, yet its use in teething powders caused a major illness with infants. It is not unreasonable to propose that exposure to ethylmercury from thimerosal (exceptionally toxic) could most likely be involved in autism and related disorders.

7. Mercury from Thimerosal in some vaccines

Our government agencies, the FDA, CDC and NIH routinely ignore the possible involvement of mercury in the cause or exacerbation of any disease. It is my opinion this shunning of mercury based toxicity studies is influenced by organized dentistry and medical interests (vaccine manufacturers) who routinely use mercury in the treatment of patients. An outrageous claim one would rationally think.

But look at the facts. In 1999 a report was published in the highly respected *Journal of the American College of Cardiology* that stated that individuals who die of Idiopathic Dilated Cardiomyopathy (IDCM) had 178,400 nanograms of mercury per gram of heart tissue, an amazing amount (Table 1). Measuring mercury is not rocket science, it is easy to accomplish if you have the proper instrument, which most research universities do. This level was 22,000 times higher than the rest of the tissues in the body, and in the heart tissue of subjects who died of other forms of cardiovascular disease (Table 1). IDCM is the named disease that young athletes unexpectedly die of and is one of the major reasons for heart transplants in many adults. Yet, with this data obviously available, neither the NIH nor the FDA has made any requests for grants to study the possible involvement of, or source of, mercury in IDCM. They have essentially ignored this just as they have ignored the obvious emission of mercury vapors from dental amalgams and the elevated mercury levels found in autistic children.

Table 1. Elevated Mercury in idiopathic dilated cardiomyopathy (IDCM). Where does Hg come from?

LEVELS ng/g	Hg	Sb
Controls[a]	8.0	1.5
IDCM[b]	178,400	19,260

[a]Controls were patients with valvular or ischemic heart disease.
[b]Athletic youth who died from IDCM.
(Frustaci et al., J. of American College of Cardiology, 33(6):1578, 1999.)

8. Major scientific studies on mercury toxicity

There have been two major studies on mercury toxicity—both involved studying the dietary mercury intake from eating fish and whale. In my opinion, these were likely funded because you cannot sue a fish and it takes the attention away from iatrogenic mercury exposures. In both the Faroe and Seychelles Island studies it was assumed that both blood and hair levels of mercury were indicative of the level of mercury exposure. I don't agree with this assumption because it ignores the fact that a subset of the population studied were possibly poor excretors and did not have a level of mercury in their hair or blood that was indicative of their mercury exposure, as demonstrated for autistic children. In both these studies there were anomalies that indicated that the erroneously assumed exposures were correct.

In the Seychelles study (see comments in M. Bauman and K. Nelson) of more than 700 children, it was implied that boys with the highest hair levels of mercury did better on the Boston Naming test and two tests of visual motor coordination. Spokespersons for the American Dental Association have used this data to claim that a little exposure to mercury is good for your brain. However, in my opinion the boys with the higher hair mercury levels were the boys that effectively excrete mercury and would likely have a lower body burden of mercury.

In the Faroe Island study it was the boys with the lower blood mercury levels (poorer excretors?) that had the blood pressure problems.

I feel it would be important to review the raw data from the Seychelles and Faroe Island studies with the understanding that blood, urine and hair mercury levels do *not* indicate level of exposure. In fact, it is not level of exposure at these low doses obtained in a fish diet that is critical, it is the lack of ability to excrete the mercury these children were exposed to that is critical. Inability to excrete causes the illnesses, not the total exposure.

9. Mercury levels in hair and nails of Alzheimer's diseased patients

I further investigated the theory of low-level mercury toxicity causing problems in just those individuals who were unable to excrete mercury. I was involved in the mercury/autism issue because of my earlier research that showed that exposure of brain tissue to mercury would cause many of the same aberrant biochemical factors found in Alzheimer's disease (AD). Therefore, I did a literature search on any relevant studies regarding mercury retention in tissues of AD versus normal controls. In doing this I found a series of studies that seem to have been forgotten. The references and quotes from the various papers are shown in Table 2.

Table 2. References and quotes regarding mercury retention in tissues

- Ehmann, Markesbery, et al. Neurotoxicology 9(2):197–208. Trace element imbalances in hair and nails of Alzheimer's diseased patients.
- Ehman, Markesbery, et al. Biological Trace Element Research, pp. 461–470. G.N. Schrauzer, ed., 1990 by the Humana Press, Inc.
- "Mercury is decreased in the nail of AD subjects compared to controls."
- "Mercury tended to decrease in nail with increasing age of patient, and with the duration and severity of the dementia."

- "This decrease is counter to the elevated levels of Hg observed in AD brain, as compared to age-matched controls."

It seems as if AD subjects have low mercury levels in their nail tissues when compared to normal age-matched controls. Also, the level of mercury in the nail tissue of AD subjects drops with increasing duration and severity of the dementia. Nail and hair tissue are very similar and it appears as if the subjects suffering from AD may have an impeded ability to excrete mercury similar to autistics.

However, autism and AD are quite different diseases and this needs explanation. First, one has to remember that the mercury exposures in autism and AD would be quite different. First, is the matter of age. In autism the infants are exposed to bolus amounts of the organic mercury compound, ethylmercury. This is while their central nervous system is developing and while they are still on a milk diet (and perhaps antibiotics). Also, their ability to excrete mercury in the bilary transport system is low because the infants are not producing adequate amounts of bile in the first few months. These are factors that prevent excretion of mercury in laboratory animals. Therefore, ethylmercury from early vaccination with thimerosal-containing vaccines likely prevents the development of normal brain neuronal connections. This situation is exacerbated in autistics that appear to be less capable of excreting mercury.

In AD the major mercury exposure is the vapor from dental amalgams and this exposure starts after the individual is mostly mature in regards to mental development and ability to excrete mercury. However, these individuals are exposed to mercury constantly from their amalgams from the time they are placed until they are removed. Mercury vapors enter the brain with a great deal of ease where the Hg^o is converted to Hg^{2+}, the toxic form. While Hg^o enters the brain with ease the Hg2+ does not cross the blood brain barrier very well in either direction. Therefore, the Hg^{2+} is trapped in the brain and is not effectively excreted. This would be increased in the elderly who seem unable to excrete mercury as easily as when they were younger, based on the mercury levels in nail tissue. Additionally, these older subjects are on the top of the priority list to obtain flu and other thimerosal-containing vaccines. This subjects them to bolus amounts of ethylmercury throughout their lives and cannot help but add to their mercury body burden and the total toxic effects of mercury.

When does the mercury start affecting the AD subject? Recent data show that individuals with mild cognitive impairment (MCI) have already started a build up of amyloid plaques, possibly before any clinical dementia has set in. An earlier study demonstrated that mercury exposure can increase the production of beta-amyloid, the protein that makes up the bulk of the amyloid plaque [6]. At the same time it disassembles tubulin from the neurofibrils [7]. The preceding publications confirm the earlier reports of mercury inducing similarities to the AD brain [8].

The bottom line is that exposure to low levels of mercury can cause tubulin to abnormally aggregate and not be found in the supernatant of a brain homogenate, preventing the natural interaction with GTP, all facts that are consistent with observations on AD brain. Since Tau protein binds tubulin protein to neurofibrils the Tau protein is now dislodged from its normal setting and can become abnormally phosphorylated as it is in AD brain. This Tau protein and neurofibrils are major proteins found in neurofibillary tangles, a major pathological diagnostic hallmark of AD. Beta-amyloid protein is produced by two proteases acting on amyloid precursor protein, a large membrane spanning protein. The increased production of beta-amyloid by Hg^{2+} exposure is quite relevant. The produced beta-amyloid peptide forms the aggregates that are called senile plaques, another pathological diagnostic hallmark of AD.

To dissolve amyloid plaques effectively one needs to use a heavy metal chelator. Therefore, the amyloid peptides are held within this plaque by interacting heavy metal linkages. This increase in heavy metals, or metals like Zn^{2+} and Cu^{2+} in the wrong place, is what would be expected if mercury levels have reached the concentration at which it has been shown to obliterate microtubulin structure and to disrupt normal homeostasis of Cu^{2+} and Zn^{2+}, etc.

Also, the disruption of the microtubulin structure impairs the transport of glutamate containing vacuoles down the axon and it is likely that these vacuoles disintegrate releasing glutamate inducing regional "excitotoxicity" and additional neuronal death. This would explain the exceptionally high levels of glutamine synthetase found in the CSF of AD versus other neurological diseases (ALS being the exception) [9]. Additionally, glutamate synthetase is a very sensitive thiol-enzyme that is rapidly inhibited by mercury.

10. Conclusions regarding mercury in brain tissue

In summary, mercury build up in the brain tissue has the ability to cause the equivalent of a biochemical train wreck. Most importantly, the axon, which contains tubulin, is rapidly and effectively disrupted by Hg^{2+}. Many pathways and many supramolecular structures are injured by mercury similar to the aberrancies observed in AD brain pathology and biochemistry. While it is possible that other environmental factors, yet unidentified, could affect brain changes similar to mercury and as observed in AD brain, it seems unquestionable that exposure to mercury vapors for scores of years and high dose vaccine-delivered thimerosal in the aged would exacerbate the disease in those who are afflicted.

Table 3 shows some data that determined the level of brain mercury and any correspondence with the number of dental amalgams in a group of nuns from the same religious order. Mercury collection in the brain of certain individuals at a higher rate than others would be expected if the "retention toxicity" of a subset of the population were a fact. A publication on the mercury levels in the brain tissue of Nuns in a study on Alzheimer's disease gives us some information on this issue. Nuns in a specific, single location were studied as they essentially had the same daily diet and roughly the same exposures to environmental mercury. In this study roughly 6% of the nuns had what would be defined as extremely mercury toxic brains of 1 micromolar level or higher and this percentage increased to about 15% when the cut-off point was a 0.5 micromolar level. This strongly indicates that certain individuals among these nuns did not have the ability to clear mercury from their brains and that this is independent of diet or amalgam exposure. According to the authors, the level of mercury in the brain did not correlate with the number of existing amalgam fillings, the major contributor to human mercury body burden. Therefore, it does appear as if the inability to excrete mercury may play a major role in the build up of brain mercury levels over many years.

Table 3. Mercury levels in the human brain

- Saxe et al., with Ehmann and Markesbery in Alzheimer's Disease, Dental Amalgam and Mercury, JADA v130, p. 191–199, 1999, determined Hg leveles in the brains of 101 human subjects, mostly Nuns, both AD and normals.
- The histogram in this paper showed 6 of 101 subjects with brain Hg leveles about 200 ng/g [wet weight; (ppb)] (C=236, 248, 319: AD=394, 622, 698). This represents between 1.2 and 3.5 micromolar, highly toxic levels of Hg in 6% of these subjects. At 100 ng Hg/g of sample, this increases to about 15% of subjects with highly toxic leveles of brain mercury.
- This indicates that certain adult individuals do not effectively excrete mercury from their brain tissue.

Figure 8 shows that addition of Hg^{2+} in the presence of excess of the chelator ethylenediamine tetraacetic acid (EDTA) still could mimic the effects seen on the brain protein tubulin in AD. This is shown where increasing Hg^{2+} decreased the binding of a GTP analog to the tubulin of normal brain; whereas, the tubulin of AD brain did not bind even in the absence of added Hg^{2+} (see band at red arrow). This is direct confirmation that Hg^{2+} exposure, if not causal, exacerbates a major biochemical flaw found in AD brain.

In earlier studies, publications from my laboratory demonstrated that the major brain protein tubulin, which polymerizes to form microtubules, was aberrant in AD brain with an average of about 80% not being viable. This lack of viability was demonstrated in two ways. First, the tubulin has to bind the natural compound GTP (guanosine-triphosphate) to be viable and polymerize. AD tubulin could not bind the GTP analog (8-azido-GTP), a proven marker for beta-tubulin. This showed the GTP binding sites on tubulin were not available or blocked. Second, normal brain tubulin is a soluble protein at 0°C and remains in the supernatant of a centrifuged homogenate. However, in AD brain the tubulin is over 80% found in the pellet indicating that it is abnormally polymerized, something effectively done by heavy metals.

Since tubulin is well known to be sensitive to heavy metals we tested all possible metals for their ability to mimic the effect seen in AD brain. One has to consider that there are considerable metal "chelation" molecules in the brain, such as citrate and other organic acids. We observed that many metals, Hg^{2+}, Pb^{2+}, Cd^{2+}, Zn^{2+}, etc.

could mimic the effects we observed in AD brain regarding tubulin. However, only one metal could do this in the presence of huge excesses of organic acid chelators (e.g., EDTA, citrate) and that was Hg^{2+}. Chelation, or binding, of heavy metals by biological organic acids is one way to decrease their toxic effects. This worked for all metals tested except Hg^{2+}.

A major question relative to autism would be the difference in the neurotoxic mechanism of organic mercury toxicity (e.g., ethylmercury) versus inorganic mercury (Hg^{2+}). To investigate this we treated normal human brain homogenates with thimerosal just as we had treated brain in Figure 8 with Hg^{2+}. The results were dramatic, with thimerosal totally inhibiting tubulin viability at very low concentrations and very rapidly (Fig. 9). Further, exposing thimerosal to light (causes a more rapid release of ethylmercury) made the thimerosal mixture more toxic or at least more rapid in its toxic effects on tubulin.

A major difference between thimerosal and Hg^{2+} was on the protein migrating just below tubulin, which was not adversely affected by Hg^{2+} levels (see Fig. 8). Thimerosal effectively prevented this protein from interacting with the GTP analog. The major protein in this band is actin, another cytoskeletal nucleotide binding protein of high abundance in brain axons. Therefore, thimerosal had a major inhibitory effect on a protein that, at the concentrations used, was not significantly affected by Hg^{2+}.

Also, these experiments were exposed to thimerosal at $0^{o}C$ for only a few minutes. This is too short of a time for the ethylmercury to be converted to Hg^{2+}. Therefore, it appears as if ethylmercury is more toxic to many proteins than is Hg^{2+} and that it does not have to break down to Hg^{2+} to cause extensive enzyme or protein toxicity (Fig. 9).

11. Conclusions

In summary, it appears as if autistics represent a subset of the population that are more susceptible to the toxic effects of mercury and thimerosal because they are not efficient excretors of these toxic materials. Further, it appears as if the sex hormones play a major role in susceptibility with the male hormones increasing susceptibility to the neurotoxicity of ethylmercury and the female hormones affording a good degree of protection. Common sense tells us that a lead toxic person would be more susceptible to mercury toxicity than a healthy, non-toxic person. Research confirms this and we routinely observe that many heavy metals increase the apparent toxicity of low levels of mercury. It is well known that a milk diet will cause the retention of mercury as does the exposure of mammals to certain antibiotics. This would make infants with ear infections prime candidates for mercury retention toxicity. Certainly, the findings of aberrant biochemistries in the autistic child that appear to correlate with mercury sensitive enzymes increases the possibility of mercury involvement in autism causation.

If certain infants are more susceptible to mercury toxicity due to their inability to excrete mercury then it seems plausible that, since this is a genetic susceptibility, older individuals may suffer from the inability to excrete mercury also. Based on the ability of mercury to mimic many of the biochemical aberrancies found in AD brain and to produce aspects of the pathological diagnostic hallmarks of AD it seems plausible that AD is a disease related to mercury toxicity. The published decrease of mercury in the nail tissue of AD versus normal age-matched individuals seems to support this possibility.

Finally, the synergistic effects of other heavy metals, diet, antibiotics, etc. on mercury toxicity make it impossible to define a "safe level of mercury exposure." Therefore it is imperative that we try to eliminate all exposure to mercury; and removal from dentistry and medicines is most important and critical for human health.

References

[1] Berlin M. Mercury in dental fillings: an environmental medicine risk assessment. A literature and knowledge summary. In: Amalgam and Health, Novakova V ed., Swedish Council for Planning and Coordination of Research (FRN), Stockholm, 1999:369.

[2] Holmes AS, Blaxill MF, Haley BE. Reduced levels of mercury in first baby haircuts of autistic children. Int. J. Toxicol., 2003 Jul-Aug; 22(4):277–85.

[3] James SJ, Cutler P, Melnyk S, Jernigan S, Janak L, Gaylor DW, Neubrander JA. Metabolic biomarkers of increased oxidative stress and impaired methylation capacity in children with autism. Am J Clin Nutr, 2004 Dec; 80:1611–7.

[4] Bradstreet J. A case-control study of mercury burden in children with autistic disorders and measles virus genome RNA in cerebrospinal fluid in children with regressive autism. Immunization safety review: Vaccines and autism. Institute of Medicine, Feb. 9, 2004.

[5] Fagan DG, Pritchard JS, Clarkson TW, Greenwood MR. Organ mercury levels in infants with omophaloceles treated with organic mercurial antiseptic. Arch Dis Child, 1977 Dec; 52(12):962–4.

[6] Olivieri G, Brack C, Muller-Spahn F, Stahelin HB, Herrmann M, Renard P; Brockhaus M, Hock C. Mercury induces cell cytotoxicity and oxidative stress and increases beta-amyloid secretion and tau phosphorylation in SHSY5Y neuroblastoma cells. J. Neurochem, 2000 Jan; 74(1):231–6.

[7] Leong, CCW, Syed NI, Lorscheider FL. Retrograde degeneration of neurite membrane structural integrity and formation of neruofibillary tangles at nerve growth cones following in vitro exposure to mercury. NeuroReports, 2001;12(4):733–7.

[8] Pendergrass JC, Haley BE. Inhibition of brain tubulin-guanosine 5'-triphosphate interactions by mercury: Similarity to observations in Alzheimer's diseased brain. In: Metal Ions in Biological Systems; 34:461–78. Mercury and Its Effects on Environment and Biology, Chapter 16. Sigel H and Sigel A, eds. , 1996. Marcel Dekker, Inc. 270 Madison Ave., N.Y., N.Y. 10016.

[9] Gunnersen D, Haley B. Detection of glutamine synthetase in the cerebrospinal fluid of Alzheimer diseased patients: a potential diagnostic biochemical marker. Proc. Natl. Acad. Sci. USA, 1992 Dec 15; 89(24):11949–53.

Figure 8. HgEDTA induces aberrant [^{32}P]8N_3GTP-β-Tubulin interactions indicative of AD

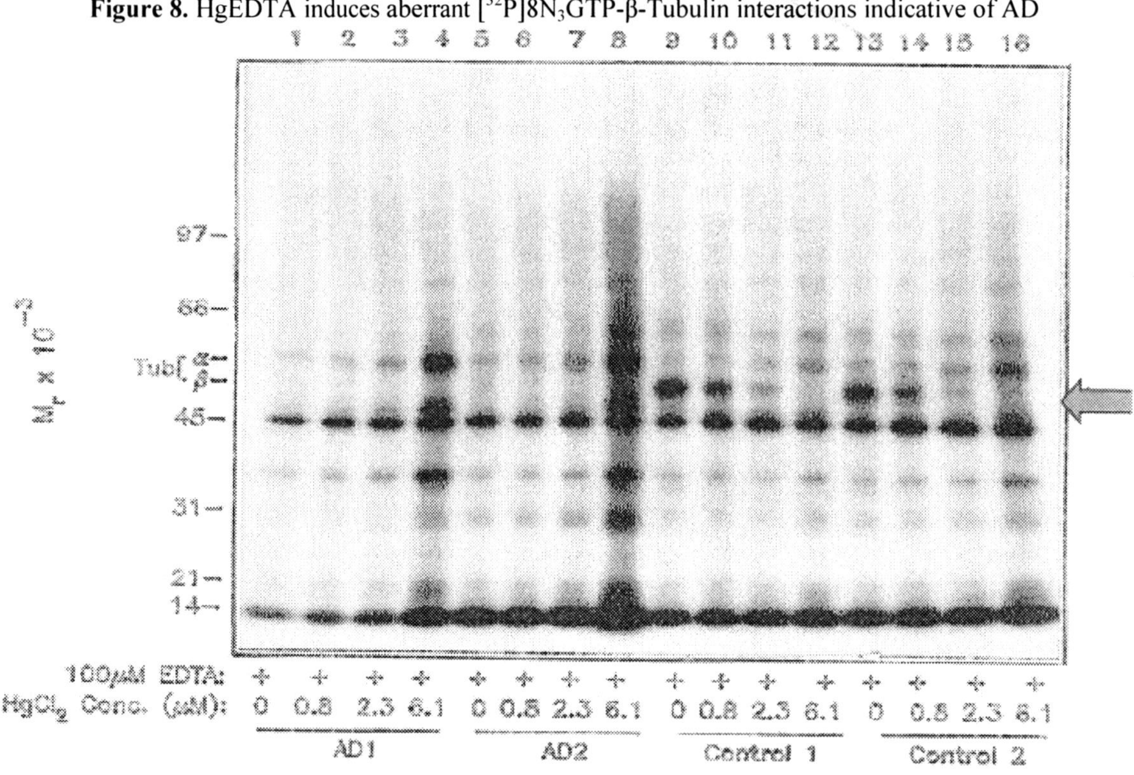

Figure 9. Autoradiogram showing Thimerosal inhibition of [γ^{32}P]8N_3GTP photolabeling of brain β-Tubulin

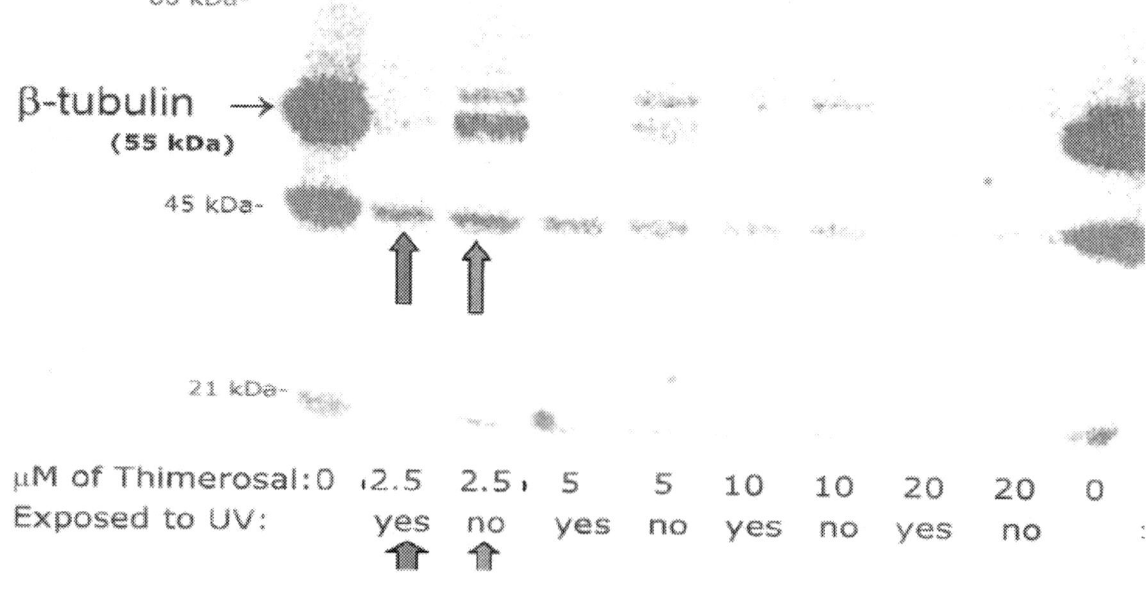

Appendix IV. Mercury in Vaccines: Institutional Malfeasance and The Department of Health and Human Services

Medical Veritas Editorial Staff
P.O. Box 847
Pearblossom, CA 93553 USA
Phone: +1 800 309 3569 Fax: +1 661 944 4483
Email: pearblossominc@aol.com Website: www.MedicalVeritas.com

Abstract

A historical perspective of the use of Thimerosal, which contains ethylmercury, in vaccines is presented. Despite the availability of evidence that mercurial compounds are toxic, public health institutions have ignored the evidence dating from the 1930s and have instead authorized acceptance of Thimerosal as a so-called "preservative." Removal of Thimerosal from several childhood vaccines in the United States was not accomplished until after the turn of the century. In its report on Thimerosal, the Institute of Medicine in 2001 commented: "The presence of mercury in some vaccines can raise doubts about the entire system of ensuring vaccine safety, and late recognition of the potential risk of Thimerosal in vaccines may contribute to a perception among some that careful attention to vaccine components has been lacking."

The CDC has a responsibility to protect the health of the American public. If there were any doubts about the neurological effects of ethylmercury in vaccines on children – and there were substantial doubts – the prevailing consideration should have been how best to protect children from potential harm. However, it appears that protecting the industry's profits took precedence over protecting children from mercury damage.

Keywords: Thimerosal, ethylmercury

In 1991, Seal et al. [1] published in the Lancet, "Thimerosal is a weak antibacterial agent that is rapidly broken down to products, including ethylmercury residues, which are neurotoxic. Its role as a preservative in vaccines has been questioned, and the pharmaceutical industry considers its use as historical." Despite such strong indictments against Thimerosal, the Food and Drug Administration (FDA) and Centers for Disease Control and Prevention (CDC) continue to allow many vaccines that contain Thimerosal to be administered to children and adults, and most recently, Thimerosal-containing influenza vaccine has been added to the required routinely administered childhood immunization schedule [2].

Evidence of ethylmercury's toxicity has been available to Federal regulators and the private sector almost since the product's inception. For far too long, both neglected this evidence. Despite evidence dating to the 1930s that ethylmercury in medicines was potentially hazardous, little was done to remove it from a number of products until the 1980s. Even then, regulatory actions to remove Thimerosal and other mercury compounds from medical products proceeded at a glacial pace. The decision to remove Thimerosal was not finalized until 1998. The removal of Thimerosal from several childhood vaccines in the United States was not accomplished until after the turn of the century [3].

For decades ethylmercury was used as a preservative or antibacterial agent in a range of products, including antiseptic ointment for treating cuts, nasal sprays, eye solutions, diaper rash treatments, and perhaps most importantly, vaccines. Several years after an FDA advisory committee found that Thimerosal was not safe for use in topical ointments, new vaccines containing Thimerosal were still being approved and added to the recommended schedule. It appears that nobody analyzed the potential impact of mercury to which young children were being exposed. In fact, if Congress had not enacted legislation in 1997 requiring the FDA to study the amounts of mercury being used in FDA-approved products, it is questionable that the FDA would have analyzed the mercury in vaccines [3].

It is no wonder that, in its report on Thimerosal, the Institute of Medicine in 2001 commented: "The presence of mercury in some vaccines can raise doubts about the entire system of ensuring vaccine safety, and late recognition of the potential risk of Thimerosal in vaccines may contribute to a perception among some that careful attention to vaccine components has been lacking [4]."

It is clear that the guiding principal for FDA policy makers has been to avoid shaking the public's confidence in the safety of vaccines. For this reason, many FDA officials have stubbornly denied that Thimerosal may cause adverse reactions. Ironically, the FDA's unwillingness to address this more forcefully, and remove Thimerosal from vaccines earlier, may have done more long-term damage to the public's trust in vaccines than confronting the problem head-on. Given the serious concerns about the safety of Thimerosal, the FDA should have acted years earlier to remove this preservative from vaccines and other medicines [5].

Eli Lilly and Company of Indianapolis licensed Thimerosal in 1930. It was marketed under the brand name 'Merthiolate.' It was used extensively both in topical ointments to prevent infections and as a preservative in a variety of medicines. Eli Lilly was not the only manufacturer of Thimerosal or other ethylmercury products. In fact, they phased-out their production of Thimerosal in 1974 [5].

In 1974, the FDA undertook a comprehensive review of the safety and effectiveness of over-the-counter (OTC) medicines. As one facet of this review, a panel of experts was assembled to review the safety and efficacy of OTC drugs containing mercury. The Advisory Review Panel on OTC Miscellaneous External Drug Products began its review in 1975. In 1980, the panel delivered its report to the FDA. It reviewed 18 products containing mercury and found them all either unsafe or ineffective for their stated purpose of killing bacteria to prevent infections. In terms of effectiveness, the panel stated, "mercury compounds as a class are of dubious value for anti-microbial use." They also stated, "mercury inhibits the growth of bacteria, but does not act swiftly to kill them." In fact, the panel cited a 1935 study of the effectiveness of Thimerosal in killing staphylococcus bacteria on chick heart tissue. The study determined that Thimerosal was 35-times more toxic to the heart tissue it was meant to protect than the bacteria it was meant to kill. In terms of safety, the panel cited a number of studies demonstrating the highly allergenic nature of Thimerosal and related organic mercury products. For instance, they cited a Swedish study that showed that 10 percent of school children, 16 percent of military recruits, and 18 percent of twins, and 26 percent of medical students had hypersensitivity to Thimerosal. They stated that while organic mercury compounds like Thimerosal were initially developed to decreased the toxicity of the mercury ion, Thimerosal was actually found to be more toxic than bi-chloride of mercury for certain human cells. By way of summary, they stated, "The Panel concludes that Thimerosal is not safe for OTC topical use because of its potential for cell damage if applied to broken skin, and its allergy potential. It is not effective as a topical antimicrobial because its bacteriostatic action can be reversed [5]."

The FDA's action on this matter was already clearly out-of-step with studies that had been conducted dating back to the 1930s showing that Thimerosal preserved vaccines (serums) were extremely toxic.

Pittman-Moore Company had conducted a study in 1935 demonstrating that Merthiolate was not appropriate for use in dogs: "We have obtained marked local reaction in about 50% of the dogs injected with serum containing dilutions of Merthiolate, varying in 1 in 40,000 to 1 in 5,000, and we have demonstrated conclusively that there is no connection between the lot of serum and the reaction. In other words, Merthiolate is unsatisfactory as a preservative for serum intended for use on dogs. Occasionally dogs do not show the local reaction, but in some instances, the reaction is extremely severe. I might say that we have tested Merthiolate on humans and find that it gives a more marked local reaction than does phenol or tricresol [5]."

Warkany and Huber reported in 1953: "In several children of our series and in some recently reported, various immunization procedures preceded the onset of acrodynia in addition to mercurial exposure... It is noteworthy that many vaccines and sera contain small amounts of mercury as preservatives which are injected together with the biologic material. These small amounts of mercurial compounds, which enter the body unnoticed, could act as sensitizing substances. This fact should be kept in mind in the analysis of future cases of acrodynia [6]."

Nelson and Gottshall from the Division of Biologic Products, Bureaus of Laboratories, Michigan Department of Public Health published in 1967, "Pertussis vaccines preserved with 0.01% Merthiolate are more toxic for mice than unpreserved vaccines prepared from the same parent concentrate and containing the same number of organisms... An increase in mortality was observed when Merthiolate was injected separately, before or after an unpreserved saline suspension of pertussis vaccine [7]." Heyworth and Truelove stated in 1979, "For many years, Merthiolate was known to have anti-microbial activity. When it was first introduced as an anti-microbial preservative, little information about the fundamental biological effects of organic mercury compounds was available. We should like to suggest that Merthiolate should now be regarded as an inappropriate preservative for anti-lymphocytic globulin preparations and other materials which are intended for administration to human subjects [8]."

In addition to evidence showing that vaccines containing Thimerosal could cause problems, a number of studies were conducted showing that Thimerosal/ethylmercury were toxic in animals and humans. Tryphonas and Nielsen conducted a study supported by the Medical Research Council of Canada to evaluate chronic low-dose exposure to ethylmercury and methylmercury compounds in young swine. The authors determined: "The resulting toxicosis was primarily related to the nervous system, in which neuronal necrosis followed by secondary gliosis, capillary endothelial proliferation, and additional neuronal necrosis due to developing degenerative arteriopathy in the blood vessels supplying injured gray matter were seen. In other systems, degeneration of hepatocytes and renal tubular cells were commonly occurring lesions in pigs given both MMD [methylmercury-containing compound] and EMC [ethylmercury-containing compound]... The results proved that the alkyl mercurial compounds MMD and EMC, if fed at low concentrations for long periods, were highly poisonous to swine [9]."

Fagan et al. in a study funded by the National Institute of Environmental Health Sciences reported that between 1969 and 1975 there were 13 cases of exomphalos treated by Thimerosal. The authors determined that 10 of the patients had died, and their tissues were analyzed for mercury content. The results showed that Thimerosal can induce blood and organ levels of organic mercury which are well in excess of the minimum toxic levels in adults and fetuses. The authors concluded, "Although Thimerosal is an ethyl mercury compound, it has similar toxicological properties to methyl mercury and the long-term neurological sequelae produced by the ingestion of either methyl or ethyl mercury-based fungicides are indistinguishable [10]." The authors also concluded that the fact that mercury readily penetrates intact membranes and is highly toxic seems to have been forgotten, and that equally effective and far less toxic broad-spectrum antifungal and antibacterial antiseptics are currently available [10].

Despite the fact that the FDA expert committee found that Thimerosal and other ethylmercury compounds were unsafe and ineffective for OTC products, the FDA would not formally require the removal of mercury from some of these products for another 18 years. The submission of the committee's report in 1980 set in motion a tortuous bureaucratic process that would not result in the banning of mercury from OTC products until 1998. The agency published Advanced Notice of Proposed Rules or Notice of Proposed Rules regarding these products in 1980, 1982, 1990, 1991, 1994 and 1995. What makes the glacial pace of these proceedings all the more mystifying is that there appears to have been no opposition to this action throughout the process. No individuals sought to appear before the advisory committee in defense of mercury-containing products, and when the FDA sought public comment along the way on proposed rules to ban certain mercury-based products, it received none. At the time of the FDA's final action, there were 20 OTC products containing mercury being marketed by eight different manufacturers. Their silence on this point is telling [5].

It is difficult to understand why it took the FDA 18 years to remove mercury from OTC products. It is equally difficult to understand why the expert panel's 1980 findings on Thimerosal's safety in topical ointments did not prompt the FDA to further and immediately review the use of Thimerosal in vaccines. Surely there must have been concern that if it was not safe to apply ethylmercury to the surface of an individual's skin, it might not be safe to inject ethylmercury deep into an infant's tissue. The Director of the FDA's National Center expressed such a concern at a 1999 meeting for Toxicological Research. Dr. Bernard Schwetz, who went on to serve as the Acting Director of the FDA for nearly a year, stated: "One thing I haven't heard discussed, the fact that we know that ethylmercury is a skin sensitizer when it's put on the skin, and now we're injecting this IM [intramuscularly] at a time when the immune system is just developing, the functionality of the immune system is just being set at this age. So now we're injecting a sensitizer several times. During that period of time, what's the impact of a sensitizer – of something that is known to be a skin sensitizer, what is the effect on the functional development of the immune system when you give a chemical of that kind repeatedly IM [5]?"

Different branches of the FDA regulate OTC products and vaccines. OTCs are regulated by the Center for Drug Evaluation and Research (CDER). Vaccines are regulated by the Center for Biologics Evaluation and Research (CBER). This, however, is little justification for the lack of coordination. The FDA's determination that mercury was unsafe and should be removed from OTC medications was published in the Federal Register no fewer than five times prior to the FDA's belated review of mercury in vaccines [5].

Despite the FDA's outright negligence concerning the dangers posed by Thimerosal as preservative in vaccines, during the 1980s and 1990s many authors published studies demonstrating the toxicity of Thimerosal, calling for vaccines with a safer preservative and also showing that Thimerosal at the concentrations present in vaccines was ineffective as a preservative to prevent bacterial contamination. Forstrom et al. published in 1980, "...reactions can be expected in such a high percentage of merthiolate-sensitive persons that merthiolate in vaccines should be replaced by another antibacterial agent [11]." In 1983, Kravchenko et al. published, "Thus Thimerosal, commonly used as a preservative, has been found not only to render its primary toxic effect, but also is capable of changing the properties of cells. This fact suggests that the use of Thimerosal for the preservation of medical biological preparations, especially those intended for children, is inadmissible [12]." Winship reported, "Multi-dose vaccines and allergy-testing extracts contain a mercurial preservative, usually 0.01% Thimerosal, and may present problems occasionally in practice. It is, therefore, now accepted that multi-dose injection preparations are undesirable and that preservatives should not be present in unit-dose preparations [13]." Cox and Forsyth recommended in 1988, "However, severe reactions to Thimerosal demonstrate a need for vaccines with an alternative preservative [14]." In 1991, Seal et al. recommended the removal of Thimerosal from vaccines [1]. Also, in August of 1998, an FDA internal "Point Paper" was prepared for the Maternal Immunization Working Group. This document recommended, "For investigational vaccines indicated for maternal immunization, the use of single dose vials should be required to avoid the need of preservative in multi-dose vials... Of concern here is the potential neurotoxic effect of mercury especially when considering cumulative doses of this component in early infancy [5]."

Additionally, Stetler et al. [one of the co-authors is Dr. Walter Orenstein who was later to become Director of the National Immunization Program (NIP), CDC] from the CDC evaluated the use of Thimerosal as a preservative in vaccines in 1985. The authors determined, "Laboratory experiments in this investigation have shown up to 2 weeks' survival of at least one strain of group A Streptococcus in multidose DTP [Diphtheria-Tetanus-Pertussis] vials. The manufacturer's preservative effectiveness tests showed that at 4°C, 4.5% of the challenge Streptococcus survived 14 days after inoculation into a multi-dose DTP vaccine vial. At currently used concentrations, Thimerosal is not an ideal preservative." The authors also warn that, "However, because Thimerosal is an organic mercurial compound, higher concentrations might reduce vaccine potency or pose a health hazard to recipients." The authors also make the following calculations and recommendations regarding the use of multi-dose vials with Thimerosal preservatives: "Single-unit packaging would approximately double the cost of DTP per dose. For example, one manufacturer charges $5.12 for a 15-dose vial of DTP vaccine or $0.34, per dose. If the $0.20 cost of a disposable syringe is added, the total cost per dose to the physician would be about $0.54. The same manufacturer charges $10.40 for a package of ten single DTP doses (needle and syringe pre-packed) or $1.04 per dose... Given the prices mentioned above and the fact that approximately 18 million doses of DTP are administered each year, the cost of switching to single-dose packing might be approximately $9 million. Neither research to develop a better preservative nor recommendations to consider single-dose packaging appear to be warranted... The Thimerosal preservative present in DTP vaccine requires substantial time to kill organisms and cannot be relied upon to prevent transmission of bacteria under conditions of practice when a vial is used over a short period. Instead, the most important means of preventing abscesses secondary to DTP vaccination is to prevent contamination by careful attention to sterile technique [15]."

What finally prompted the FDA to review mercury in vaccines was not its own regulatory process, but rather an act of Congress. In 1997, Congress passed and the President signed into law, the Food and Drug

Administration Modernization Act (FDAMA). Among other things, this law required the FDA to compile a list of foods and drugs that contained intentionally-introduced mercury, study its effects on the human body, and restrict its use if found to be harmful.

Once the FDA did initiate its review of mercury in vaccines, it kicked off a vigorous debate among Federal regulators over the dangers of using Thimerosal in childhood vaccines. This debate, which at times pitted one health-care bureaucracy against another, has spanned more than four years. Given the fact that almost twenty years had passed since an expert panel had determined that Thimerosal was unsafe in topical ointments, it is surprising that there was any further debate at all.

There was tremendous reluctance on the part of some officials to admit that a mistake had been made in allowing ethylmercury to be used in vaccines. However, the institutional resistance to change was counter-balanced by the growing realization that there was more ethylmercury in childhood vaccines than previously thought, and that nobody had thought to calculate the cumulative amounts. The essence of the debate was captured in a 1999 e-mail from a former FDA official weighing the pros and cons of taking action. He opined that hastening the removal of Thimerosal from vaccines would "...raise questions about FDA being 'asleep at the switch' for decades by allowing a potentially hazardous compound to remain in many childhood vaccines, and not forcing manufacturers to exclude it from new products. It will also raise questions about various advisory bodies regarding aggressive recommendations for use. (We must keep in mind that the dose of ethylmercury was not generated by 'rocket science'. Conversion of the percentage Thimerosal to actual micrograms involves ninth grade algebra. What took the FDA so long to do the calculations? Why didn't CDC and the advisory bodies do these calculations when they rapidly expanded the childhood immunization schedule?) [5]"

It is clear that each time an important decision had to be made, the factions that were skeptical of Thimerosal's dangers and favored a "go-slow" approach, were able to water down the actions. In 1999, when the Federal government could have ordered Thimerosal removed from vaccines by a specific date, or stated a preference for Thimerosal-free vaccines, a statement was instead issued asking for a commitment from vaccine manufacturers to eliminate or reduce mercury in vaccines as expeditiously as possible. As a result, almost two years passed before the three major Thimerosal-containing vaccines–DTaP, Haemphilous influenza Type b (Hib), and hepatitis B–were being manufactured in Thimerosal-free formulations. In 2001, when the CDC and its influential advisory committee could have stated a preference for Thimerosal-free vaccines, they chose not to do so. As a result, Thimerosal-containing vaccines that remained in stock in doctors' offices continued to be used. In point of fact we have no proof that in 2003, some children in the United States were still not receiving Thimerosal-preserved vaccines that have lingered in medical offices or clinics. The CDC's decision not to endorse Thimerosal-free vaccines in 2001 is particularly troubling. With the exception of the influenza vaccine, all major childhood vaccines were being manufactured without Thimerosal at that time, so there was little threat of shortages. Their failure to state a preference was an additional abdication of their responsibility [5].

The task of analyzing the amount of mercury in vaccines and its ramifications was assigned to Dr. Leslie Ball, and pediatrician employed at the FDA, and her husband and colleague Dr. Robert Ball, a medical office at FDA's CBER. The pair developed two working conclusions following their review: (1) The recommended guidelines for exposure to methylmercury were a good starting point for reviewing exposure to ethylmercury; and (2) the amount of ethylmercury in children's vaccines exceeded the EPA's guidelines for exposure to methylmercury. An exchange of e-mails in October of 1998 makes clear that Dr. Leslie Ball was already leaning toward the removal of Thimerosal from vaccines. It also makes clear that there was internal resistance to such an action. Dr. Marion Gruber of the Office of Vaccine Research and Review forwarded an internal memo to Dr. Ball, which concluded, "...no scientific data to take regulatory actions and to recommend to take Thimerosal either out of vaccines or to leave it in." Dr. Ball's response on October 15, 1998 was sharp, "I disagree about the conclusion regarding no basis for removal of Thimerosal... However, there are factors/data that would argue for the removal of Thimerosal, including data on methylmercury exposure in infants and the knowledge that Thimerosal is not an essential component to vaccines. In addition, the European community is moving to ban Thimerosal [5]."

An important part of the FDA's review was a comparison of the amount of ethylmercury in vaccines to the recommended safe levels for exposure to methylmercury established by the EPA and the FDA. In 1999 (June 28, 1999), a consultant to the FDA, Dr. Barry Rumack, developed a pharmacokinetic model to analyze the amount of mercury to which infants were being exposed. The charts developed by Dr. Barry Rumack demonstrated that most children in the 1990s received doses of ethylmercury in their vaccines that exceeded the EPA's limits for exposure to methylmercury (0.1 micrograms per kilogram per day) for at least the first six months of their lives. Even more significantly, the charts also indicated that most children received doses of ethylmercury that exceeded the FDA's less-restrictive limits (0.4 micrograms per kilogram per day) for at least the first two months of their lives. It is noteworthy that the charts produced by Dr. Rumack, and the FDA's analysis in general, failed to take into consideration background levels of mercury to which children were exposed from other sources. Dr. Ball pointed out this weakness in her June 1999 e-mail, "These calculations do not account for other sources of Hg [mercury] in the environment. Even infants can have additional exposures, e.g., breast milk." One document written by Dr. Ball estimated that exposure to mercury from other sources than vaccines could total roughly 80 to 100 micrograms per year. Background levels were included in all calculations prepared by the European Medical Evaluation Agency (EMEA), which was at the time reviewing Thimerosal in vaccines in Europe [5].

In mid-June of 1999, CBER's findings came to the attention of Dr. Neal Halsey, Director of the Johns Hopkins Institute for Vaccine Safety. Halsey is a pediatrician and highly respected vaccine expert. When he learned of the CBER findings, he was finishing up a four-year term as chairperson of the AAP Committee on Infectious Diseases, the committee that determines AAP vaccination policy and edits the Red Book. Long before he heard about the Thimerosal findings, Halsey had become worried about the progress of vaccination protest groups in the United States. In May, Congress had held a contentious hearing on the dangers of vaccination. Halsey feared that the tide was turning against childhood vaccination, with potentially dangerous consequences. Halsey confirmed CBER's calculations and did his own research on mercury, consulting with experts around the country. He became convinced that the findings were worthy of alarm, and he worried if they became public prematurely, vaccination protesters would use them to stage yet another attack on the nation's immunization programs. Halsey met with officials as CBER on June 22nd and then called Dr. Walter Orenstein, director of the CDC's NIP [16].

The next day, on June 23, 1999, Dr. Halsey wrote a letter to the members of the AAP's Committee on Infectious Diseases that stated, "In the past few days, I have become aware that the amount of Thimerosal in most hepatitis B, DTaP and Hib vaccines that we administer to infants results in a total dose of mercury that exceeds the maximum exposure recommended by the EPA, the FDA, CDC, and WHO... [5]"

The EMEA, which is responsible for establishing guidelines for the use of drugs and biologics in the European Union, issued a report on June 29, 1999, following an initial meeting in London on April 19, 1999 (Dr. Norman Baylor of the FDA attended this meeting), encouraging the removal of Thimerosal from childhood vaccines: "Vaccines: The fact that the target population for vaccines in primary immunization schedules is a health one, and in view of the demonstrated risks of Thimerosal and other mercurial-containing preservatives, precautionary measures (as outlined below) could be considered...For vaccination in infants and toddlers, the use of vaccines without Thimerosal and other mercurial preservatives should be encouraged [5]."

On June 30th, NIP staff flew to Washington to meet with FDA, AAP, and vaccine manufacturers. From the start Halsey and his colleagues at AAP, including the new chairperson of the Infectious Disease Committee, Dr. Jon Abramson, took a strong proactive stance. They argued that physicians should be told – soon – about the amount of mercury in vaccines and the conflict with a federal guideline. CDC was surprised by the urgent and undoubting position taken by Halsey and his colleagues at AAP. CDC officials argued that there was no need for precipitous actions. They were loath to undermine confidence in existing vaccines by labeling some vaccines "bad" (Thimerosal-containing) and "good" (Thimerosal-free). But, in further discussions through the first few days of July, it became clear that Halsey and AAP would not retreat - they believed that immediate action was needed [17].

In a July 2, 1999 e-mail, Dr. Ruth Etzel of the Department of Agriculture also noted the Public Health Service's resistance: "We must follow three basic rules: (1) act quickly to inform pediatricians that the products have more mercury than we realized; (2) be open with consumers about why we didn't catch this earlier; (3)

show contrition. As you know, the Public Health Service informed us yesterday that they were planning to conduct business as usual, and would probably indicate no preference for either product. While the Public Health Service may think that their 'product' is immunizations, I think their 'product' is their recommendations. If the public loses faith in the Public Health Services recommendations, then the immunization battle will falter. To keep faith, we must be open and honest and move forward quickly to replace these products [5]."

Within AAP the issue ascended quickly from Halsey's committee to the executive board. AAP executives felt that their members needed more than just information about Thimerosal – they also needed a way to reduce mercury exposure in their tiny patients. They feared that pediatricians who continued to administer Thimerosal-containing vaccines could face a flurry of lawsuits, perhaps claiming that children had acquired learning disabilities from mercury exposure [17].

The discussion quickly veered toward pushing vaccine doses back from the first six months of life to a later time, when infants' bodies were larger and better able to tolerate mercury. Delaying vaccinations against DTP or Hib was not practical or could expose children to serious infections. It soon became evident that the delayed vaccine would have to be hepatitis B. Only two single-antigen pediatric hepatitis B vaccines exist on the United States' market. Energix-B (SmithKline Beecham) and Recombivax HB (Merck). Both contained Thimerosal and 12.5 micrograms of mercury per 0.5 ml dose. AAP pressed CDC to agree to a delay of the hepatitis B vaccination series, usually started at birth for children born to hepatitis surface antigen (HBsAg)-seronegative mothers. The Academy argued that the delay would only be temporary because both Merck and SmithKline Beecham had promised that they could quickly shift manufacturing to Thimerosal-free vaccine perhaps in just a few months. FDA had already promised to review applications for Thimerosal-free hepatitis B vaccine rapidly – within 30 days. At the CDC Hepatitis Branch in Atlanta, Dr. Harold Margolis, Chief of the Branch, and staff epidemiologist Eric Mast saw trouble. Margolis and Mast began working furiously to build a case against delaying hepatitis B vaccination [17].

Negotiations continued with AAP nearly around the clock. Everyone was becoming exhausted. AAP insisted on a six-month delay of hepatitis B vaccination of HBsAg-negative moms. CDC resisted. As the groups continued negotiations over days, worries increased that the story would leak to the press in an uncontrolled way, triggering a general vaccination scare. "Everyone worried that with the vaccination protest groups looking over our shoulders, if they got the sense that some [toxicological] standard was broken, all hell would break loose," said a senior official who worked on the issue. Finally, after a week of late night meetings involving the AAP executive board, Surgeon General Dr. David Satcher, CDC Director Dr. Jeffrey Koplan and other CDC officials, FDA, the manufacturers, and others, the exhausted group, struck a compromise. An AAP-USPHS joint statement was issued on July 7 at 4:15 PM [17].

Dr. Johns Clements, a physician from the World Health Organization (WHO) said at the NIH workshop regarding the United States' policy of removing Thimerosal from vaccines, "the U.S. has gone on its due process to identify a problem and correct it. But there is a knock-on effect which the world must bear as a consequence." Clements pointed out that only multi-dose, multi-puncture vials can be used in developing countries because of cost and cold-chain considerations. Removing Thimerosal from these vials is not an option for WHO, at least for the next several years, he said. In an August interview, Dr. Halsey defended the Thimerosal decision-making process used by AAP and CDC. It would not have been possible to deal with Thimerosal in the usual public forums like Advisory Committee on Immunization Practices (ACIP), Halsey said, because the presence of vaccination protestors would have made rational discussion hopeless. Deliberations were handled in the only way possible he said. But Halsey acknowledged that many of his immunization colleagues are angry with him and miffed about the way the issue was handled [17].

The joint statement that was released on July 7, 1999 by the AAP and the USPHS included the following points: (1) acknowledged that some children may have been exposed to levels of mercury that exceed one Federal guideline on methylmercury during the first six months of life; (2) asserted there is no evidence of any harm caused by Thimerosal in vaccines; (3) called on vaccine manufacturers to make a clear commitment to reduce as expeditiously as possible the mercury content of their vaccines; (4) urged doctors and parents to immunize all children, even if Thimerosal-free vaccines were not available; and (5) encouraged doctors and parents to postpone the hepatitis B vaccine (which contained Thimerosal at the time, and was generally given immediately after birth) until the child was two to six months old, unless the mother tested positive for hepatitis B [5].

Given the information that the Federal agencies had at the time, the plan of action laid out in the joint statement was inadequate. They could have, but did not, acknowledge that the amount of Thimerosal vaccines exceeded every Federal Guideline for exposure to methylmercury for the majority of infants. They could have, but did not, require vaccine manufacturers to remove Thimerosal from vaccines by a specific date. They could have, but did not urge pediatricians to choose Thimerosal-free vaccines when both Thimerosal-containing and Thimerosal-free vaccines were available. As a result of the limited steps taken in 1999, vaccines containing Thimerosal remained on the market for nearly two years. GlaxoSmithKline's hepatitis B vaccine did not become Thimerosal-free until March of 2000, and Aventis Pasteur's DTaP vaccine did not become Thimerosal-free until March 2001. In addition, Thimerosal-containing vaccines on the shelves in doctors' offices around the country continued to be used in spite of the fact that Thimerosal-free versions were available [5].

The fact that more forceful action to remove Thimerosal from the vaccine marketplace was not taken in 1999 is disappointing. Just as disappointing, and even more difficult to understand, is the fact that the CDC on two separate occasions refused to publicly state a preference for Thimerosal-free vaccines.

In June of 2000, the CDC's Advisory Committee on Immunization Practice met in Atlanta. Among other things, the Advisory Committee was called upon to recommend whether the CDC should issue a public statement of preference for Thimerosal-free vaccines. At the time, the industry was in the midst of transition to Thimerosal-free childhood vaccines, and several vaccines containing Thimerosal were still on the market. Of particular concern was the DTaP vaccine. In June of 2000, three of the four DTaP manufacturers (Aventis Pasteur, North American, and Wyeth) were still producing DTaP with Thimerosal. Only SmithKline Beecham produced a Thimerosal- free DTaP. In addition, because manufacturers of the Hib and hepatitis B vaccines had just recently converted to formulas that were Thimerosal-free or contained trace amounts of Thimerosal, older versions of these vaccines containing Thimerosal were still in inventories and being used around the country. A statement of preference by the CDC would have been a clear signal to pediatricians not to use vaccines containing Thimerosal, when Thimerosal-free versions were available. This action would have substantially reduced the exposure to ethylmercury for many infants. Despite this knowledge the advisory committee voted unanimously not to state a preference [5].

CDC officials guided the Advisory Committee toward this conclusion. For example, while three different options were presented to the Advisory Committee members, a detailed policy statement to be issued to the public had been prepared for only one of these options - as statement of no preference. In describing the three options, Dr. Roger Bernier of the CDC clearly indicated the CDC's desire not to state a preference for Thimerosal-free vaccines. He said, "We believe that such a policy would be consistent with the evidence that we have at this time. This policy seems to be working... As I said the policy seems to be working. So this indicates that on this particular factor, this policy is moving us in an upward direction towards-it's a positive thing [5]."

In rejecting a statement for preference of Thimerosal-free vaccines, the Advisory Committee considered a number of factors. These included a desire to avoid confusion, and a concern that immunization rates might fall, allowing for an outbreak of diseases such as pertussis or hepatitis B. However, one of the factors that was also considered was the financial health of the vaccine industry. In describing the pros and cons of each option, Dr. Bernier returned several times to financial issues: "We think that having this type of a more staged transition reduces the potential for financial losses of existing inventories, and is somewhat akin to what was done in the transition form oral polio to inactivated polio. It could entail financial losses of inventory if current vaccine inventory is wasted. It could harm one or more manufacturers and may then decrease the number of suppliers. The evidence justifying this kind of abrupt policy change does not appear to exist, and it could entail financial losses for all existing stocks of vaccines that contain Thimerosal [5]."

The financial health of industry should never have been a factor in this decision. The financial health of vaccine manufacturers certainly should never have been more important to the Federal health officials than the health and well being of the nation's children. The CDC has a responsibility to protect the health of the American public. If there were any doubts about the neurological effects of ethylmercury in vaccines on children - and there were substantial doubts – the prevailing consideration should have been how best to protect children from potential harm. However, it appears that protecting the industry's profits took precedence over protecting children from mercury damage [5].

In opting not to state a preference for Thimerosal-free vaccines, the Advisory Committee shrugged off two sensible proposals that were presented during the meeting. A representative of SmithKline Beecham stated that her company could supply sufficient amounts of Thimerosal-free DTaP vaccine to ensure that the youngest infants receive Thimerosal-free doses, "I think it's important that you know that, although we cannot supply the entire U.S. market right now for all five doses immediately, we would be able to supply the vast majority of the U.S. market for the primary series, that is with targeting of the first three doses." Given the repeated concerns expressed about the effects of mercury on the developing central nervous system in very young babies, ensuring Thimerosal-free doses for the first three doses of DTaP would seem to merit serious consideration. However, this suggestion was passed over without any comment. Later in the discussion, Dr. Neal Halsey made another suggestion that would limit the exposure of infants to ethylmercury. He suggested that the Advisory Committee adopt a policy that no children should receive more than one Thimerosal-containing vaccine per day, "Roger you said that after July, the maximum exposure will be 75 micrograms. My understanding from the manufacturers is that there really is some Hib out there in the market that is being used that does contain Thimerosal as a preservative. There also is hepatitis B out there that does contain it. So there's no guarantee the maximum exposure would be 75 micrograms. What I proposed last October was that they put a limit of one Thimerosal-containing vaccine as a preservative per visit which would then guarantee what you're looking for. And I think that's the right policy because that allows for the continued use, though very limited. It eliminates the maximum exposure, but you do have the problems of what's in the pipeline." Again, it appears that this seemingly sensible proposal received no serious consideration [5].

In July 2000 the Government Reform Committee of the United States Congress held hearings on mercury. Congresswoman Helen Chenoweth-Hage (R-ID) eloquently expressed the view of many: "...I have a staffer who is in the Navy Reserve right now, but he used to be active with the airborne divisions, and he was in for a test in one of the medical military hospitals, and upon taking his temperature, they broke a thermometer, and mercury splattered across his glasses and some got in his eye. Well, the first thing they did was cutoff his clothes. The second thing was call in OSHA to clean up the mercury. And then they worked on him to make sure his eyes were irrigated, and you guys, you witnesses, absolutely amaze me. I wonder where the disconnect is, for Pete's sake. You listened to the testimony just as I did, and you are willing to, with a straight face, tell us that you are eventually going to phase this out after we know that a small baby's body is slammed with 62 times the amount of mercury that it is supposed to have, and OSHA reacts like they did in the case of this accident of this naval man. It doesn't make sense. No wonder people are losing faith in their government. And to have one of the witnesses tell us it is because mothers eat too much fish? Come on. We expect you to get real. We heard devastating testimony in this hearing today, and we heard it last April. And this is the kind of response we get from our government agencies? I am sorry. When I was a little girl, my daddy talked to me about something about a duck test. I would ask each one of you to read this very excellent work by Sallie Bernard and Albert Enayati, who testified here today. My daddy used to say if it walks like a duck and talks like a duck and sounds like a duck, for Pete's sake it is a duck. I recommend that you read this, side-by-side, page after page of analysis of the symptoms of people who are affected with mercury poisoning compared to autism, this is the duck test, and you folks are trying to tell us that you can't take this off the market when 8,000 children are going to be injected tomorrow; 80 children may be coming down, beginning tomorrow with autism? What if there was an E. coli scare? What if there was a problem with an automobile? Their recall would be like that. We are asking you to do more than analyze it. We are asking you to tell this body and the American people that it is more than inconclusive. It passes the duck test, and we need you to respond. We need that to come off the market now because you think that we are elevating the case today? Just wait until it gets in the courts. This case could dwarf the tobacco case. And we would expect you to do something now before that circus starts taking place. Denial is not proper right now. You know, I still go back to the fact–I still want to talk about the duck test, Mr. Egan [FDA], I will address this to you. You know, it was shown in the last panel that autistic symptoms emerge after vaccination. It was shown that vaccines contain toxic doses of mercury. It was shown that autism and mercury poisoning, the physiological comparison is striking. There is altered neurotransmitter activity, abnormal brain neuronal organization, immune system disturbance, EEG abnormalities. It goes on and on and on, the comparisons. That is why I say, I back up what the Chairman and the ranking members are all asking you, that we cannot wait until 2001 to have this pulled off. You know, if a jury were to look at this, the circumstantial evidence would be overwhelming. Let's do something before we see it in the courts [5]."

One year later, in June of 2001, the Advisory Committee again rejected the idea of expressing a preference for Thimerosal-free vaccines, despite the fact that all manufacturers of Hib, hepatitis B and DTaP had shifted to Thimerosal-free products at that point. The CDC's decision not to express a preference for Thimerosal-free vaccines, and the Advisory Committee's concurrence in this policy, was an abdication of their responsibility. As a result of their inaction, children continued to receive vaccinations containing ethylmercury at a time when there were serious doubts about its safety [46].

What makes the CDC's decision even more vexing is that just prior to the Advisory Committee meeting in 2000, a study conducted by the CDC suggested that there was at least a weak correlation between exposure to Thimerosal and several types of neurological disorders. The study initiated in 1999 reviewed the medical records of 110,000 children in the CDC's Vaccine Safety Datalink (VSD). The VSD is a massive database that tracks the medical records of hundreds of thousands of patients belonging to seven major health maintenance organizations. Phase I of the study was designed to screen data for potential associations between Thimerosal-containing vaccines and selected neurological disorders. Phase II was designed to test the hypotheses generated in the first phase. Phase I produced a statistically-significant association between exposure to Thimerosal during the first three months of life and tics, attention deficit disorder, language and speech delays, and general neurodevelopmental delays. The study did not find a correlation between Thimerosal and autism because the sample size of children diagnosed with autism was in all probability not large enough [5].

The findings of Dr. Verstraeten, the primary author of the study, set off a fierce debate within the Federal health agencies when they were internally released in June 2000. Enough concern was generated that a closed-private conference of medical experts was assembled at the Simpsonwood Retreat Center near Atlanta. Among those in attendance included representatives from CDC, FDA, Aventis Pasteur, Wyeth, Merck, SmithKline Beecham, and North American Vaccine. The following are some statements that were recorded as part of the official transcript, and illustrate the conspiratorial acts committed:

Dr. Bernier: Page 113: "We have asked you to keep this information confidential... So we are asking people who have done a great job protecting this information up until now, to continue to do that until the time of the ACIP meeting...That would help all of us to use the machinery that we have in place for considering these data and for arriving at policy recommendations."

Dr. Verstraeten: Page 31: "It is sort of interesting that when I first came to the CDC as a NIS officer a year ago only, I didn't really know what I wanted to do, but one of the things I knew I didn't want to do was studies that had to do with toxicology or environmental health. Because I thought it was too much confounding and it's very hard to prove anything in those studies. Now it turns out that other people also thought that this study was not the right thing to do, so what I will present to you is the study that nobody thought we should do."

Dr. Verstraeten: Page 40: "...we have found statistically significant relationships between the exposures and outcomes for these different exposures and outcomes. First, for two months of age, an unspecified developmental delay which has its own specific ICD-9 code. Exposure at three months of age–Tics. Exposure at six months of age–an attention deficit disorder. Exposure at one, three and six months of age–language and speech delays which are two separate ICD-9 codes. Exposure at one, three and six months of age–the entire category of neurodevelopmental delays, which includes all of these plus a number of other disorders."

Dr. Weil: Page 75: "I think that what you are saying is in term of chronic exposure. I think that the alternative scenario is that this is repeated acute exposures, and like many repeated acute exposures, if you consider a dose of 25 micrograms on one day, then you are above threshold. At least we think you are, and then you do that over and over to a series of neurons where the toxic effect may be the same set of neurons or the same set of neurologic processes; it is conceivable that the more mercury you get, the more effect you are going to get."

Dr. Chen: Page 151: "One of the reasons that led me personally to not be so quick to dismiss the findings was that on his own Tom independently picked three different outcomes that he did not think could be associated with mercury (conjunctivitis, diarrhea and injury) and three out of three had a different pattern across different exposure levels as compared to the ones that again on a priority basis we picked as biologically plausible to be due to mercury exposure."

Dr. Johnston: Page 198: "This association leads me to favor a recommendation that infants up to two years old not be immunized with Thimerosal containing vaccines if suitable alternative preparations are available… My gut feeling? It worries me enough. Forgive this personal comment, but I got called out a eight o'clock for an emergency call and my daughter-in-law delivered a son by C-Section. Our first male in the line of the next generation, and I do not want that grandson to get a Thimerosal containing vaccine until we know better what is going on. It will probably take a long time. In the meantime, and I know there are probably implications for this internationally, but in the meantime I think I want that grandson to only be given Thimerosal-free vaccines."

Dr. Weil: Page 207: "The number of dose related relationships are linear and statistically significant. You can play with this all you want. They are linear. They are statistically significant. The positive relationships are those that one might expect from the Faeroe Islands studies. They are also related to those data we do have on experimental animal data and similar to the neurodevelopmental tox data on other substances, so that I think you can't accept that this is out of the ordinary. It isn't out of the ordinary."

Dr. Brent: Page 229: "The medical legal findings in this study, causal or not, are horrendous and therefore, it is important that the suggested epidemiological, pharmacokinetic, and animal studies be performed. If an allegation was made that a child's neurobehavioral findings were caused by Thimerosal-containing vaccines, you could readily find a junk scientist who would support the claim with 'a reasonable degree of certainty.' But you will not find a scientist with any integrity who would say the reverse with the data that is available. And that is true. So we are in a bad position from the standpoint of defending any lawsuits if they were initiated and I am concerned."

Dr. Clements: Page 247: "I am really concerned that we have taken off like a boat going down one arm of the mangrove swamp at high speed, when in fact there was not enough discussion really early on about which way the boat should go at all. And I really want to risk offending everyone in the room by saying that perhaps this study should not have been done at all, because the outcome of it could have, to some extent, been predicted, and we have all reached this point now where we are left hanging, even though I hear the majority of consultants say to the Board that they are not convinced there is a causality direct link between Thimerosal and various neurological outcomes. I know how we handle it from here is extremely problematic. The ACIP is going to depend on comments from this group in order to move forward into policy, and I have been advised that whatever I say should not move into the policy area because that is not the point of this meeting. But nonetheless, we know from many experiences in history that the pure scientist has done research because of pure science. But that pure science has resulted in splitting the atom or some other process which is completely beyond the power of the scientists who did the research to control it. And what we have here is people who have, for every best reason in the world, pursued a direction of research. But there is now the point at which the research results have to be handled, and even if this committee decides that there is no association and that information gets out, the work that has been done and through the freedom of information that will be taken by others, will be used in ways beyond the control of this group. And I am very concerned about that as I suspect it is already too late to do anything regardless of any professional body and what they say … [18]"

It was clear in subsequent documents that Dr. Verstraeten was not pleased with the response to his study. During the Simpsonwood conference he stated, "When I saw this, and I went back through the literature, I was actually stunned by what I saw – because I thought it was plausible." A month later he sent an e-mail to Dr. Phillippe Grandjean, the author of several groundbreaking studies on the toxicity of mercury. Dr Verstraeten wrote, "I know that much of this is very hypothetical and, personally, I would rather not drag the Faeroe and Seychelles studies into this entire Thimerosal debate, as I think they are as comparable as apples and pears at the best. Unfortunately, I have witnessed how many experts, looking at this Thimerosal issue, do not seem bothered to compare apples to pears and insist as if nothing is happening in these studies, then nothing should be feared of Thimerosal. I do not wish to be the advocate of the anti-vaccine lobby and sound as if I am convinced that Thimerosal is or was harmful; but at least I feel we should use sound scientific argumentation, and not let our standards be dictated by our desire to disprove an unpleasant theory [5]."

It appears that many who participated in the Thimerosal debates allowed their standards to be dictated by their desire to disprove an unpleasant theory [5].

Phase II of the VSD study, which provided enough data to analyze only speech delay and attention deficit disorder, did not detect an association between those disorders and Thimerosal, as had Phase I. In part, Phase II of the VSD study failed to confirm the findings of Phase I because of the small sample size employed (16,000 as opposed to 110,000 children in Phase I) [5]. Additionally, at the time that the Phase II data was brought in from a Massachusetts HMO (Harvard Pilgrim, HP): HP was in receivership by the state of Massachusetts; its computer records had been in shambles for years; it had multiple computer systems that could not communicate with one another; it used a health care coding system totally different from the one used across the VSD; and there are significant questions relating to a significant underreporting of autism in the state of Massachusetts [19].

In November 2003, an article was published by Verstraeten et al. in *Pediatrics* reporting on the CDC results of their VSD analysis of Thimerosal and neurodevelopmental disorders [53]. On October 31, 2003, Congressman Dr. Weldon wrote a letter to Julie Gerberding, Director of the CDC, stating, "I have reviewed the article and have serious reservations about the four-year evolution and conclusions of this study." The Congressman continued: "I am a strong supporter of childhood vaccinations and know that they have saved us from considerable death and suffering. A key part of our vaccination program is to ensure that we do everything possible to ensure that these vaccines, which are mandatory, are as safe as possible. We must fully disclose adverse events. Anything less than this undermines public confidence. I have read the upcoming *Pediatrics* study and several earlier versions of this study dating back to February 2000. I have read various e-mails from Dr. Verstraeten and coauthors. I have reviewed the transcripts of a discussion at Simpsonwood, GA between the author, various CDC employees and vaccine industry representatives. I have found a disturbing pattern… A review of these documents leaves me very concerned that rather than seeking to understand whether or not some children were exposed to harmful levels of mercury in childhood vaccines in the 1990s, there may have been a selective use of the data to make the associations in the earliest study disappear… Furthermore, the lead author of the article, Dr. Thomas Verstraeten, worked for the CDC until he left over two years ago to work for GlaxoSmithKline (GSK), a vaccine manufacturer facing liability over TCVs [Thimerosal-containing vaccines]. In violation of their own standards of conduct, *Pediatrics* failed to disclose that Dr. Verstraeten is employed by GSK and incorrectly identifies him as an employee of the CDC. This revelation undermines this study further. The first version of the study, produced in February 2000, found a significant association between exposure to TCVs and autism and neurological developmental delays (NDDs). When comparing children exposed to 62.5 :g [micrograms] of mercury by 3 months of age to those exposed to less than 37.5 :g, the study found a relative risk for autism of 2.48 for those with the higher exposure levels… For NDDs the study found a relative risk of 1.59 and a definite upward trend as exposure levels increased. A June 2000 version of the study applied various data manipulations to reduce the autism association to 1.69 and the authors went outside of the VSD database to secure data from a Massachusetts HMO (Harvard Pilgrim, HP) in order to counter the association found between TCVs and speech delay. At the time that HP's data was brought in, HP was in receivership by the state of Massachusetts, its computer records had been in shambles for years, it had multiple computer systems that could not communicate with one another, and it used a health care coding system totally different from the one used across the VSD. There are questions relating to a significant underreporting of autism in Massachusetts. The HP dataset is only about 15% of the HMO dataset used in the February 2000 study. There may also be significant problems with the statistical power of the dataset. In June 2000 a meeting was held in Simpsonwood, GA, involving the authors of the study, representatives of the CDC, and the vaccine industry. I have reviewed a transcript of this meeting that was obtained through the Freedom of Information Act (FOIA). Comments from Simpsonwood, meeting include: (summary form, not direct quotes): We found a statistically significant relationship between exposures and outcomes. There is certainly an under ascertainment of adverse outcomes because some children are just simply not old enough to be diagnosed, the current incidence rates are much lower than we would expect to see (Verstraeten); we could exclude the lower exposure children from our database. Also suggested was removing the children that got the highest exposure levels since they represented an unusually high percentage of outcomes (Rhodes); the significant association with language delay is quite large (Verstraeten); this information should be kept confidential and considered embargoed; we can push and pull this data anyway we want to get the results we want; we can alter the exclusion criteria any way we want, give reasonable justifications for doing so, and get any result we want; There was really no need to do this study. We could have predicted the outcomes; I will not give TCVs to my grandson until I find out what is going on here. Another version of the study – after further manipulation – finds no association between TCVs and autism, and no consistency across HMOs between TCVs and NDDs and speech delay. The final version of the study concludes that "No consistent significant associations were found between TCVs and neurodevelopmental outcomes," and that the lack of consistency argues against an association. In reviewing the study there are data points where children with higher exposures to the neurotoxin mercury had fewer developmental disorders. This demonstrates to me how excessive manipulation of data can lead to absurd results. Such a conclusion is not unexpected from an author with a serious, though undisclosed, conflict of interest. This study increases speculation of an association between TCVs and neurodevelopmental outcomes. I cannot say it was the author's intent to eliminate the earlier findings of an association. Nonetheless, the elimination of this association is exactly what happened and the manner in which this was achieved raises speculation. The dialogue at the Simpsonwood meeting clearly indicates how easily the authors could manipulate the data and have reasonable sounding justifications for many of their decisions. The only way these issues are going to be resolved – and I have only mentioned a few of them – is by making this particular dataset and the entire VSD dataset open for independent analysis. One such independent researcher, Dr. Mark Geier, has already been approved by the CDC and the various IRBs to access this dataset. They have requested the CDC allow them to access this dataset and your staff indicated to my office that they would make this particular dataset available after the *Pediatrics* study is published. Earlier this month the CDC had prepared three similar datasets for this researcher to review to allow him to reanalyze CDC study datasets. However when they accessed the datasets – which the researchers paid the CDC to assemble – the datasets were found to have no usable data in them. I request that you personally intervene with those in the CDC who are assembling this dataset to ensure that they provide the complete dataset, in a usable format, to these researchers within two weeks. The treatment these well-published researchers have received from the CDC thus far has been abysmal and embarrassing. I would be curious to know whether Dr. Verstraeten, an outside researcher for more than two years now, was required to go through the same process as Dr. Geier in order to continue accessing the VSD [19]."

The lead author, Dr. Verstraeten has subsequently published a letter to the editor in which he concluded that his study was neutral (i.e., could neither accept nor reject a causal relationship) regarding the relationship between Thimerosal and NDDs [21].

A report prepared by the staff of the Subcommittee on Human Rights and Wellness, Committee on Government Reform of the United States' House of Representatives, concluded following a three-year investigation: The Food and Drug Administration's (FDA) mission is to "promote and protect the public health by helping safe and effective products reach the market in a timely way, and monitoring products for continued safety after they are in use." However, the FDA uses a subjective barometer in determining when a product that has known risks can remain on the market. According to the agency, "at the heart of all FDA's product evaluation decisions is a judgment about whether a new product's benefits to users will outweigh its risks. No regulated product is totally risk-free, so these judgments are important. FDA will allow a product to present more of risk when its potential benefit is great – especially for products used to treat serious, life-threatening conditions." This argument – that known risks of infectious diseases outweigh a potential risk of neurological damage from exposure to Thimerosal in vaccines – is one that has continuously been presented to the Committee by government officials. FDA officials have stressed that any possible risk from Thimerosal was theoretical, that no proof of harm existed. However, the Committee, upon a through review of the scientific literature and internal documents from government and industry, did find evidence that Thimerosal did pose a risk. Thimerosal used as a preservative in vaccines is likely related to the autism epidemic. This epidemic in all probability may have been prevented or curtailed had the FDA not been asleep at the switch regarding the lack of safety data regarding injected Thimerosal and the sharp rise of infant exposure to this known neurotoxin. Our public health agencies' failure to act is indicative of institutional malfeasance for self-protection and misplaced protectionism of the pharmaceutical industry [5].

Additionally, the U.S. Office of Special Counsel (OSC), an independent federal agency, has issued a letter to Congress stating: "I have recently received hundreds of disclosures from private citizens alleging a widespread danger to the public health, specifically to infants and toddlers, caused by childhood vaccines which include Thimerosal, a mercury-containing preservative... The disclosures allege that Thimerosal/mercury is still present in childhood vaccines, contrary to statements made by HHS agencies, HHS Office of Investigations and the American Academy of Pediatrics. According to the information provided, vaccines containing 25 micrograms of mercury and carrying expiration dates of 2005 continue to be produced and administered. In addition, the disclosures allege, among other things, that some datasets showing a relationship between Thimerosal/mercury and neurological disorders no longer exist, that independent researchers have been arbitrarily denied access to the Centers for Disease Control and Prevention (CDC) databases, and that government-sponsored studies have not assessed the genetic vulnerabilities of subpopulations. Due to their heightened concern that additional datasets may be destroyed, these citizens urge the immediate safeguarding of the Vaccine Safety Datalink database and other relevant CDC information so that critical data are not lost. The disclosures also allege that the CDC and the Food and Drug Administration colluded with pharmaceutical companies at a conference in Norcross, Georgia, in June 2000 to prevent the release of a study which showed a statistical correlation between Thimerosal/mercury exposure through pediatric vaccines and neurological disorders including autism, Attention-Deficit/Hyperactivity Disorder, stuttering, tics, and speech and language delays. Instead of releasing the data presented at the conference, the author of the study, Dr. Thomas Verstraeten, later published a different version of the study in the November 2003 issue of *Pediatrics*, which did not show a statistical correlation. No explanation has been provided for this discrepancy. Finally, the disclosures allege that there is an increasing body of clinical evidence on the connection of Thimerosal/mercury exposure to neurological disorders which is being ignored by government public health agencies... I believe that these allegations raise serious continuing concerns about the administration of the nation's vaccine program and the government's possibly inadequate response to the growing body of scientific research on the public health danger of mercury in vaccines. The allegations also present troubling information regarding children's cumulative exposure to mercury and the connection of that exposure to the increase in neurological disorders such as autism and autism-related conditions among children in the US [22]."

Acknowledgement

The Editorial Staff of *MedicalVeritas* wishes to thank David Geier for his contribution of sources and information that proved invaluable to this article.

References

[1] Seal D, Ficker L, Wright P, Andrews V. The Case Against Thimerosal. Lancet 1991;338:315–6.

[2] http://www.aafp.org/x7666.xml

[3] Subcommittee on Human Rights and Wellness, Government Reform Committee. Mercury in Medicine Report. Washington, DC: Congressional Record, May 21, 2003:E1011–30.

[4] Institute of Medicine (US). *Immunization Safety Review: Thimerosal-containing Vaccines and Neurodevelopmental Disorders*. Washington, DC: National Academy Press, 2001.

[5] *Mercury in Medicine Report*, 2003.
[6] Warkany J, Hubbard DM. Acrodynia and mercury. J Pediatr 1953; 42:365–86.
[7] Nelson EA, Gottshall RY. Enhanced toxicity for mice of pertussis vaccines when preserved with mertiolate. Appl Microbiol 1967;15:590–3.
[8] Heyworth MF, Truelove SC. Problems associated with the use of merthiolate as a preservative in anti-lymphocytic globulin. Toxicology 1979;12:325–33.
[9] Trypohonas L, Nielsen NO. Pathology of chronic alkylmercurial poisoning in swine. Am J Vet Res 1973;34:379–92.
[10] Fagan DG, Pritchard JS, Clarkson TW, Greenwood MR. Organ mercury levels in infants with omphaloceles treated with organic mercurial antiseptic. Arch Dis Child 1977;52:962–4.
[11] Forstrom L, Hannuksela M, Kousa M, Lehmuskallio E. Merthiolate hypersensitivity and vaccination. Contact Dermatitis 1980;6:241–5.
[12] Kravchenko AT, Dzagurov SG, Chervonskaia GP. Evaluation of the toxic action of prophylactic and therapeutic preparations on cell cultures paper III: The detection of toxic properties in medical biological preparations by the degree of cell damage in the L-132 continuous cell-line. Zh Mikrobiol Epidemiol Immunobiol 1983;3:87–92.
[13] Winship KA. Organic mercury compounds and their toxicity. Adv Drug React Ac Pois Rev 1986;3:141–80.
[14] Cox NH, Forsyth A. Thimerosal allergy and vaccination reactions. Contact Dermatitis 1988;18:229–33.
[15] Stetler HC, Garbe PL, Swyer DM, Facklam RR, Orenstein WA, West GR, Dudley J, Bloch AB. Outbreaks of Group A Streptococcal abscesses following Diphtheria-Tetanus Toxoid-Pertussis vaccination. Pediatrics 1985;75:299–303.
[16] Shaw FE (ed). *Hepatitis Control Report – Uproar over a little-known preservative, Thimerosal, jostles U.S. hepatitis B vaccination policy*. Summer 1999;4(2).
[17] *Hepatitis Control Report*, 1999.
[18] Simpsonwood Transcript. June 7-8, 2000 in Norcross, Georgia. Obtained under the Freedom of Information Act (FOIA).
[19] Congressman Dr. Weldon Letter to Julie Gerberding, Director of the CDC, October 31, 2003. Journal of Law, Ethics and Medicine, September 22, 2000.
[20] Verstaeten T, Davis RL, DeStefano F, Lieu TA, Rhodes PH, Black SB et al. Safety of Thimerosal-containing vaccines: a two-phased study of computerized health maintenance organization databases. Pediatrics 2003;112:1039–48.
[21] Verstraeten T. Thimerosal, the Centers for Disease Control and Prevention, and GlaxoSmithKline. Pediatrics 2004;113:932.
[22] Special Counsel Scott Bloch's Letter to Congress, May 20, 2004.

Appendix V. Shaken Baby Syndrome (SBS): General Commentary

Harold E. Buttram, MD, FAAEM
Woodlands Healing Research Institution
5724 Clymer Road
Quakertown, Pennsylvania 18951
Email: hbuttram@woodmed.com

Abstract

On August 16, 2003, I received the following communication from a grandmother, whose first name is Sharon, somewhat in the fashion of a desperate plea for help on behalf of her daughter, who has been accused of injuring her infant daughter by Shaken Baby Syndrome (SBS). As a poignant example of what I consider to be ill-advised administration of vaccines to a highly fragile and vulnerable infant, I thought that this story needs to be told, which I am now doing with the permission of the grandmother and her daughter. My response to the letter can in no way be construed as a medical report but rather as a general commentary on my observations in reviewing numerous cases of the SBS during the past four years.

Keywords: Shaken Baby Syndrome (SBS), retinal hemorrhages, fragile infants

Introduction

The information about the case includes the following message from the grandmother:

> My daughter had 'Twin Transfusion Syndrome.' It was diagnosed in her twenty-fifth (25th) or twenty-sixth (26th) week. She had an amniocentesis three or four times, as Baby B was stuck to the wall of the uterus. The syndrome progressed. It took its toll, and at twenty-nine weeks we lost Baby B.
>
> Her…ObGyn physician wanted her to continue her pregnancy until thirty-five weeks to ensure that Baby A was developed and that her lungs matured. That was the safest thing to do, I felt as well. However, we were told to watch for any discharge with dark color, foul odor, things of that nature. When my daughter developed a dark brown discharge, the doctor on call did a full pelvic exam, including use of a speculum. Two hours after returning home from the examination her water broke.
>
> I then took her back to the hospital and she was admitted. She stayed in the hospital five days after which labor was induced with delivery of a baby girl weighing 2 lbs and 14 ounces. The baby's APGARs were 1 at one minute, 5 at five minutes, and 6 at six minutes. The baby stayed in a newborn intensive care unit for 2 months and was, for example, diagnosed with milk pulmonary valve stenosis, ventricular septal defect, anemia of prematurity, apnea and bradycardia, suspected necrotizing enterocolitis-medical, bloody stools, and hyperbilirubinemia.
>
> After discharge from the hospital the baby was visited two or three times a week by a visiting nurse. At approximately two months of age the baby was administered four shots - the DTaP, Hib, IPV, and Prevnar vaccines. She did not do well after the shots. She wasn't eating well. She was fussy and cried with high-pitched screams. Her mother took her to the doctor because she was jerking the second day following the vaccines, but he was not concerned. She then took her to the sitter where the baby became lifeless. The sitter did not summon help, nor did she call my daughter until it was time to get off work. My baby granddaughter was taken to the ER that night where she was having seizures back-to-back and was

> admitted to the hospital. Three days later the attending physician said he thought the baby had been injured by Shaken Baby Syndrome.
>
> An MRI confirmed she had a brain they expected to see from a baby that weighed less than 3 pounds. There was no blood on the brain or in the spinal fluid. There were no rib fractures. She had no bruises or broken bones. She has never missed a doctor's appointment. She was on a heart monitor which showed no motion artifacts. *All she had were retinal hemorrhages...*
>
> My granddaughter was a 30-week gestation baby, small for gestational age...will this SBS stuff ever fade away?

As a sequel to the story, based on the lone finding of retinal hemorrhages, the baby was removed from custody of the mother and placed in a foster home. The grandmother, who is now disabled and unable to work, is trying to gain custody of the baby.

Analysis and General Commentary

In the next 25 years or so, when there is greater knowledge about the adverse reactions and aftermath from current childhood vaccine programs, physicians and scientists, as well as the lay public, may look back on these programs with embarrassment if not worse. This is not to say that vaccines do not have a proper role in preventive health, which they do, but not with neglect of safety considerations, of which in my opinion this case serves as an example.

The rationale for these statements is based largely on the work of Dr. Archivedes Kalokerinos, who worked as a medical officer among the Australian aborigines in the "outback" in the 1960s and 1970s. Being troubled by very high infant mortality, in some areas approaching 50%, he began to investigate possible causes. Having noticed signs of scurvy in some of the infants, and observing that the children often died following immunizations, especially if they had colds or minor respiratory infections, the thought occurred to him that there might be a connection between vitamin C deficiency and deaths following vaccines. With improved nutrition, routine oral vitamin C supplementation of children and infants, *avoidance of immunizations during minor illnesses, even if just a runny nose,* and large doses of injectable vitamin C during crises, infant mortality was virtually abolished. Although Kalokerinos was awarded the Australian Medal of Merit in 1978 for his work, it has never been acknowledged by mainstream medicine. What is worse, it has never been subjected to systematic, meaningful scientific study.

With the work and clinical observations of Dr Kalokerinos in mind, I would next like to turn to the work of attorney Toni Blake of San Diego, who specializes in defending parents and caretakers accused of shaken baby syndrome, and who has described a pattern he has noted with these infants. They tend to have the following characteristics: (1) All babies came from problem pregnancies including prematurity, low birth weights, maternal diabetes or toxemia of pregnancy, maternal drugs or alcohol, (or other prenatal risk factors involving immaturity or compromise of the liver, kidneys, and immune system); (2) all had subdural brain hemorrhages; (3) many had fractures; (4) infant complications occurred in clusters around 2 months, 4 months, and 6 months of age; (5) most infant complications and collapses occurred with 11 or 12 days of vaccinations. (Personal communications 2000 and 2002)

In my opinion, the observations of attorney Toni Blake may hold a key to what is happening in many of these infants now being (mis)diagnosed as victims of shaken baby syndrome; that is, the ill-advised vaccination of fragile infants, as described above, and/or the vaccination in the presence of minor viral or bacterial infections. What is happening in these infants?

In contrast to classical scurvy of earlier times in the days of wooden sailing ships, when scurvy was characterized by a total lack of Vitamin C, what we may be seeing today is something quite different. As described by Dr. Kalokerinos [1] and Alan Clemetson, MD [2] subclinical scurvy is a condition in which apparently healthy infants with marginally low but adequate levels of Vitamin C in unstressed conditions may be suddenly thrown into states of critical Vitamin C depletion by combinations of stresses from common infections and toxins, including the toxins found in vaccines. As one example of marginal Vitamin C deficiency on the modern scene, in a study of people attending an HMO (Health Maintenance Organization Clinic) in Tempe, Arizona in 1998, 30% were found to be depleted with plasma Vitamin C levels between 0.2 and 0.5 mgs/100 ml and to be deficient in 6% with levels below 0.2% [3]. In regards to infants, it is true that infant formulas have been mandated to include Vitamin C at levels providing the required 30 mgs per day. However, this is a maintenance level and makes no allowances for additional stresses which may bring about many-fold increases in need for Vitamin C. Common colds, for instance, have been shown to reduce Vitamin C levels up to 50%[4]. No one knows the effects of vaccines on Vitamin C levels in infants, because before-and-after studies of this type have never been done, but Vitamin C is known to neutralize the toxins of diphtheria [5-8], tetanus [9], typhoid endotoxin [10], and four varieties of gas gangrene [11]. As will be described below, in the process of neutralizing these toxins, Vitamin C is necessarily used up and depleted.

(Note: If the reader will consult with these references, which were extracted from an article by A Clemetson [12], it will be found that most of these studies are quite old and some published in foreign languages. To me that is the pity of it, as our own scientific and medical system has never recognized their importance or followed through with further investigations.)

It is seldom appreciated that vaccines contain a variety of toxins. In addition to bacterial endotoxins and attenuated live viruses, depending on the vaccines, vaccines may also contain formaldehyde, mercury, aluminum phosphate, antibiotics, phenols, alcohols, mineral oils, animal serums, animal DNA, chicken embryo, aborted fetal tissue (in measles, mumps, rubella, and chicken pox vaccines), Simian Cytomegalo Virus (CMV) in oral polio vaccines, and Mycoplasma. (This list of ingredients has been compiled from current *Physicians' Desk Reference* manuals and from report in the medical literature in the cases of Simian CMV and Mycoplasma).

Returning to the importance of vitamin C in relation to vaccines, one of the prime roles of Vitamin C in the body is its action as an antioxidant in donating electrons to quench free-radial inflammatory damage from infections and/or toxins, with our consideration here being vaccine toxins. However, in the process of donating electrons, Vitamin C necessarily becomes depleted. Once the level of Vitamin C is reduced to the point that it can no longer protect the brain, which is unduly susceptible to toxic and infectious damage, it (the brain) may become subject to free-radical damage. By definition "free-radicals" consist of oxygen molecules with an odd number of electrons in their outer orbits. When uncontrolled, these can be very destructive to the body, such as may take place when exposed to harmful radiation. Vitamin C is critically important in protecting against free-radical proliferation because, in donating electrons, it neutralizes the unpaired electrons in the "free-radical" oxygen molecules. Of all the organs of the body, the brain appears to be most vulnerable to this type of damage because of its relatively high fat content.

For these reasons, the combination of ill-advised vaccines given to fragile infants, as in the present case, with highly immature detoxification organs (liver and kidneys) and immature immune systems, or as often takes place, in the presence of viral or bacterial infections, is in my opinion an invitation to disaster with the brain being potentially subjected to a firestorm of free-radical inflammatory damage. I believe that this is what is likely happening in many of these infants. Once this pattern has been set in motion, there is a variable latent period with gradual progression of inflammatory brain swelling commonly complicated by brain and retinal hemorrhages. As the brain continues to swell, the breathing center, located at the base of the brain, may become herniated into the spinal canal and become constricted, this in turn resulting in respiratory arrest and collapse. In other instances there may be seizures, as in the present case. Among the cases of SBS that I have reviewed, I have found these to be common patterns, too frequent to be coincidental.

As described in his autobiography, Dr. Kalokerinos describes the mechanisms involved in the production of brain edema with retinal and brain hemorrhages in much the same fashion:

1. Endotoxin (endogenous and/or from vaccines) damages the endothelial linings of the brain's blood vessels.
2. Endotoxin then 'leaks' through to the surrounding brain tissue. This includes the retina that is an extension of the brain.
3. The brain tissue is damaged.

4. The blood supply to the portions of the brain involved is reduced.
5. Insufficient oxygen, glucose, and Vitamin C follows.
6. Parts of the brain are 'rich' in 'bound' (controlled) iron. This is released.
7. Violent free radical reactions result and these cannot be controlled because of a lack of immediately available Vitamin C and other antioxidants.
8. So further, and rapid, brain tissue damage results, with more free radical reactions.
9. Hemorrhages occur in the area/areas involved.
10. After a variable period (depending on a host of factors) some of the red blood cells in the hemorrhages break down and release their stores of iron and copper.
11. This results in a further cascade of free radical reactions and tissue destruction.
12. Cerebral edema (brain swelling) occurs.

By way of comparison, in Vienna in the 1840s, long before recognition of the importance of sanitation and the role of microbes in causing disease, a doctor named Ignaz Semmelweis was assigned to an obstetrical post at a birthing center which was notorious for its high maternal mortality rates. Based on simple observation, Semmelweis deduced that doctors and nurses were carrying infections from one patient to another and subsequently required that they wash their hands between patients. As a result, the mortality rate among maternity patients under his care was reduced from nearly 30% in other wings of the hospital to less than 2% for patients under his care or supervision.

Was Semmelweis honored by his peers for this discovery? No, at least not at that time. Instead he was dismissed from the hospital staff because his procedures did not conform to the medical thinking of the time. In the case of Dr. Archivedes Kalokerinos, could history be repeating itself?

References

[1] Kalokerinos, A. *Medical Pioneer of the 20th Century, an Autobiography,* Dr. Archivedes Kalokerinos, Biology Therapies Publishing, Braeside, Melbourne, Victoria, Australia, Fax 011-61-39587-1720, Publ.2000.

[2] Clemetson CAB. *Vitamin C,* Volume I in a 3-volume set, CRC Press, Boca Raton, 1989, pages 215–21.

[3] Johnston CS, Thompson MS. Vitamin C status of an out-patient population, *J Amer Col Nutr,* 1998; 17:366–70.

[4] Hume R, Weyers E. Changes in the leucocyte ascorbic acid concentration during the common cold, *Scot Med J,* 1973; 18:3.

[5] Zvirbely JL, Szent-Gyorgyi A. The chemical nature of vitamin C, *Biochem J,* 1932; 27:279–85.

[6] King CG, Waugh WA. The chemical nature of vitamin C, *J Science,* 1932; 75:357–8.

[7] Harde E. Acide ascorbique (vitamin C) et intoxications, *CR Acad Sci,* 1934; 119:618–20.

[8] Parrot JL. Richet. Accroissement de la sensabilite a histamine chez le cobaye sournis a un regime scorbutogene, *CR Soc Biol,* 1945;139:1072–5.

[9] Dey PK. Efficiency of vitamin C in counteracting tetanus toxin toxicity, *Naturwissenchaften,* 1966; 53:310.

[10] Fukada T. Koyama T. Prevention by ascorbic acid of liver glycogen depletion in endotoxin intoxication, *Nature* (London) 1963;200:1327.

[11] Buller Souto A, Lima C. Activity of L-ascorbic acid on the toxins of gas gangrene, Vol 12, Sao Paul, Brazil: Memorias do instituto Butantan, 1939:265–95.

[12] Sircus MA. Clemetson A. Barlow's disease, *Medical Hypothesis*, 2002; 59(1):52–6.

Appendix VI. Interview with Dr. Mark Geier and David Geier concerning Thimerosal, Testosterone, and Autism Treatment Hypothesis

Mark R. Geier[a], MD, PhD; David A. Geier[b], BA; Teri Small[c]
[b]Genetic Centers of America
[b]MedCon, Inc.
[c]AutismOne Radio
1816 Houston Ave.
Fullerton, CA 92833 USA
Phone: +1 714 680 0792
Email: tsmall@autismone.org Website: www.autismone.org

Abstract

In this transcript of an interview given by Dr. Mark and David Geier, these researchers provide insight into the growing proof of Thimerosal toxicity manifesting in children after routine vaccinations, as evidenced within the CDC's own Vaccine Safety Datalink (VSD) database. The interview conducted on January 13, 2005, gives indication of cover-ups on the part of senior public health officials, who have found within the statistics of VSD such compelling evidence that they are unable to obfuscate it with statistical manipulations. Topics broached include illegal collusion of authorities with industry; perjury from experts in sworn testimonies before Congress; and non-cooperation with Congressional orders that independent bodies (namely the Geiers) access the critical VSD data. The public health ramifications for the nation are discussed, as well as the possible mechanisms of Thimerosal's adverse neurodevelopmental outcomes, and—if this assessment turns out to be accurate—some potential steps that might be taken to assuage the widespread damage now being observed in children. The Geier's treatment hypothesis was developed based on their observation of testosterone-mercury toxicity.

Keywords: Thimerosal, testosterone, mercury, precocious puberty, institutional malfeasance, adverse vaccine reactions, autism, neurological developmental disorders

My guests today are Dr. Mark Geier, President of the Genetic Centers of America (Silver Springs, MD), and David Geier, President of MedCon, Inc. They are the first and only researchers to be allowed to examine the CDC Vaccine Safety Datalink (VSD) database. Their findings surprised even them. But they have had the courage, integrity and no-nonsense approach to keep telling it like it is. Their renowned published study, Thimerosal in Childhood Vaccines, Neurodevelopment Disorders, and Heart Disease in the United States, in the Journal of American Physicians and Surgeons of Spring, 2003, provided "strong epidemiological evidence for a link between increasing mercury from Thimerosal-containing childhood vaccines and neurodevelopment disorders" saying, "a causal relationship between Thimerosal-containing childhood vaccines and neurodevelopment disorders and heart disease appears to be confirmed." They will not tolerate more of America's children becoming needlessly debilitated or kept debilitated by autism. And their latest published paper, The Potential Importance of Steroids in the Treatment of Autistic Spectrum Disorders and other Disorders involving Mercury Toxicity, in the current issue of Medical Hypotheses may help do just that—prevent many of our children on the autism spectrum from remaining needlessly debilitated.

Dr. Geier has been an invited expert before the House Government Reform Committee; the Geiers have twice in the last year been invited to present to the Institute of Medicine (IOM) of the National Academy of Sciences on vaccine issues; the Geiers have been involved in vaccine cases for the no-fault National Vaccine Injury Compensation Program (NVICP) and in civil litigation.

It was a Sunday in 2002, you were in the midst of vacation playing tennis, minding your own business, as the saying goes, and you received a call from a Congressional staff person asking you to be there on Tuesday to render an opinion on the connection between Thimerosal and autism and to investigate the secret Vaccine Safety Datalink database. Who called you, and why did they choose you to call?

In 2002, Congressional staff person, Beth Clay in Congressman Burton's office [Burton who was Chairman of the Government Reform Committee, U.S. House of Representatives] called [us] to attend an upcoming meeting to render an opinion between the connection between Thimerosal and autism and to help investigate the secret Vaccine Safety Datalink (VSD) database. I think we were chosen because we had been essentially the only independent group that had been investigating vaccines. We had been working with the CDC—they had been supplying us with databases and numbers in order to investigate the issue. Congress wanted an independent group to look at the secret database. I guess our names came up and they wanted to hear what we had to say.

What were your findings?

We only got to see the VSD—the Vaccine Safety Datalink--under very difficult conditions. It took us from the time that we were called, another year and a half almost in order to get to see it. Because although Congress had agreed to a compromise that CDC would allow independent researchers into their database, CDC did not make it particularly easy to go there to see it. In fact, it took weekly conference calls with Congress people on the line to finally force them to allow us to see it. And when we saw it, we saw in their database, the same thing we've seen in all the other databases, which was that the more mercury from Thimerosal-containing vaccines children received, the more likely they were to have autism and other neurological disorders.

Initially, when we first started off looking at Thimerosal in late 2001, early 2002, we were very, very skeptical that Thimerosal could be causing autism. It did not make a whole lot of sense—after all Thimerosal in vaccines was very, very low level. We are taking about children that weigh several pounds and the amount of mercury in the micrograms. It didn't make a whole lot of sense how that could be toxic. So parents said, "Well, if you look around, the amount of autism went up with the amount of immunizations being given." They said that the two must be linked. And our first response was that the amount of television watching has gone up in the last 10 or 15 years and we don't say that that's linked with autism. But autism parents wouldn't leave us alone, "You are studying vaccines—you are looking at the Vaccine Adverse Event Reporting System (VAERS), surely there must be some kind of study that you can do on this." I personally got so upset, I said, "Leave me alone and if you keep doing this, I will testify against you guys." Because I said there were genuine safety concerns and I thought that we were addressing them through peer-reviewed scientific publications. But parents of these children with autism were distracting away from the genuine study of vaccine safety concerns.

In working with CDC, analyzing the VAERS database, they provided us a key that allowed us to be able to look at the Thimerosal question. The way in which we looked at it was that when they provided us with the number of doses administered not only by vaccine type, but also by vaccine manufacturer, because it turns out that there were manufacturers of Diphtheria, Tetanus and acellular Pertusis vaccine during the 1990s that did not use Thimerosal as a preservative—they used an alternate preservative called 2-Phenoxyethanol. So now we had a group that had received Thimerosal in the DTaP vaccine—millions of children, and we had a group of children that did not receive Thimerosal—they received the 2-Phenoxyethanol. So we went to the VAERS database to compare the rate, almost positive that there would be no difference in the rate of neurodevelopmental disorders. But when we did that in our first study, we found the rate of autism was six times higher in those who got Thimerosal-containing DTaP versus Thimerosal-free DTaP. Then we went and looked at other kinds of neurodevelopmental disorders—things like mental retardation, speech disorders, and found that they too were also statistically significantly elevated with the Thimerosal-containing DTaP vaccine. So our first thought was "these results surely must be biased." Maybe parents with children that received Thimerosal-containing vaccine were so upset that they went and contacted their doctors to file VAERS reports. We went and looked at things that we did not think could be linked to Thimerosal in the vaccine—things like fever, injection site pain, rashes, and we found that they were similar in both groups. We were seeing just a neurodevelopmental disorder effect. We put this together in our first paper which was written in December 2002, accepted some time after the Congressional hearing convened in December, and the manuscript was not published until June, 2003 in *Experimental Biology in Medicine*.

In the interim, while we were waiting, this was right around the time of the Congressional hearing, Lyn Redwood contacted us from SafeMinds and what she showed us was that the CDC had been studying this Thimerosal question via the Vaccine Safety Datalink (VSD) database. And she showed us graphs that showed a dose response effect of Thimerosal—meaning that the more mercury children got, the more risk they had of developing neurodevelopmental disorders—including autism. This is a very, very powerful way to show an effect in science. If you noticed, we asked the question, "Did you get Thimerosal-containing vaccines?" It was "yes or no." They asked, "Did you get a little bit of Thimerosal, did you get a little bit of effect? If you got a lot of Thimerosal, did you get a lot of effect? The answer was "Yes." This was the first time we got very scared that maybe, indeed, Thimerosal really was contributing to a large number of autism cases out there. So we went back and did a second study in the *Journal of American Physicians and Surgeons* where we decided that we were really going to do an in-depth analysis of this subject. And what we did in that paper was to look at several different important points. First, we looked to see how much mercury children were receiving. We read [that] CDC claimed children received mercury from the vaccines that might have exceeded safety guidelines ever so slightly. So what we did was go to the Environmental Protection Agency (EPA) which established the limit for methylmercury exposure orally of 0.1 micrograms of methylmercury exposure orally ingested per kilogram body weight per day and used that as the limit for the ethylmercury in the vaccine—which is what the CDC did.

That means that an average newborn weighs about 3 kilograms, about 7 pounds, so they were allowed 0.3 micrograms of mercury. They got a Hepatitis B vaccine that had 12.5 micrograms of mercury, so they were 40-fold in excess of the safety guidelines on the day of birth. Then at two months of age, children got another Hepatitis B vaccine, with 12.5 micrograms, they got a *Haemophilus influenzae* type B (or Hib) vaccine and they got a DTaP vaccine, each with 25 more micrograms. So now they got 62.5 micrograms. The average child weighed about 5 kilograms, so they were allowed 0.5 micrograms. Now they were 129-fold in excess of the safety guidelines. And this is a trend that continued. At 4-months they were many, many fold over again, at 6-months again, and so on. Through most of the first year of life, children were over the safety guidelines. And those safety guidelines, now in retrospect that we mention in our paper, actually were a considerable underestimate of the true exposure to mercury children received. Because in our estimates, we assumed that there was no environmental mercury. Clearly children were exposed to between 80 and 100 micrograms of mercury just breathing the air, drinking the water, eating food—and that is per the CDC's own numbers. And then on top of that, when you give a shot, let's say the Hepatitis B at birth, that shot, the amount of mercury has a half life, it doesn't all go away immediately. Some is going to be remaining at 2- months and some from 2-months will remain at 4-months. So these estimates, even though we said there was 129-fold over, are a considerable underestimate of true exposure. Then we went back to VAERS and we analyzed, just like the CDC, the dose response effect of Thimerosal. So we saw that the more mercury children got, Thimerosal-containing DTaP compared to those getting the Thimerosal-free one, the more risk you had of getting a neurological disorder. Then, thirdly, we went to the U.S. Department of Education database—which is independent—and did a cohort prevalence—which means we calculated when children were born; we looked at the average amount of mercury they got from their vaccines and we plotted that versus the prevalence of autism in the Department of Education. And what we found was a striking correlation that the more mercury children got in their vaccines, the more prevalence of autism. Then we went to look and see what others had reported in the literature. This is something anybody can do. You go to *www.pubmed.com* or *Medline* and simply type in the word "Thimerosal." And what you'll find is that there are hundreds of articles published on the toxicity of Thimerosal in peer-reviewed publications dating back to the 1950s and 1960s.

You have established causality here; a good background for reason to be suspicious and to think that there is a connection between Thimerosal and neurodevelopment disorders. And one of the things that I really appreciated about your paper, Thimerosal in Childhood Vaccines: Neurodevelopmental Disorders and Heart Disease in the United States, was that I got the sense that you had gone into this being actually skeptical that you would find a connection. So you sort of went into it with an open mind and you did find the connection. You were willing to stand by that finding and defend and protect these children.

Now, Dr. Geier, we know there was a cover up of the statistically significant correlation between Thimerosal and adverse neurodevelopmental outcomes. Was there even another report that the general public does not know about that showed an even higher correlation—any sort of preliminary report?

Yes, we got some information on what the CDC did initially--when they first looked into this. And it was looked into by Dr. Verstraeten. And he looked into it probably the same way we would have, except he used their own private database. In his initial look, he found that the relative risk of autism was statistically significantly elevated with the increasing amounts of Thimerosal. This is in contradiction to what the CDC people and the FDA people and the American Academy of Pediatrics have been testifying under oath--that they have never found a statistically significant correlation. And in fact they did. In fact we also have e-mails where the initial author is writing to various people like Bob Davis and [Frank] DeStefano and they keep saying that well, we have to find another way to look at it to make this go away. And the next e-mail will say, "It just won't go away" or that we tried that...we did something else. The next e-mail says, "It all came back" or it seems to really be there. And they spent a considerable length of time trying to find a way to manipulate the data so that the effect would become smaller and smaller. And when they got it down to about 2-1/2 times relative risk, they wrote a paper—a complete paper—never sent it. But we have a copy of the paper. It has references; it has an introduction; it is a completely finished paper saying that they found Thimerosal was associated with neurodevelopmental disorders, speech disorders, developmental delays, and autism. We also have their memo saying that we must publish this right away. But they didn't publish it. What they did is they had a secret illegal meeting at a place called Simpsonwood, Georgia. And in this meeting they invited CDC, FDA, and members of the industry. And there's a law in this county--you can have a meeting among CDC people privately—no problem. But the minute you invite the industry, it has to be an open meeting. It has to be announced in the Federal register; it has to be announced to Congress; there is a whole list of things they have to do. They have to put all documents they are going to discuss out for public display. They did none of this. They had a secret meeting. And in the meeting, just to make sure you knew it was secret, they kept a transcript--which was foolish on their part--because we got to see what they said. And in the transcript they say, "Now everybody understand, we have to keep this completely secret."

And in the meeting the author Dr. Verstraeten stands up and states that he thinks there is a significant relationship between Thimerosal and neurodevelopmtnal disorders. And others at the meeting say that Well, we can't let this happen—we can't let this get out. And others say that you can play with this data all you want, (they talk about how they can play with it to make it go away) it is statistically significant. And another gentleman, Dr. Johnston, gets up and says that he's going to make a phone call—he doesn't want his grandson to get this—he was just born. They never tell the public—they hide this. And in fact, two weeks later Dr. Bernier, who was at the meeting, who was the one who said that make sure you keep this secret, gets up in a sworn testimony before Congress and he says that we've never seen any data whatsoever that indicates that there is a problem with Thimerosal, which is of course perjury. Unfortunately, no one pursues it. He can do that because no one is going to charge him.

Yet, they are still letting him speak at IOM meetings. Is that correct?

He speaks at IOM meetings; he sets policy. I have been involved with [him] since the 1980s and at that time he was opposing the switch between DTP vaccine and DTaP. The Japanese had used it on 60 million Japanese children and they had gotten rid of all the problems. And there was many conferences discussing that we could buy it from Japan and have a better vaccine. For 20 years he dragged his feet and finally we switched. And by the way, do you know how we switched? We buy it from Japan. But during those 20 years, many, many—probably tens of thousands of children--died or were damaged by the fact that they dragged their feet. This is the same gentleman that now is getting up and trying to drag his feet on getting rid of Thimerosal even though their own internal memos show, and in fact even their public announcement said, it should be out of the vaccines as soon as possible.

And you must put this in perspective for all our listeners. You must understand what we are taking about. We are not talking about DTP here. We are talking about the worst catastrophic event that has ever happened to the United States and probably the industrialized world. We are talking about, according to the CDC's own estimates, the rate of autism now has risen from in the 1980s, it was something like 1 in 2500, they say now 1 in 166, and it is probably much higher than that. And worse than that, there has been a massive rise in neurodevelopmental disorders, speech delays, mental retardation, so that according to their own A.L.A.R.M.[1] it is now 1 in 6. And according to some other experts that have recently published in the *Washington Post*, it is as high as 1 in 3. The United States of America will not survive as a first rate nation if 1 in 3 of our children are brain damaged. That would mean if it continued, there would be 100 million Americans with brain damage.

We are not going to be the leading country in the world if we don't stop this. In fact, in some ways it is too late already. We have done it to a whole generation. This affects males far more than females. This is something the CDC is hiding. They are not only hiding what happened, but they are continuing to introduce Thimerosal-containing vaccines. This year the flu vaccine was introduced as a required childhood vaccine and it contains a full dose of Thimerosal. And in addition by hiding it, they are stopping any funds going into any kind of research that will help treat these children. And they are pretending that these children don't have mercury poisoning. And if you don't recognize that they have mercury poisoning, then you are not going to design a rational treatment that is going to help it. And so these kids now fill our school systems. And we visited some of the schools. There are many schools now in the country that have more special education kids than they have normal kids—ADD, ADHD, behavioral disorders filling our schools—which were never there before. No matter how much they try to hide it, every parent knows, they just have to go to school, they were not like that. When these kids grow up--this began to happen in 1990/1991 when the United States tripled the amount of vaccines and tripled the amount of mercury—they are not going to be able to work. They are going to need institutionalized care or special care and the bill to this country is going to be so devastating; this country is going to have trouble surviving the way we know it. The estimate from the Congressional committee which had a 3-year hearing, all of which agreed first of all that the evidence was overwhelming—that Thimerosal caused the current epidemic. Secondly, they agreed that CDC and FDA were asleep at the switch and they could have prevented it or curtailed it. "Asleep at the switch," by the way, is in their own memos where they said "we were asleep at the switch." And they also said that FDA and CDC are guilty of "institutional malfeasance for self-protectionism and misplaced protection of the industry." This kind of thing is going to absolutely devastate the United States, and it is happening at just the worst moment. This is the moment in about 4, 5 or 6 years when the baby boomers are going to start to retire. We already had a problem that we don't have enough people to work to support our social security in our whole society. And now these people that are coming up, a good number of them are not going to be able to work. And just to throw on top of that, they are now killing off some more of them in Iraq. This country is in for big trouble. They are hiding it to some extent now--they are not going to be able to hide it when these kids grow up and they need to be put in institutions.

Plus the parents won't always be around to take care of them because they are aging. But part of the reason that we have you here today, a main reason, is so that we can prevent our children from having to be put into an institutionalized setting. So let's move on to your new treatment hypothesis. You've given us the background on your findings of the relationship between Thimerosal and adverse neurodevelopmental outcomes. What is the scientific background between your new treatment theory for Thimerosal and how this may mitigate mercury toxicity?

Let me give you a little background. I am an MD, Ph.D. and I practice obstetrical genetics. I don't take care of children. So you might think, well, the Geiers have been involved with vaccines all the back to my 10 years at the NIH which goes back to the 1970s, so it might be surprising that we would be also contributing a new treatment method. The way this happened was that we were attending various conferences. And at the conferences were many doctors who treat Thimerosal-damaged children. And they had meetings where they discussed the current therapies. And they kept inviting us to come to the meetings. And my first reaction was, "Well, you know, I don't treat children—no offense, but I'll probably fall asleep at your meeting because that is not what I do." But they kept insisting, so I kept going. David and I both kept going. And we started seeing that indeed some of these children were helped by various therapies. And so let me go over a few of these therapies and how they made sense to me.

The most obvious one that makes sense is "if children have too much mercury, you should try to get rid of the mercury." So a number of these treaters were using various methods of chelation. Chelation is a method of using a chemical that binds heavy metals. There is a chelator that is approved for lead toxicity. They were trying to use this chelator to get some of the mercury out of the kids. And they were able to show, in fact, these kids had a lot of mercury and that they could release mercury. In some cases some of the kids responded very well to this and got quite a bit better.

There is another group of doctors who try to manipulate the glutathione pathway. This is the pathway by which mercury is eliminated naturally and it has been shown by us and others in the publications coming out all the time now that one of the reasons that children who are affected by the mercury as opposed to those who are not, is that they have poor ability to get rid of mercury and have problems with the glutathione pathway. So people were starting and trying to manipulate that pathway and again occasionally they would get some good success—the child would get a lot better by giving various elements of this pathway.

Then we ran into people that were giving Secretin. Secretin is a substance that is given primarily because these children have bowel problems. Secretin controls the function of the bowel. But some of these kids not only got better with their bowels when they got Secretin, they got better mentally.

Then we talked to some people that gave growth hormone. Some of those kids got better. Then we found some people that gave antibiotics that kill yeast—they were trying again to help the bowel. Again some of these kids got better.

So I am taking home that, first of all, these are hardworking honest clinicians. There are some amazing stories of how kids got better. But it did not make a whole lot of sense to me: how could these treatments that had nothing to do with each other make kids better? Now, the other thing is that I started getting interested—because my background is in obstetrics, in fertility, and in vitro fertilization, and I'm a biochemical geneticist—I decided I did not know much about the glutathione pathway, but I would look at the testosterone pathway because it had been shown that, first of all, males are far more affected than females by mercury. Not just in this autism epidemic, but wherever mercury poisoning appears it often affects males more than females. Also Boyd Haley and some other people had done experiments where they throw Thimerosal/mercury in and they kill neurons. And if you throw in testosterone, it kills 100 times better, whereas estrogen tends to ameliorate Thimerosal/mercury toxicity.

So I said, "See if you can figure out how that happens." So I started writing out the testosterone synthesis pathway which begins with cholesterol, it goes to testosterone and then some breakdown products. Then I got to a crucial point in the pathway which is DHEA. This is something you can buy in any health food store—it is not yet a steroid. In DHEA, either the synthesis goes on towards testosterone or most of it actually goes on to DHEA-S, which is adding a sulphur. There is an enzyme which makes DHEA into DHEA-S and I was reading about this enzyme. And I found that it was known that this enzyme is inhibited by mercury and its cofactor is glutathione. So a light bulb went off in my head, and I said, "You know, maybe these kids are not getting better maybe not just because they are removing the mercury." These kids are aggressive, this type of autism often leads to aggression, and testosterone may have something to do with aggression. What if the DHEA step, when there is mercury around, doesn't go to DHEA-S, but instead it goes to testosterone and raises the testosterone, then you remove the mercury to allow the production of DHEA-S and you lower the testosterone. You add glutathione or things related to glutathione, again you allow DHEA-S to be made and you lower the testosterone. So two of the main therapies not only have to do with mercury, but they lower testosterone.

Then I started thinking, well how about the others—how about the secretin and the Nystatin® which is the antibiotic that kills yeast, and the growth hormone—clearly how could those have anything to do with testosterone? Then I started to think about it. Testosterone is controlled by the pituitary axis. The pituitary makes FSH and LH which in girls causes the cycle and in boys causes testosterone. And anything that inhibits that pathway will turn off FSH and LH. In fact, it is a feedback loop. That is, when girls have periods, during their period they make substances that turn it off and that is how it is cyclical. And so I look at the pathway, and guess what is on the pathway? Growth hormone and secretin--both inhibit the pathway. So if you give secretin, you lower FSH and you lower testosterone. And if you give growth hormone, you lower FSH and you lower testosterone. In fact, much to my surprise, Nystatin®, the antibiotic, also affects that pathway and lowers testosterone. There are many publications on this. So I started keeping score and every single therapy that we could find that has had any success, there is one thing in common—they all lower testosterone.

If fact, some of the things that are given in traditional medicine, like Strattera® and Ritalin®—Ritalin® is a surprising drug—because if a normal person takes Ritalin® it makes them worse, but some autistics, some ADD and ADHD, it makes them better. And it was unexpected, but it has been observed. But guess what—that may lower testosterone, too.

So in addition, some people now, we have just been reading, are finding that autistics and neurodevelopment disorder kids have a low level of serotonin which is a brain transmitter. Guess what? The more testosterone you have the less serotonin you have. It is well known, well published, there is a link between the two. **So I came up with the idea that the problem here is not just mercury, but it is the interaction between mercury and testosterone.** And that if you just try to remove the mercury, it will move around—it will react to the testosterone. And there is more data. The mercury actually binds to the testosterone sites in the brain—testosterone receptor sites. So again we found publications for that. Then we found an x-ray crystallography study that showed that actually testosterone itself directly binds to mercury and makes the testosterone form a big sheet which may be why the testosterone level goes higher and higher.

Now when I gave this presentation to some of these doctors, light bulbs went off in their head and they said, "You know, a lot of our patients have precocious puberty." That's what you get when you have too high testosterone. So we came up with the idea that you should lower the testosterone and then remove the mercury. That's the new idea and that's what is coming out in the publication in Medical Hypotheses.

In addition, if you start thinking about this, we all live in a mercury toxic environment. Many people have amalgams in their teeth, they have a lot of mercury--there is mercury in the air, there is mercury in the fish, and, in fact, we calculated almost everybody in our society may be near or over the EPA limit—even if you don't get vaccines—and there is not much we can do about it—short term, not much—long term maybe we can help the environment. So we have got to live with mercury problems.

We started looking at some of the other chronic disorders that go on. We found that testosterone affects the bowel with mercury. And, therefore, that may be the reason why there is a bowel problem in autism. And, then we found that in Alzheimer's many people have observed that mercury levels are higher in the brain. And, by the way, estrogen protects against Alzheimer's disease. And, then there are some forms of heart diseases where it involves testosterone and mercury, and then there are strokes that involve testosterone and mercury. And it looks like a lot of chronic diseases... ALS is another one, Lou Gehrig's disease. There are publications that talk about the effect of testosterone and the effect of mercury. So it looks like a number of these chronic diseases that are sort of overwhelming our society involve testosterone and mercury. And we might well learn how to manipulate the testosterone-mercury combination if we are going to try to help some of these kids.

We need to treat the problem directly. Giving growth hormone does turn off the FSH and LH--but very indirectly and very unreliably. The good news is that we have FDA-approved drugs that can do that kind of thing—that have been used for things like precocious puberty and various other things. So if we really want to turn it off, we can really turn it off.

My idea was that we need to study this to find out which testosterone process is causing the problem. We gave the talk and we suggested that probably nobody should do this treatment, but we should find a way to do this research. Of course, the NIH is not going to fund it.

But what happened is, apparently somebody heard this talk, and within two days they called us and one of the doctors said that a patient "accidentally" gave a medicine that lowered testosterone to her child. But anyway, the child got much better for a few days and then as the medicine wore off, got worse.

So we had a friend that had a very severe autistic and she begged us to try it. So she had a developmental pediatrician who was willing to help. We actually found a regimen to lower the testosterone and the child had a remarkable improvement. He never said a word, and now he speaks—this is about five weeks later. He didn't interact and now he is interacting. Within days his bowel problems completely cleared up. So what we are doing is lowering his testosterone and then we are chelating out the mercury.

You can't keep the testosterone level in these kids down to zero forever, they have to go to puberty. But you can keep it down for years. Let's say the kid is 8, you can keep it down from age 8 to 10 while you remove the mercury.

That also brings up another thing that I need to mention. We've got a ticking time bomb here. I believe that once the children reach puberty and their testosterone levels go very high, the damage if the mercury is still there is going to be massive. This problem began in 1990/1991. The oldest kids are starting to get toward puberty. The time bomb is ticking. If we are going to try to ameliorate this, we've got to do it very soon. And if this therapy is going to work and we are really are going to do something about our society we have an unbelievable problem. We have got hundreds of thousands--maybe millions of children who would need to be treated this way. It would take a massive government program to do it. We can do a handful of our friends. But if you wanted to do a million people you would have to have as many treatment centers as there are *McDonalds*® across the country. It would take billions of dollars of investment and only the government has that kind of money. However that would be a wonderful investment because it wouldn't save billions, it would save trillions. And it might save our society and everything that we know.

But, of course, there is a problem, and that is, the Federal people if they support this in a certain way are going to hang themselves. Because to support this program you sort of have to admit that mercury has something to do with it and if mercury has something to do with it--*they* have something to do with it—and that makes it their fault and they don't want to hear about it.

This is a totally experimental treatment, everybody has to understand our experience is very small.

Have you run up across any other roadblocks in trying to do further research in so far as the VSD goes? I know that you were mentioning the clandestine Simpsonwood meeting and I know that Congressman Weldon became concerned about those transcripts and he wanted to look into this. Could you tell us more about that?

Basically what happened, when we started to try to look at the database, Congress was trying to help us to be able do that. I think it came about as a result of the fact that every time that we made a request to CDC—we want to look at this data, we want to look at this HMO's data in the VSD—CDC would basically balk at that kind of idea—so Dr. Weldon and his staff interceded and tried to help do what we needed to do. That went on for a year and a half. When we finally went in and had this brief look at the data, CDC got very, very upset because we reported our preliminary results from that to the Institute of Medicine where we announced that the Vaccine Safety Datalink appears to confirm our other results. CDC's response was, and this was in February of 2004, within one week of our testimony, CDC sends a letter to all the HMO's alleging that we had violated patient confidentiality with VSD. Now you have to understand VSD is assembled for external researchers--it has no names, addresses, phone numbers or any other kind of identifying information. Patients in that database are assigned a randomly assigned number. Then it is has some information about what vaccines they had and what kinds of outcomes.

So they did that. The first response was the HMOs terminated our ability to access the VSD. So we spent months, from February through about August, writing letters, having attorneys write letters to the HMO's stating we did not do anything wrong. As I said, you couldn't violate patient confidentiality if you wanted to. We did not even want to--we are not that kind of people that would even violate it even if we could. Finally when the HMOs met and had discussions about it, a number of HMOs re-approved us, showing that the CDC has raised false, basically malicious kinds of accusations. And what has happened since that time now is that CDC, or what we are really referring to is the National Immunization Program of the CDC, has given up the responsibility of the VSD, even though they bought it for CDC and they're the ones that analyze it, they have decided they are going to wash their hands clean of VSD and passed it on to the National Center for Health Statistics. So we have now been trying to work with the National Center for Health Statistics and there has been terrible problems dealing with them. First they have been very unresponsive. And second, they have the problem, that while I think some of the employees there might like us to actually see the data—they don't even understand what the Vaccine Safety Datalink is and the potential very damaging material it has in it—they don't have the database. Even though the National Immunization Program says they are no longer in charge of it, they still house the VSD database. So when the National Center for Health Statistics wants the database, they have to go back to the CDC.

---

[1]*Autism A.L.A.R.M.* document, a joint publication by CDC and others. Please see below.

Autism A.L.A.R.M.

Autism is prevalent

- 1 out of 6 children are diagnosed with a developmental disorder and/or behavioral problem
- 1 in 166 children are diagnosed with an autism spectrum disorder
- Developmental disorders have subtle signs and may be easily missed

Listen to parents

- Early signs of autism are often present before 18 months
- Parents usually DO have concerns that something is wrong
- Parents generally DO give accurate and quality information
- When parents do not spontaneously raise concerns, ask if they have any

Act early

- Make screening and surveillance an important part of your practice (as endorsed by the AAP)
- Know the subtle differences between typical and atypical development
- Learn to recognize red flags
- Use validated screening tools and identify problems early
- Improve the quality of life for children and their families through early and appropriate intervention

Refer

- To Early Intervention or a local school program (do not wait for a diagnosis)
- To an autism specialist, or team of specialists, immediately for a definitive diagnosis
- To audiology and rule out a hearing impairment
- To local community resources for help and family support

Monitor

- Schedule a follow-up appointment to discuss concerns more thoroughly
- Look for other features known to be associated with autism
- Educate parents and provide them with up-to-date information
- Advocate for families with local early intervention programs, schools, respite care agencies, and insurance companies
- Continue surveillance and watch for additional or late signs of autism and/or other developmental disorders

Medical Veritas Editor's Comment

The Geiers and their insights into the behind-the-scenes machinations by public health authorities reveal the latter's foremost allegiances in a very clear way. It demonstrates that as far as these institutions are concerned, their priority seems to be to protect professional and industrial interests over and above their superficial *raison d'être*, namely the protection of the public's health. The confidential meetings with industry, and the attempted thwarting of efforts of independent parties to truly investigate the data, illustrate that the legal frameworks that are supposed to bind the operations of these organizations are at times seemingly treated with pure contempt.

It is an understatement to note that this is very alarming and should be taken as a "red alert" to all who are concerned with maintaining any semblance of democracy as regards health care in a modern society. It should be deeply disturbing to health practitioners around the world who dispense medical advice and services on the basis of the information that these authorities provide. It should be distressing to health consumers, who have trusted that these authorities act in accordance with their directives rather than serve some professional or economic motive that is abjectly foreign to medicines' supposed aims.

This episode should also be disquieting to everyone who maintains the romantic notion that science is inviolate, that its arguments are automatically untainted by "the non-scientific", and that trust can be implicitly maintained in peer-reviewed scientific publications. This brewing Thimerosal debacle is a lesson in politics of science that needs to be heeded throughout the world.

The Geiers courageously give us some idea of the violations of ethics and corruption of mandates that are occurring at the highest levels of the medical establishment. It should make us wonder how much of the published research of these public health authorities are merely contrived apologetics, rather than attempts to provide medical veritas to the populations of whom they are supposed to serve. If these organizations do not serve the populations in the manner in which their very formation had intended, perhaps this calls for a radical rethinking by bodies such as the *House Government Reform Committee*, regarding the form of, the independence of, and the very authority given to such bodies.

Appendix VII. Interview with Dr. Mark Geier and David Geier: Decreasing Trends in Autism and Neurodevelopmental Disorders following Decreasing Use of Thimerosal-Containing Vaccines

Mark R. Geier[a], MD, PhD; David A. Geier[b], BA; and Teri Small[a]

[a]Genetic Centers of America

[b]Graduate Student, Department of Biochemistry, George Washington Unviersity.

[c]AutismOne Radio

1816 Houston Ave.

Fullerton, CA 92833 USA

Phone: +1 714 680 0792

Email: tsmall@autismone.org Website: www.autismone.org

Abstract

Thimerosal is an ethylmercury-containing compound (49.55% mercury by weight) that has been historically added to many vaccines. Starting in the early 1990s the amount of Thimerosal administered to American infants roughly tripled with addition of hepatitis B and *haemophilus infleunzae* type b (Hib) vaccines. Additionally, at the same time, Thimerosal-containing Rho-immune globulin began to be routinely administered to all Rh-negative mothers at 28 weeks gestation. Concurrently, significant epidemic trends in autism and other neurodevelopmental disorders were observed in the United States. On July 7, 1999 the U.S. Public Health Services (USPHS) and the American Academy of Pediatrics (AAP) issued a joint-statement calling for the immediate removal of Thimerosal from all vaccines citing theoretical risks posed by the cumulative mercury doses contained in routine childhood vaccines. The most recent epidemiological research has shown a significant correlation between the reduction of Thimerosal from childhood vaccines post-1999 and the rate of new cases of autism and other neurodevelopmental disorders in three independent databases in the United States. In the last several years, the Centers for Disease Control and Prevention (CDC) has undertaken a campaign to rapidly expand the required U.S. childhood vaccine schedule to include additional Thimerosal-containing vaccines, so that under the immunization schedule, children may be exposed to greater than 50% of the mercury dose children were exposed to prior to the July 7, 1999 USPHS and AAP recommendation to remove Thimerosal from vaccines. All told under the new influenza vaccine immunization schedule that calls for the administration of at one influenza vaccine to all pregnant women (at any trimester during pregnancy), and subsequent administration of 6 influenza vaccines during the first 5 years of life, today's children may be exposed to greater than 125 micrograms of mercury from Thimerosal-containing influenza vaccines. It is clear given recently emerging scientific evidence that mercury has no place in pharmaceuticals administered to human populations.

Keywords: autism, ethylmercury, speech disorder, Thimerosal-containing vaccines,

We welcome Dr. Mark Geier and David Geier. Dr. Mark Geier is president of the Genetic Centers of America and has been in clinical practice for more than 20 years. He was a researcher at the National Institutes of Health for ten years. Dr. Geier has authored almost 100 peer-reviewed scientific-medical publications. Most recently, he has co-authored about 30 peer-reviewed scientific medical publications on vaccine safety, efficacy and policy.

David Geier is the president of MedCon. David has co-authored approximately 30 peer-reviewed scientific-medical publications on vaccine safety, efficacy and policy. He has recently received critical acclaim from his colleagues for his research on vaccines by winning the Stanley W. Jackson Prize given to authors having the best paper in the preceding three years in the Journal of the History of Medicine and Allied Sciences, published by Duke University.

Dr. Geier has been an invited expert before the House Government Reform Committee. The Geiers have presented to the Institute of Medicine of the National Academy of Sciences on vaccine issues. The Geiers are the first and only researchers to be allowed to examine the CDC's Vaccine Safety Datalink database. Their studies include "Thimerosal in Childhood Vaccines, Neurodevelopment Disorders, and Heart Disease in the United States" in the Journal of American Physicians and Surgeons of Spring 2003 (Vol. 8, No. 1). "Neurodevelopmental Disorders Following Thimerosal-Containing Childhood Immunizations: A Follow-Up Analysis," published in The International Journal of Toxicology, and their recently published paper, "The Potential Importance of Steroids in the Treatment of Autistic Spectrum Disorders and Other Disorders Involving Mercury Toxicity" in Medical Hypotheses.

Today, we are discussing their most recently published paper entitled, "Early Downward Trends in Neurodevelopmental Disorders Following Removal of Thimerosal-Containing Vaccines" in the Journal of American Physicians and Surgeons (Vol. 11, No. 1, Spring 2006).

Gentlemen, thank you for joining us.

Mark Geier: Thank you for having us.

Since many people know of background on the autism epidemic, but some listeners may not, I'd like to start with a little bit of background information. Is there a true epidemic of autism? Have agencies such as the American Academy of Pediatrics, the Department of Health and Human Services, and the CDC formally recognized an increase in autistic disorder and other developmental or behavioral disorders?

Mark Geier: It seems that it depends on the day. There are many members of those organizations that on certain days agree that there's an epidemic, and other days they say they're not sure. Other days they say there's no epidemic. This is all part of their disinformation campaign. There is no doubt whatsoever that there's an epidemic and it's an enormous epidemic. It's such a big epidemic that it is a threat to the very existence of the United States of America as a first-rate country. The epidemic, by the CDC's own official *Autism A.L.A.R.M.,* which was issued in January of 2004, stated that 1 in a 166 children have Autism Spectrum Disorder, and far worse 1 in 6 children have a neurodevelopmental or behavioral disorder. To pretend that that rate has been going on indefinitely in the past and that we were just missing the diagnosis is completely ridiculous. Because if it's 1 in 6 – and there are almost 300,000 million Americans – there would have to be 50 million brain damaged people in this country. There are not 50 million brain damaged people in this country.

Additionally, the estimates that I just read to you, in my opinion and many other people's opinion, do not actually reflect the magnitude of the problem. I think at the peak, which was probably around 1998 – as far as when the children were born – I think the true rate of autism was something like 1 in 30. I think the true rate of neurodevelopmental disorder or behavioral disorder is somewhere around 1 in 3, although there are people that are even more aggressive than that— like Dr. Weldon, a Congressman from Florida, who thinks that probably all of our children were damaged. It's just the other two out of three weren't damaged enough to be clinically noticeable. This kind of damage, the level of damage, can easily be confirmed by any parent, anybody that wants to look. You merely have to go to our local school system. Our school systems that used to have a very rare child with a neurological problem, now many of them have more special education buses than normal children's buses.

Almost every classroom is full of ADD/ADHD, autism. They cannot cover this up.

In addition, if the children had been affected in the past and we simply didn't diagnose them – which incidentally is an insult because 60% of them never speak—so what they're saying is we never noticed that they never spoke—you know, they were just sitting in the classroom and we never noticed it. Where is the hidden horde? In other words, there should be the same number of 40-year-old autistics as there are 10-year-old autistics. There should be the same number of 50-year-old autistics. It's a complete joke. There are almost no autistics of that age. We're in the midst of an absolutely threatening epidemic. The U.S. Congress held three years of hearings on this. Their estimate is the damage that has been done to the United States exceeds $20 trillion – that's with a T. To put that into perspective, the current war in Iraq has not yet reached one-half a trillion. So it's more than 40 times the war in Iraq. In fact, it's more damage than has ever happened to the United States in anything. More damage than World War I, World War II, Korea, 9/11, the AIDS epidemic.

People are still sitting around and saying, "What happened?" This denial will no longer be tolerated. We cannot tolerate this. These kids are filling our school systems. When they get to be 21, they're not going to go into our workforce. The other thing that people who don't have an autistic child have to understand is these autistics are not the "Rain Man." Everybody thinks of the movie, the character the Rain Man. The autistic that sits in the corner, who's kind of quiet. The autistics that we're talking about in this epidemic are what's called regressive autism. These kids are not autistic at birth but they become – they have a first year of normal development, maybe a year and a half, and then they regress. Regressive autism, actually there almost is no such disease—it's actually mercury poisoning. These kids, just like people who are mercury poisoned, are aggressive. They have high testosterone and they're so aggressive that they hit their mother and fathers. They break the chandelier. They break the wall. They threaten everybody. When these kids come out, which is going to be starting to happen probably in another five or six years, our society is going to be different than you've ever seen before. The reason it's going to start happening in another five or six years is everybody needs to understand what happened and why the epidemic began.

In 1990 approximately – 1990, 1991 – the United States went from giving a series of DTP shots – that's diphtheria, tetanus and pertussis – to a series of DTP shots plus hepatitis B plus Hib. Now we're pro vaccine and I'm not arguing that those were not good vaccines, but each one of those contained mercury. Basically what we did when we increased the vaccine schedule is we tripled the amount of mercury. As the FDA's own memo says, we were "asleep at the switch." Additionally, around 1990, women who were Rh negative began to be given – at the recommendation of the American College of OB/GYN – routinely during pregnancy at 28 weeks a RhoGAM shot to prevent Rh incompatibility disease. Again, a very bad disease, a very good treatment, but unfortunately that product also contained Thimerosal.

So we went way up in the amount of Thimerosal and the epidemic went straight up and it went up and up and up, and it continued up. Actually it continued up until the CDC, the FDA, the U.S. Health Department in 1999 made an unprecedented and unrequested – no one forced them to do it – press release in which they were asking the vaccine manufacturers to voluntarily remove Thimerosal from the childhood vaccines. This happened in 1999 and although they probably should have required an immediate recall, many of the vaccine companies over the ensuing few years began to actually remove Thimerosal from a number of the childhood vaccines—not all of them, but some of them.

Our most recent paper studies the pattern on the amount of autism in three different databases. What it shows is that in all three databases—the database from the State of California, from VAERS, which is our nationwide vaccine adverse event reporting system, and from the U.S. Department of Education—autism went straight up in the early 1990s when we introduced the vaccines. We had predicted that about three years following the beginning of the withdrawal of Thimerosal from the vaccines and the RhoGAM, that if we were right, there would begin to be a decline in the rate of new cases of autism. In fact, people at the CDC said if we were right that would happen, but it would never happen. Well, that's what happened in 1999 – the reason for the three years is it takes about that long to start getting diagnoses. Now all of a sudden in our recent papers we have observed, as many others have observed, this cannot be denied; that there had begun to be a drop in all three databases, just as predicted, and the fact that there's a drop in other state databases. In fact, these drops can be confirmed because these databases are available to anybody online. This doesn't need statistics. We did some statistics. You can argue about them. This passes the eyeball test. The issue is over. They've got to stop giving our children this poison.

The CDC response has been first of all to deny all three databases. This one's no good for one reason. That one's no good for another reason. Their further response is that they're going to increase the amount of Thimerosal in the vaccines because the influenza vaccine that is recommended for children only has been recommended since 2004. They recommended three shots in the first year and a half. Now, just recently, they're now giving shots at age 2, 3, 4 and 5 and they're also giving them to pregnant women with full-dose Thimerosal. So they're putting back the Thimerosal even though they've seen that there was a drop. This is unacceptable. This is totally out of touch with reality. Last week the EU – European Union – banned Thimerosal in all of Europe. It has already been banned in most of the countries. Meanwhile, our CDC has gone from in 1999 a position of saying that we should remove Thimerosal to be prudent, to 2004 when their IOM said we shouldn't care, to the current position which is, "We're actually making an attempt to put as much Thimerosal in as possible."

I'm a physician, so I buy from Sanofi Pasteur some of the influenza vaccine. They sent me a notice: "Dr. Geier, you can now buy your 2007 influenza vaccine." This is eight years after they said they were going to remove it. About three weeks later, I got another letter: "You can now buy your 2007 influenza vaccine, but we're all out of the ones with Thimerosal. But we have plenty of the vaccine without Thimerosal." They are actually instructing the local health departments to preferentially buy the one with Thimerosal. We the people of the United States are not going to tolerate this anymore. Already we've had six states ban Thimerosal. A seventh one just banned it about two weeks ago, which is Washington state. The first state was Iowa, then it was California. Missouri, Delaware, Illinois, and New York.

Now hopefully this week, Maryland will ban it. We are not going to tolerate this anymore. These people are not above the law. Our representatives are voting to get rid of it. There's a bill in Congress that I think, last I heard, had 77 co-sponsors. We do not want the poison in the vaccines, and we are not going to be dictated to. This is going to stop. The jig is up. Now the U.S. Senate and House have passed a resolution to investigate and they've said that the CDC is no longer believable and they can't do the investigation. It was followed up by a letter by a bunch of U.S. senators and representatives. There's a major investigation in Europe. This is not going to be tolerated anymore. They're not going to harm our children any further. The evidence is overwhelming.

In addition in the last year or so, there have been numerous NIH-sponsored studies showing damage in monkeys, showing damage in tissue cultures, showing damage everywhere you look. Thimerosal causes birth defects, it causes cancer. There are 5,000 papers. Anybody can confirm that there are papers that show that this is a deadly substance. It cannot be used in vaccines, and we cannot have Dr. Julie Gerberding keep getting up in front of Congress and saying, "There's not one single paper ever published that showed it ever caused any damage." When anybody can go to MedLine, type in the word "Thimer-osal", and see what pops up. This kind of lie will not be tolerated anymore in the future.

Well Dr. Geier, thank you for that overview. I'd like to backtrack a little bit and break the steps down in our discussion a bit more. So in your overview, you did mention that there was an Autism A.L.A.R.M., and that was back, I believe, in January 2004. So that would speak to the fact that agencies such as the American Academy of Pediatrics, CDC and HHS did formally recognize that there was an increase in autistic disorder and other behavioral and developmental disorders. So you also mentioned about better diagnoses, or changes in diagnostic criteria being ruled out as the cause. Is that correct: diagnostic criteria, better diagnosis, and population shift—have all of those explanations been ruled out for this increase?

Mark Geier: Yes. Those have been studied and those do not account for the increase. They've been studied in California. There are several publications showing that; that it's not increased diagnosis or population shift. In reality, as I said, this is one of those things you don't need a study for. You can go to any school system anywhere in this country and they're just overwhelmed. You can't be overwhelmed by differential diagnoses. They're not making diagnoses. What happens is they have the new kids of kindergarten, first grade, second grade – show up and the kids are abnormal. They can't exist in the classroom. That has nothing to do with diagnosis; the kids are different.

And you mentioned that Congressman Weldon believes that all children have been damaged to some extent, it's just that some you can't recognize clinically. Is that what you said?

Mark Geier: That's what I said. A very disturbing thing that's been coming out is that the average boy now – and I'm not talking about autistic, I'm not talking about any other diagnosis – the average boy in the public school system is now 2½ years behind the average girl. What you start hearing is, you know, "Boys have always been stupider than girls." Well I'm a big supporter of women's lib. I went to school and that wasn't true. The reason that the boys are behind the girls is that males are much more susceptible to mercury poisoning than females. We're now in a position where there are more girls in college than boys, more girls in medical school than boys, more girls in graduate school than boys. I love to see the women doing well, but it's not that the women are doing well, it's that the boys have been damaged. It's so obvious, and we have absolutely decimated a generation and a half of particularly males. There are some females affected.

Now the females may be affected in a different way. When they go to reproduce – and they're not quite old enough yet – they may have a very high rate of malformations, problems with pregnancies. Also females with mercury have a problem of autoimmune diseases and other things, but they're quite a bit less sensitive to brain damage. But I think that we've done something that is unprecedented. I mean we all are aware that the CDC and the FDA have been asleep at the switch in some of the drugs, like Vioxx. I mean after all, it killed an estimated 50,000 to 150,000 people. Sounds like a big number, but compared to the thing we're talking about here, this is much worse because no medicine is taken by everybody; not everybody took Vioxx. But with the vaccines, virtually every child in the country is vaccinated. You cannot make mistakes on vaccines or you'll decimate a country. Unfortunately, that's exactly what has happened here.

And you mentioned that the boys have been more affected than the girls; that boys' scores aren't as good as girls'—not as many boys entering college. Is that what you said?

Mark Geier: Yes, and of course just back a generation and a half ago it was far more boys than girls who were in college.

All right. So that would tend to speak to the fact that estrogen has a protective effect in the presence of mercury, and that one's susceptibility to the toxicity of Thimerosal is dramatically increased by testosterone. Is that the case?

Mark Geier: That's the case and that has been known for a long time. It's been shown in recent studies in tissue culture, where Thimerosal kills tissue culture cells. If you throw in testosterone, you kill them a hundred times faster. If you throw in estrogen, you protect. But this has been known. In fact, there are publications in the '80's from the CDC that have shown in animals at low to moderate doses, females are far more resistant than males, and it's also been studied in human poisonings, where there were spills. Males are affected much more than females and, in effect, we think we have a biochemical explanation. We think we know exactly where the mercury and the testosterone interact, and it's involved in our new therapy. But there is no doubt that this is another one of the things that the public health is trying to cover up. They say they don't know what causes it. Some of them are denying that they don't even know there are more boys than girls. This is the ostrich head in the sand thing. It's published all over the place that there are more boys than girls. This is exactly what's going on and it's, as I said, undeniably known that mercury poisoning damages more boys than girls.

So we've established that agencies know and have recognized that there has been an increase in autistic disorder, an increase in other developmental and behavioral disorders. We've established that changes in diagnostic criteria, better diagnosis and population shift have been ruled out. We've established that this is going to be very bad for the country because of so many affected individuals, so many affected males. We've established that this is a true epidemic. Dr. Geier, could it be a genetic epidemic?

Mark Geier: Not in the way that they're trying to imply. I'm a board certified geneticist. There are no epidemics that are caused by genetics. That's a no-brainer. The definition of an epidemic is a rapid rise in human disease. The fastest known change in genetics is one percent per hundred years. So no epidemic in history has ever been caused by genetics. Now that being said, that doesn't mean there isn't a genetic component to virtually every epidemic. For example, when Christopher Columbus came to the United States, within 100 years, 99% of the New World people had died. They didn't die of Spanish cannon – a few of them did – they died of measles and smallpox. Were the people of the New World more sensitive genetically to measles and smallpox than the Europeans who'd been exposed and selected for survival for a thousand years? Of course they were. Was that a genetic epidemic? Of course it wasn't. That was an infectious epidemic on a susceptible population.

We now know very well that there is a genetic susceptibility in a certain percentage of our population that makes them susceptible to mercury. This has been worked out by numerous investigators published all over the place. Basically, there are several susceptibilities. One is, you can't get rid of your mercury because you make low glutathione. Glutathione is the substance that allows you to get rid of mercury. Then if you don't get exposed to mercury, you'll be fine but if you're exposed to mercury, you'll be susceptible to a much lower dose of mercury than someone who has a normal or a fully functioning glutathione pathway. There are genetic studies that show that almost 100% of autistics have some genetic changes in their glutathione pathway. Did the changes cause the autism? No. The changes made susceptibility and then when we threw in the extra mercury, we caused the disease.

There's also good evidence that families that tend to have high testosterone are also susceptible. Did the high testosterone cause the disease? No. But when we threw in the mercury, those families that had high testosterone and low glutathione were susceptible. By the way, the discovery that David and I have made is that there's a link between glutathione and testosterone. Anybody who has high testosterone will have low glutathione, and anybody who has a low glutathione will have high testosterone.

There's a genetic component. But it is not a genetic cause as they're saying. There has to be an environmental stimulus and the environmental stimulus here was one thing and one thing only—and that is the mercury in the vaccines and the RhoGAM. I get misquoted on this all the time. They say, "Oh, I've got a case of autism. It wasn't caused by the vaccines or the RhoGAM." That's right. I didn't say – and I'll say it again – I didn't say all the cases were caused by Thimerosal in the vaccines and the RhoGAM. I said the epidemic – that is the rapid rise – was caused by that. There are a number of other low-level, rare causes that existed before we threw in the vaccines. They still exist but they didn't go up with the increase in mercury. What went up was regressive autism and that is mercury poisoning. The epidemic was caused by the mercury in the vaccines and the RhoGAM. There's certainly bad damage done by mercury in the teeth, mercury in the environment, mercury in the smokestacks, mercury in the fish. None of those things caused the rapid rise. None of those things went up as a matter of fact. The number of amalgams placed has gone down. The amount of mercury coming out of the smokestacks has gone down. Not as fast as it should have. The only thing that went up was the Thimerosal in the vaccines and RhoGAM. The only thing that went down right when the epidemic began to decline were those things. This epidemic was caused virtually exclusively by the Thimerosal increase in the vaccines and the Thimerosal in the RhoGAM. It should never have happened, and our health authorities are aware of it.

Anybody can read this. You can go on NoMercury.org or any one of numerous other websites, or you can read David Kirby's book, *Evidence of Harm*. You can read their own documents where they had secret meetings; no one has challenged the correctness of the transcripts. In the transcripts they say, "We know what caused it and we have to keep it a secret." They had illegal meetings and there was a fight within the organization. There's still a fight within the organization. There's still those that want to disclose it. Those who wanted to hide it won. It has been hidden and it can no longer be hidden. This cannot be tolerated any further. In fact, the truth of the matter is a good number of the people who wanted to hide it have been fired. The National Immunization Program that has been in charge of vaccine safety for 30 years is no longer in charge of vaccine safety.

However, for reasons that I don't fully understand, the local health department – and no one is blaming them, they just did what they were told – choose to strongly support the handful of studies that were manipulated out of the small group that has since been fired. I don't understand why they don't just get up now and say – the American Academy of Pediatrics doesn't say, "Gee, we were fooled. We want good vaccines for our kids," and the local health department doesn't get up and say, "Well, look. Maybe we can't buy the ones that you want us to buy, but to the extent we can buy them, we'll buy them. Give us more money, we'll be happy to cooperate." Instead, they choose to cover up for the small group of the National Immunization Program who have been fired. That group was fully aware that it caused – you can read their transcripts. There are numerous memos. There's no doubt they were aware. No study will ever convince them because there's one group of people you cannot convince and that's somebody who already knows.

Now Dr. Geier, does mercury cause many similar behavioral and physiological disturbances as those shown in autism?

Mark Geier: Absolutely. There's been a published publication by Lyn Redwood and some of her colleagues which simply documented about 100 signs and symptoms of mercury poisoning, and about 100 signs and symptoms of autistic disorder. There's almost an exact match between the symptoms because, as I said, a regressive autism basically isn't a disease, it is mercury poisoning. It can be demonstrated by laboratory testing. It can be demonstrated in many, many ways. It is mercury poisoning. They're one in the same.

What is Thimerosal?

Mark Geier: We want to ask David that. He's really good at that.

David Geier: Thimerosal is half mercury by weight. The kind of mercury that's in Thimerosal is ethylmercury, which means that it's organic mercury. Thimerosal, when it's injected in the vaccines, goes rapidly into the bloodstream, crosses the placental barrier, crosses the blood brain barrier, causes significant amounts of mercury to enter into the brain. The problem with organic mercury, one is that it crosses into the brain; the second is that it has been shown to become inorganic mercury fairly rapidly in the brain. Once this process happens, it results in mercury that's sort of trapped in the brain and basically doesn't leave over time so that people my age who got Thimerosal-containing vaccines, we still carry inorganic mercury in our brains from our childhood shots. Unfortunately the autistics, who have a much decreased ability to excrete mercury, got much, much higher levels into their brain and they got to a level where it caused neurological damage.

Mercury, once it gets into the brain, is very insidious in that your body can't do anything with it. Mercury is an element; it can't be decomposed. By definition, an element is the most basic thing. And as Mercury sits in the brain, it causes inflammation, it causes the neurons to die and to degenerate, and causes terrible problems in development. The problem with these shots in the routine childhood vaccine schedule is that they're given at a period in the first year, year and a half of life, when the brain is rapidly going through normal development. Once mercury gets lodged into the brain at high levels, it's going to interfere with the wiring connecting one part of the brain with another one. It's going to cause connectivity disorders and selective death of certain kinds of neurons that are crucial for neuronal development. Hence, these children appear to develop normally in the first year of life. Mercury's coming in from the shots; eventually it reaches a high enough level where the children reach their toxic tipping point and then all of a sudden development either stops or, in some cases, it even goes backwards because the mercury starts killing or damaging the neurons.

David, in the 1990's, which Thimerosal-containing vaccines were added to the routine immunization schedule for babies? And I know Dr. Geier began to address this, but I want to address it following the explanation of what Thimerosal is and what it did.

David Geier: The vaccine that existed at the time, from the '70's and the '80's, was a vaccine called DPT, as my father said. Those had 25 micrograms of mercury. People my age who were born back in the 1980's got four or five shots of DPT vaccine. So they got between 100 and 125 micrograms of mercury as a total. Beginning in the early '90's, the hepatitis B vaccine was added in and the first dose of that vaccine was given on the day of birth. The old DPT vaccines would be given – their first dose was at two months of age. So starting on the day of birth, children got a hepatitis B shot with 12½ micrograms of mercury. They subsequently got two or three more of those shots. In addition, the *haemophilus influenza* type B, or Hib shot, was added in. Hib shots, by and large, had 25 micrograms of mercury also and they were given four times in the first 18 months of life. So in effect, the amount of mercury was tripled in the shots. Children went from getting 100 to 125 micrograms of mercury all the way up to between 200 and 300 micrograms in the first 18 months of life.

In addition, as my father said, RhoGAM shots were given during pregnancy at 28 weeks to Rh negative moms, which represent about 10% of the population. So 400,000 fetuses were exposed to mercury that way. Those ranged in concentration between about 10½ micrograms of mercury all the way in the most severe examples such as the Bayer product that may have had over 40 micrograms of mercury per dose. Those were given routinely at 28 weeks. In addition, if you were Rh negative and you had an amniocentesis or you bled during the pregnancy, you could get additional shots of RhoGAM, so that one was sort of a minimum; some people had two or three. In addition, it was given after birth to Rh negative moms who had Rh positive babies. So if those mothers breastfed their newborn babies, those babies were getting exposed to mercury that way.

In addition, towards the late '90's as flu vaccines started becoming more and more prevalent and being recommended to an ever-increasing number of infants. Those shots have 12½ micrograms of mercury and all told, if you factor that vaccine in plus the other ones, infants could have gotten almost 300 micrograms of mercury in the first 18 months of life plus RhoGAM exposure. In addition, infants were exposed to environmental sources such as by breathing the air or drinking the water, or from fish. These children were over all of the safety limits that were set for mercury. To give you an idea as to how much the mercury safety limits are, the EPA has set a limit of 0.1 micrograms of mercury per kilogram body weight per day. To translate that into how much mercury children got from their vaccines, a newborn infant on the day of birth got a hepatitis B vaccine with 12½ micrograms of mercury. An average newborn weighs about three kilograms – that's about seven pounds – so three kilograms times 0.1 means that that infant was allowed 0.3 micrograms of mercury on the day of birth. The hepatitis B shot, as I said, had 12½ so they were approximately 40 times over the safety limit on the day of birth.

Additionally, things got much worse for infants. At two months of age, the routine childhood vaccine schedule called for another hepatitis B shot with 12½ micrograms of mercury, a DPT shot with 25 more and a Hib vaccine with 25 more on top of that. At two month's of age an average infant weighed about 12 pounds – or five kilograms – so they were allowed 0.5 micrograms of mercury. They received 62.5. They were now approximately 129 fold over the safety limit. Maybe another way to think about that for people who can't picture what 129-fold over means, Dr. Neal Halsey suggested you should think of like the children got the maximal allowable dose, which was in this case 0.5. They were allowed that for day one, day two, day three, day four, etc. They got 129 days' worth of exposure at the limit in a single day from their shots. So that in effect it's like – Dr. Haley often gives the example about getting drunk – maybe if you can handle one drink a day and so you take 129 days' worth of one drink and you take them all in one day, you're going to get drunk and you're probably going to kill yourself. That's what was going on in these shots. They were bolus doses of mercury and mercury, as I said, has this nasty habit of having a half-life in the body so that when an infant – let's take that two-month-old infant again – when they got the 62.5 micrograms of mercury, it went into their body and it persisted.

If you allow sort of a generous half-life, assuming that it went down – as I said, some of the mercury never goes down in the body – so let's say that the half-life was 30 days. That means in 30 days half of the mercury in the body got excreted so that that would mean at three months of age, that infant would have about 31 micrograms of mercury. At four months of age, you have a second half-life, now there would be 16 micrograms of mercury. At four months of age, they would come in and they would give the next part of the childhood vaccine schedule – a DPT shot and a Hib – so potentially 50 micrograms of mercury plus the 16 that was left over from two months, and a smaller fraction would be left over from birth. So each time these children went in, starting from birth and then two months, four months, six months and so on, they kept getting more and more mercury into their body. These autistic children, because they had decreased ability to excrete mercury, it kept building and building and building much more rapidly than those children who went on to be normal, and they reached their toxic tipping point by between first and second year of life.

Plus, a baby on the day that he is born can't even excrete it in bile, can he?

David Geier: Yes, that's very true. Even normal children have diminished capacity to detoxify mercury. Historically, people know that the younger the baby or into the fetal period, the younger they are the more sensitive they will be to mercury because they have less ability to excrete it through their bile, and, also as you get smaller and smaller, your brain becomes a much bigger percentage of your body, so that proportionally more and more mercury is ending up in the brain of a younger and younger infant or fetus.

So we've established that the amount of mercury that babies received in their routine infant immunizations exceeded agency guidelines?

David Geier: Yes. The way I did it was as an instantaneous excess. Some people question the validity of that. They say that you need to average over days. Even if you take your infant in the first six months—I'll give that example—an average infant weighs maybe 5 kilograms during that time – so that they allow 0.5 per day and at six months they are 180 days old, so they were allowed let's say 90 to 100 micrograms of mercury according to the EPA guideline. From the shots, the children could have theoretically gotten up to 200 micrograms of mercury, so they were more than two-fold in excess of the limit. Even if you average it over every day in their first six months of life, they were still two-fold over the limit, and that's giving the best way possible to look at it from the point of view of minimal toxic effect. They were still more than twice over the EPA limit.

Now David, I think you may have addressed this earlier but is Thimerosal-derived ethylmercury safer than fish-derived methylmercury?

David Geier: Well, they are very similar. The way for laypeople to think about this is mercury, as I said, is an element. What's happened in methyl and ethyl mercury is that some carbons have been added on to the mercury. Carbon of course is what makes up your body; we're all made out of carbon. We're organic. By putting carbons onto the mercury, it makes the mercury into an organic substance. Methyl, ethyl and propyl – so that's one-, two- and three-carbon—all of those are considered to be what are called short-chain alkyl mercury compounds. They all have a tremendous ability to penetrate through membranes, meaning if you had the substance in your hand and you sort of grasp it, all three of those would go right through your skin—which acts as a membrane—goes right through the blood brain barrier, right through the placental barrier. So that organic; your body can't differentiate that from self. They all have the property that once they get sort of imbedded into tissue like the brain or many other organs in the body, the only way your body can slowly respond to them is it can try to remove the carbon. As it removes the carbon, the mercury changes from organic mercury into inorganic mercury.

What has been shown with Thimerosal is that it has a very interesting dual property meaning that when you inject it initially, it has organic properties which means that it behaves a lot like methylmercury – goes into the brain, goes into the organs – and then the two carbons are cut off to make it into inorganic mercury. Once that step happens, the inorganic mercury cannot be excreted out of the tissues. So that while methylmercury may cross more effectively into somewhere like the brain, it has the ability to cross back out because the carbons aren't removed as fast as in ethylmercury. So that with ethylmercury, you get slightly less mercury in the brain relative to methyl, but that the ethylmercury persists for a much longer period of time relative to the methylmercury.

That's an excellent explanation, David. It doesn't sound to me as if Thimerosal-derived ethyl mercury is safer than fish-derived methyl mercury. Is that a fair assessment?

David Geier: That's a very fair assessment. Let me just mention one other thing which is that these safety limits that were set for methylmercury, that's for orally ingested methylmercury which in many ways is very, very different than vaccine exposure. First, it's in something like fish so that it's bound up to the proteins in fish and you're taking it orally so that a significant amount of that mercury – even though you can put it in a chemical analyzer and derive a certain amount of mercury in the fish – only a fraction of the mercury in the fish comes off. The fish are also full of selenium and other nutrients that help you to naturally excrete mercury. Also in your gut – because for many eons humans have been eating fish and things with mercury in it – your gut is full of sulfhydryl groups and things that help excrete the mercury to try to make it so you don't absorb it. So then in many ways the limits that have been set for methylmercury are sort of overestimating the amount of mercury. If they say 0.1 is safe, if you inject the vaccine directly into you, you're getting 100% uptake, so that the vaccine in some ways is much more dangerous because it's a 100% absorbed.

Let me just mention something else about Thimerosal that's not very widely known. In chemical reactions, which is how you synthesize Thimerosal, which is you take ethylmercury and thiosalicylate and try to bind them together. When you do a reaction like that, there's always a certain amount of impurity. People have done experiments now in animals where they've injected Thimerosal, like the vaccine, and they showed that there was ethylmercury in the tissues. They showed inorganic mercury got into the tissues, and they showed methylmercury got into the tissues, because in the synthesis reaction to make the ethylmercury that binds up with the thiosalicylate, even if they're extremely good at it, one, two, three percent impurity, that would be a wonderful chemical reaction for purity's sake— if you have 1 to 3% methylmercury in there, which is naturally going to happen—these children were over the methymercury safety limit.

Let me just give you the same example we were talking about before. You take your two-month-old infant again. If they got 62.5 micrograms of mercury at that point, and let's say it was just one percent methylmercury in Thimerosal, that would mean that you would have as an approximate number about 0.625 micrograms of methylmercury. As I said, the EPA safety limit was 0.1 times 5-kilogram body weight. So they were allowed 0.5 micrograms and they got 0.625. They were over the EPA safety limit at that time using the methylmercury part of Thimerosal, let alone all the ethylmercury in there.

Well David, can you tell us about the timing and the rigor of the portions of the childhood immunization schedule that included administration of Thimerosal-containing vaccines in the United States, for example, as opposed to that used by some European or Scandinavian countries. Was that an important factor?

David Geier: Yes. The rigors of the U.S. vaccine schedule are like no others in the world. For whatever reason, the stars aligned and people were so asleep here that we unfortunately in this country ended up with the worst of all possible worlds. No other country routinely gave Thimerosal-containing RhoGAM to all Rh negative women. No other country gave Thimerosal-containing hepatitis B on the day of birth. Nobody had the kind of exposure to mercury that existed in this country from vaccine. Everywhere else, something was better. If it was in Denmark, they gave it later in infancy and they gave much less, and they didn't have the RhoGAM exposure. Nobody was doing what we did and nobody has our kind of autism problem.

So the epi studies that are oft quoted in Scandinavian countries, is that kind of like comparing apples to oranges to compare it to the United States?

David Geier: The European studies that have been done – and there's a study out of Sweden, a couple out of Denmark, there's one out of England – have extremely little applicability to the U.S. experience. That being said, now that we have seen a lot of the internal CDC documents, day by day as we read more and more of the emails and more and more of the discussion, it becomes more and more upsetting as to what happened. The CDC, if you interviewed them, would say that these are well-designed, well-controlled studies done by independent researchers.

And what we see is that that is not the case at all, that these studies where they discussed with CDC about how to do the studies, in many cases CDC themselves designed the protocols, looked over the results, modified the results to get the desired outcome. We've read – as an example, there's a series of emails between Elizabeth Miller – she's the person, the head author, on the United Kingdom studies on Thimerosal– she wrote an email describing that she wanted to do a study in England. Dr. Verstraeten, believe it or not, wrote back an email to her discussing basically the severe limitations to her study where he described that the dose of Thimerosal in England was not going to be high enough to see the effects he was seeing in the VSD (Vaccine Safety Datalink) database. He also severely criticized the database that she wanted to look at saying that the data was so muddled that she'd never be able to see the effect. He suggested as a conclusion that maybe we don't want to give the money to her.

The next email that came back from Elizabeth Miller said, "Does that mean that I have to give the money back to do the study?" Our CDC people were involved in funding the English study. Our own CDC people, the honest ones, were criticizing that there wasn't enough mercury, the database was no good. Despite all of these limitations, the next email to come back is, "Studies going ahead anyways," and now Elizabeth Miller is asking Robert Chen from our CDC exactly what they did in the VSD and how to take the effects that they're seeing in the VSD and try to make them appear in this English database, and then how to make them go away. Then in the final study, Elizabeth Miller – you can see this reflected in the published Verstraeten study which claims that there is no significant effect – one of the outcomes that they found linked to Thimerosal was tics in the published study. You look at the published Elizabeth Miller study where she showed across the board Thimerosal seemed to significantly prevent neurodevelopmental disorders. But you get down to tics, tics was significantly elevated in her results.

Well David, even though the United States had such a rigorous childhood immunization schedule with more vaccines given and earlier timing – and by the way, am I correct in saying that?

David Geier: Yes, that's certainly true.

Notwithstanding all of that, have some children regressed into autism or other neurodevelopmental disorders even receiving Thimerosal-containing vaccines a little or a lot later in life?

David Geier: There are stories. I mean, this is anecdotal but I certainly have talked to many parents; that their children were sort of on the edge of the toxic tipping point and that at age 10 or 11, or even older, some of them regressed into autism at that time. So that I think it's sort of a function of how susceptible you are, how much mercury you have in your body, and when it's given. All of those things are applicable here. This is kind of off-topic here, but we even see some adults who get these Thimerosal-containing vaccines who develop neurological problems. It looks somewhat like autism, but isn't exactly autism because the sequence of events in development is so different in adults. I think that Thimerosal, as Boyd Haley would say, is a poison anywhere. You can show it in tissue culture, people, animals; any kind of system you want. It's just a question really of do you have enough on board to reach your individual toxic tipping point, and that no amount of mercury is really safe.

We talk a lot about trace vaccines and clearly we applaud CDC for trying to encourage that, but it's just a question of how many people you're going to damage. At the 25 micrograms per shot, it's clearly totally unacceptable. If you make it trace you'll damage a lot less, and if you make it sort of sub-trace you'll damage even less. The ultimate absolute answer here is we need no mercury at all in the vaccine.

So can even decreased amounts of mercury combine synergistically with other toxins and contaminants to create a harmful effect? It sounds like you're implying that, as well.

David Geier: Well, I think that mercury interacts with other things in the body. What I'm saying though here is that for many poisons, there is an acceptable level. You can show at such-and-such a level that nobody will be harmed. In the case of mercury, all you can do is reduce the amount of harm done to less and less people. As long as mercury is present, there's a very high probability someone will be adversely affected somewhere. It's just a question of numbers. It's sort of like the reverse of the autism epidemic. What we did was we went to such a high level we were starting to pick off significant numbers of children. As we look back historically into the record of the mercury in the shots, and as less and less were given, there was less and less with autism until we reach a point of very, very low levels.

So it's something basically we need to eliminate altogether. The only way you can make mercury safe is to remove it from the equation.

Good point. Is there any idea of how much of the population is even more susceptible to mercury toxicity?

David Geier: I think there's a fair percentage of the population that's susceptible to mercury, but what's very unusual about the vaccine exposure is how rigorous and soon it happens. It's very unlike anything else in human history in many ways. I mean the closest that you can come by is poisonings of mercury where somebody ate contaminated grain or contaminated seafood. But even that is not really the same thing because in the case of the vaccines, this was mandated, a required thing that basically upwards of 95% of the people in this country took, and they took it year-in/year-out, year-in/year-out. So that's very unlike any kind of other poisonings. Poisonings are usually localized, a small group of people, and you see that there are people damaged. We've never seen such a broad-based kind of exposure to such a harmful chemical to go on – I mean maybe one time, one year – this went on year after year after year.

As my father said, we're up to two generations' worth of children that have been exposed. So our society is like a chemistry project. We're doing our clinical trial on ourselves. God only knows what the long-term outcomes will be. We know acutely that it caused neurodevelopmental disorders and neurological damage in an extreme number of children. But what happens when the children in the Thimerosal generations who were unaffected when they reach 30, 40, 50 and they have all this inorganic mercury sitting in their brains? Are they going to develop Alzheimer's at 40 instead of 60 or 70? Are they going to develop breast cancer at age 30 when they should never have had it? All of those are things that we can only speculate on based upon what's been previously reported with mercury. I can't give you a definite answer of the association between exposure to mercury from vaccines and any of those outcomes, and that's really scary to think about because we may have a ticking time-bomb waiting to explode in the Thimerosal generation.

Well it's certainly a valid question to think about, David. Now I know that you said that no amount of mercury could be considered a safe amount of mercury. Even with trace amounts you just damage fewer people. But if you do have trace amounts and that combines with something like lead or PCBs, would a low amount of mercury tend to have a synergistic effect with other contaminants or toxicants?

David Geier: It's been shown in animal poisonings and even in human poisonings that mercury will interact with other kinds of poisons. Famous example, you throw mercury and lead together; you don't get just mercury toxicity and lead toxicity and add them together. There's a synergistic kind of toxicity meaning that the sum of two is greater than the individual, so that – I mean we want to limit mercury exposure as much as possible to people. That being said, I'm not a non-practical person. I recognize that there are limitations in manufacturing vaccines and we are talking about a transition so that for the moment, we want to make sure that at least all the vaccines have trace amounts. But as the long-term objective, we want to make sure that all the vaccines are completely mercury-free.

Is autism increasing in foreign countries where recently there's more rigorous use of Thimerosal-containing vaccines?

David Geier: There's some indication of that. There are reports that China is entering the midst of an autism epidemic that seems to mirror the introduction of western vaccines. There's no controlled study really looking at that. There's only anecdotal stories like we hear that vaccines are now being used in this population and autism seems to be going up. Unfortunately, one of the things that's happening in the world is that everybody is trying to scramble, especially the countries who were trying to hide things, trying to scramble to make their rate of autism the same as the U.S. Kind of an amazing phenomena to see. I mean you take somewhere like Denmark where all the experts said the rate of autism was less than 1 in 1,000. So we announced in the '90's it was 1 in 500 and they tried to adjust their numbers to 1 in 500. Then the *Autism Alarm* came out suggesting maybe 1 in 150, then they came out with studies trying to get it up to 1 in 200 or 300. Our rate keeps going up and they keep trying to adjust it to follow suit. I don't believe that a lot of these other countries have the same kind of rates as we do. I think that they're trying to just manipulate numbers.

Before we move on to your study specifically, Dr. Geier and David, I just want to double check one thing that David said. David, you said that there was an interesting phenomena with the Thimerosal-containing vaccines and that there was some methylmercury present, and that methylmercury even exceeded the guidelines.

David Geier: Yes, that's very true. It has been shown in animals that methylmercury levels go up with the injection of ethylmercury-containing Thimerosal because of impurities.

Wow. That kind of zaps that argument that we hear sometimes, doesn't it?

David Geier: Unfortunately, the people who are running the public health departments around the country, the people at the CDC and FDA, they really are not trying to analyze – to review – the historical information. As my father said, there are thousands of articles out there on Thimerosal and ethylmercury, and these people don't read them, they don't want to know about them. All they want to know about is how to try to cover this over and not look at what's there. They attack any piece of evidence that comes out. That's their sort of 'business as usual.' They're not actively looking out for the interests of the children. They're looking out for their own interests and how they think they can maybe survive this big debacle.

Now gentlemen, let's move on to your recent study entitled, "Early Downward Trends in Neurodevelopmental Disorders Following Removal of Thimerosal-Containing Vaccines." With regard to neurodevelopmental disorders, which databases did you look at to see if there was a rise, and are either of those databases used by government agencies from which to derive their own information?

David Geier: The databases we looked at were the Vaccine Adverse Event Reporting System, California Department of Developmental Services. We also looked at data from the U.S. Department of Education. All three of these databases are state or federal databases. They're used to track trends in diagnoses. The California database is the source of several publications out of the State of California showing that the autism rate is indeed significantly increasing and that it can't be explained away. The VAERS database is a federal source of monitoring vaccine reactions. The CDC and the FDA have published numerous studies out of the VAERS database and have even shaped U.S. vaccine policy. As an example, about the Rotavirus vaccine, it was shown that it caused intussuception based upon analysis of the VAERS database. Once CDC found that association, the vaccine was withdrawn from the U.S. market. So that it is a valid surveillance tool and the CDC even developed the techniques that we routinely use to analyze that database. U.S. Department of Education, another federal database—That's how we keep track of the people in our schools.

All three of these databases show the same phenomena, meaning that from the early 1990's through about mid-2002 – roughly a 12-year period – that there was a significant increase in the rate of new cases of autism and other neurodevelopmental disorders coming into the system. And what we've seen is that since mid-2002, when there was a peak, that the number of new cases or the changes in the populations in these databases has significantly changed from the past. Numbers that had been going up, up, up, all of a sudden started going down in total number. So what we're saying here is that while the overall prevalence of autism in the United States continues to rise because autistic children are not dying, the rate of new cases or the incidence rate of autism is dramatically changing, and it's changing in a way where it's going down.

Now the databases that you used for this study, are they independent of each other?

David Geier: Yes, these are independent databases. Different reporting tools. California Department of Developmental Services is, as it suggests, a specific branch of the California government that tracks, as they call them, consumers in this program which pays for lifetime care of autistics. The VAERS database tracks vaccine-associated adverse events, and U.S. Department of Education tracks educational status of children and their needs around the country. Three different data sets entirely.

Do the majority of the VAERS reports come from parents according to what the CDC has said?

David Geier: Historically, the CDC has published less than 5% of reports come from parents according to the CDC. It's kind of interesting that one of the most recent studies, which tries to criticize our work in VAERS, said that we were just looking at time trends in autism, what they called a longitudinal study in VAERS, which we've never done up until this new one. But they claim that when you look at VAERS that supposedly it's the lawyers who are reporting to VAERS and so that they're manufacturing an increase in autism in VAERS. What's very ironic about our new publication is that at the same time they published that, within about one month before our new study came out, we published that the rate of autism is actually going down in VAERS. When they're saying that it's being driven by the lawyers and it's pushing it up, we're reporting that it's going down.

That's interesting,

David Geier: Very interesting.

Yes.

Mark Geier: In addition, it should be pointed out that we did our studies in a way to rule that out. We looked at trends in 1994 when there were no lawyers. We looked at effects that no one could possibly have known about. It is not being done by the lawyers, and in fact the lawyers don't push it up. Most lawyers tell their clients not to report to VAERS. This is ridiculous. Even if you think that there are weaknesses in each of the three databases, the odds that we would predict that three years following the withdrawal of Thimerosal you would start to see that children born at this time would have less autism, and that autism would go down at the same time in all three databases. You don't need any statistical analysis, but we did some. This is the eyeball test. Anybody can get on these – you can go to the journal line. They have links there for the databases. You can go look at it yourself. We have no control over those databases. The odds that three databases, good or bad, would go down exactly at the same time and exactly as predicted, defies logic. Yet they think they can convince anybody that this isn't related to the vaccines when we ourselves said that this would happen. They said if we're right it would happen, and they would believe it if it happened but it would never happen. Now that it happens, they're not going to believe it. They're going to have to eat this one. This is the final nail in the coffin. Anybody can understand this. It's totally transparent. It's over. Their lies will no longer be acceptable.

David Geier: And as you know personally, Teri, I mean we presented at your autism conference in the Spring of 2003, which is when we had our first articles accepted in the *Journal of American Physicians and Surgeons* and *Experimental Biology in Medicine* – those were written in the summer of 2002 – predating any decrease in autism. We said in those articles that based on our epidemiological studies that as Thimerosal was removed from the vaccines beginning in 1999, that the new children being born in mid-1999 on were going to have less autism. We've come back now three years to the exact issue in the *Journal of American Physicians and Surgeons* and reported that it's exactly what happened in all three of those databases. They did indeed go down, and it looks like the children born from mid-1999 on, as Thimerosal was gradually reduced from some of the childhood vaccines, low and behold they have less autism than the children born before that recommendation. People are starting to look at other databases and what do they see? Exactly the same thing.

One of the databases – I'll just briefly mention it here – is they're looking in the Minnesota data. Minnesota has good accurate records about autism and speech disorders, and you look at that data—just like what you see in VAERS, U.S. Department of Education, California Department of Developmental Services—the Minnesota databases show that beginning in 2002 to 2003, there's been a significance decline in the number of new cases of autism and speech disorders. The decline is almost exactly of the magnitude we saw in those other three databases.

So conceivably, parents could try to find out in every one of their states what these figures look like.

David Geier: What we see across the board, I believe, in this country is that at the very least, the curve that had been going up tremendously fast has either flattened out in the states or is going down. Either way, it's a success story for Thimerosal because if you look at the curve, there was no indication at all that it should go down. As many people had predicted – and there were doomsayers out there – I mean it was up to 1 in 150 and you do the mathematical models, in another 10 or 15 years it was going to 100% of the children had autism in this country, so that a flattening out, as we show in our article, by itself is significant. We're not only seeing it flattening out, we're seeing it going down now in many of the states.

Right. Let me ask you a question about the California Department of Developmental Services data. Does CDDS only provide regional center services based upon professional diagnosis of full-syndrome autism?

David Geier: Yes, that's correct. The California data, those are—and we've even had experience now—we've talked to a number of the psychologists and pediatric neurologists out in California. They are very, very nitpicky in California and they've been for a very long time. In California, as I said, if you get a diagnosis of full-syndrome DSM IV-autism, the State of California will pay for your lifetime care, all medical expenses, everything. So that they have forever been very careful to make sure that the children really have full-syndrome autism. We've heard stories about if you do willy-nilly diagnoses, there's no way those kids are going to make it into the system— now or in the past—you must be full-syndrome autism.

I would observe that full-syndrome autism is hard to miss.

David Geier: I think that that's certainly the case, and I think based on what's going on in this country, it doesn't make any sense of why it should go down. If you look at California population as an example, it has continued to rise. As people have talked about California and their paying for lifetime care, if anything people have begun to migrate into California. Certainly there hasn't been a mass exodus; if anything, people have gone in. So those numbers, like I said, if it had leveled off and was flat line, it was a tremendous triumph. In reality, we're seeing that data go down, so that as we show in our paper, if you extrapolate based on where the numbers should have gone, they were continuing at the same rate of increase as they always had been at versus where they are today, there are 350 fewer cases of autism in the system per reporting quarter now than you would have expected based on the lines that have been going up. We looked from '94 through 2002, so that comes out to over 1,000 fewer autistics per year.

So, David, can you remind us when mercury was, to a large extent, phased out of the routine infant vaccination schedule?

David Geier: It was begun to be removed in mid-1999, and based on the three-year lag as a minimum to get a diagnosis of autism, that means 2000, 2001, 2002. Mid-2002 should be the peak because that goes back to mid-1999, when children were born. Subsequent to that time, you should start seeing that as mercury was withdrawn from some of the shots, they also recommended that, as an example, the hepatitis B vaccine should be delayed away from birth outside of the first six months of life; that all of those kinds of things extrapolate from mid-1999, mid-2002, from that period on there's a significant decrease in autism and other neurodevelopmental disorders.

So basically, the graph followed the prediction?

David Geier: The exact prediction that if there was a direct correlation – which the increase looks like it follows. As an example, if you look at Mark Blaxill's graph looking at California of coverage of

Thimerosal-containing vaccines versus the rate of autism, you see that the two went up at the exact same time. Now what we're seeing is, just like the old graph, we have a point where mercury should start going down and that's exactly where autism starts going down.

So this is kind of an overview and I want to backtrack and break it down a little bit. What reporting quarters did you analyze?

David Geier: We analyzed in VAERS and California Department of Developmental Services starting January 1, 1994 so that those are children born in 1991, right at the beginning of the epidemic. We tracked the first section of increase from that period through January 2003 in both California and VAERS so that we would capture the theoretical peak within the window of 2002 to 2003, assuming that Thimerosal had an affect here. We then did a second reporting window from January 2002 through just about the end of 2005 in both VAERS and California data. I forget the exact quarter, but it was towards the end of 2005. We showed statistically in both databases that there was a significant rise in autism from 1994 through 2003 and then we showed that the line significantly decreased from 2002 to the end of 2005, and then we compared the slopes, meaning the rate of change, in both of the two periods and showed statistically that they were very different – significantly different. We did this for autism in California, autism in VAERS. Then in the VAERS database, because you have additional outcomes that are unavailable in California, we showed that speech disorders followed the same kind of pattern. Then as a third database, we looked at the young children with autism coming into the U.S. Department of Education and showed that for the last several years that there was an increase in those young children. Then in the last year or two, there was a significant decrease in the number of new cases coming in there as well.

Mark Geier: Just one comment to your listeners. To those that are intimidated by statistics – although we did the statistics and they're right – you don't need statistics. This is one of those things that passes the eyeball test. Anybody can look at those dots on the graph. No one has ever disputed that they're plotted correctly. With your eyes you can easily see that there's been a major change in the same place in all three graphs. You don't really need a statistical thing. Although of course as scientists we do that. This one passes what I call the eyeball test.

David Geier: You see it went up and it went down; that's what my father is referring to.

David, what were you referring to earlier that was different? Do you remember? You said something was different and when I eyeballed these things, the lines looked as if they roughly paralleled each other to me.

David Geier: Yes, what I'm saying is that in California and in VAERS for autism, we followed the same kind of exact procedure to track autism. We did it on a quarterly basis in the change in autism in each of the quarters. We saw that they went up for the same period and then they went down for the same period.

Okay. Now what about these graphs roughly paralleling each other for things like speech disorders?

David Geier: That shows that the effect is expanded beyond just autism. As the title of our paper suggests – and we've said since the very beginning – the association is between Thimerosal and neurodevelopmental disorders, of which autism is a type of neurodevelopmental disorder, there are many others such as Attention Deficit Disorder, such as ADHD, such as speech of language delay, tics. There's a whole list of these things that are in that spectrum. Autism – maybe another way to more easily consider it – is the top of the iceberg. As you go down the iceberg to these less severe conditions, you find that more and more children are affected, but they become less and less severe. That's where as Congressman Weldon says, perhaps all the children are in someway affected. As you get down towards the base of the iceberg, you reach a point where maybe children only lost two I.Q. points due to the mercury exposure. You'd never be able to really quantify that, but they are affected in some way.

Haven't they needed to decrease the qualification criteria for college and such – college entrance?

David Geier: They've had to adjust many of the standardized tests. There's an example, by definition the I.Q. test says that average is 100, but they've had to adjust the scores to keep 100 at the same place. They've had to adjust them downwards because unfortunately the children today are not performing as well as they did in the past. Same kinds of things with the SAT score. They've had to adjust for the fact that children aren't performing as well as they did a decade or 20 years ago.

Did you figure out confounding factors in your study?

David Geier: The way in which we tried to adjust confounding and biasing factors is the consistency of the effect. As we said, the graphs are similar both in California, VAERS and U.S. Department of Education, that argues against that there is some confounding artifact causing this. Additionally, we looked at other neurodevelopmental disorders like speech disorders to show that the affect was broad-based, not particular to one outcome or another. Then the most important aspect for confounding is that this was a prospective assessment, meaning that it's not something we came back years and years after the fact and said, "Oh look, autism went up and it went down, and we know what Thimerosal did in that time." If we saw that, even by itself, this is powerful evidence. But this is what we had predicted, we and other researchers who had said Thimerosal was a causal factor in neurodevelopmental disorders and autism. We said that when mercury was begun to be removed from the shots, that autism and neurodevelopmental disorders would go down.

As my father said, and everybody who's sort of been on the other side, they said, "If you could show us that autism and neurodevelopmental disorders went down, we would believe you." That would be the deciding factor here. What we've shown now in this first study in the *Journal of American Physicians and Surgeons* – and we now have a second study that's accepted in the *Medical Science Monitor* which is sponsored by Eli Lilly themselves, they're the developers of Thimerosal – is that autism and other neurodevelopmental disorders went up with the mercury in the shots and now that mercury has been reduced from some of the childhood shots, that autism and neurodevelopmental disorders have gone down. Let me make an additional prediction, because we predicted this before. If they were to remove the mercury completely, the levels would go down to very, very low levels. Not zero because there still are some background causes like fragile-X and fetal alcohol syndrome. That's the good prediction. The bad prediction is if they keep putting it back in, which is what they're obviously trying to do, they're going to make this drop be temporary. I think that's what they're trying to do, unfortunately.

Let me quantify about the current exposure, because this is in some ways the most scary thing of all. Very quietly CDC, FDA, public health officials have moved to get the mercury back in the shots. My father said that, I've said that, a bunch of us have said that. Let me tell you how much mercury we're talking about, and to a certain extent even how unknown the effect of that will be. One aspect of it – and this is the most troubling one – is that they now recommend, and American College of Obstetrics and Gynecology is carrying this out, to give all pregnant women a flu shot. In the past, the story was that only Rh negative moms would get a RhoGAM shot and we knew generally it was at 28 weeks so it was one specific window in pregnancy. The new recommendation is, as I said, all pregnant women. So it's not 400,000 Rh negative moms a year; it's four million moms. Beyond that, the recommendation is not in one specific window. They've now approved it for the first trimester, second trimester, third trimester—anywhere in pregnancy. I have no idea, and nobody knows, what giving it in let's say the first month of pregnancy versus the fifth month—what the difference will be in risks to the fetus. Each of those flu shots almost exclusively is going to have 25 micrograms of mercury.

Isn't the fetus like a sponge?

David Geier: The fetus, yes. Clearly, and there are excellent studies on this, the mercury from the flu shot is going to be taken up much more by the fetus relative to the mom. In some ways they call it like the toxic waste dump; all the nasty chemicals go into the fetus. It's been shown and reported that the ethylmercury is much more readily taken up by the developing fetus than methylmercury. It's been shown if you make the mercury radioactive that the ethylmercury will go into the fetus and it goes into the fetus' central nervous system. When you measure using the radioactive label that the amount in the fetus' central nervous system relative to the mom's central nervous system is much, much higher. I can't even begin to assess how much damage that may do.

Yes, it's pretty grim. I think some real prudence is called for here.

David Geier: Let me just say, historically what we know about Thimerosal and pregnancy – and this is not available in the influenza vaccine package inserts that has Thimerosal – what they claim is that it's a class C meaning that you only are supposed to give it in pregnancy under dyer emergency and that it's never been tested in people or animals prior to its use. Well it turns out Thimerosal has been tested. Thimerosal has been shown to cause fetal abortions, fetal malformations, fetal – any kind of mess you want to see possible in fetuses. I mean these stories and these experiments in animals – we have pictures of fetuses exposed to Thimerosal where they developed cleft lip, cleft palette. They exposed chicken embryos to low levels of Thimerosal. They showed the feet became cock-eyed and crooked because it interferes with bone ossification. They showed that the beaks in these fetal chickens became abnormal and crooked. These are horrifying things.

Then in humans—believe it or not, people have studied Thimerosal in pregnant humans—and this is a study by the NIH, CDC and the FDA published in 1977 – they showed putting some Thimerosal on your skin, a of couple drops, significantly raised the rate of birth defects approximately three-fold in humans. So this is not available in the flu package insert even though it has been shown. So this is very, very bad. On top of the mercury in-utero exposure, they now recommend three influenza shots in the first 18 months of life. Each one of those can have 12½ micrograms of mercury. So that's on top of the 25 in-utero. Then the children are supposed to, from age two to five, each year get flu vaccines and each of those flu shots can have 25 micrograms more. So when you add all of this up, the total is about 125 micrograms of mercury, slightly more than that. The old total maximal exposure I said was between 200 and 300 micrograms. When you assess this, we're now over 50 percent as high in the first five years of life as we were back in 1999 before the recommendations to get it out. When you evaluate on a per-kilogram basis how much mercury – because now you're giving it routinely to fetuses – the level is almost exactly what we were giving pre-1999 recommendation to get it out. This is horrific. Horrifying. They have plans on the drawing board to approve new Thimerosal-containing vaccines. They have every intention, if they're not regulated and society doesn't keep putting the pressure on them, of having as much or more mercury in these shots than they did pre-1999 recommendation to get it out.

Mark Geier: And as Dr. Offit said in his interview, "You can bet on it, that the new vaccines are going to have Thimerosal, and there's nothing you can do about it." I think there's something we can – and we are – going to do about it.

All right. That's really some awful news there. To recap a bit, in 1994 we had stable diagnostic criteria in the DSM4, and did you say that there was a rise in each database from 1994 to 2002 in autism, neurodevelopmental disorders, and speech disorders?

David Geier: Yes, that's what we said in our studies.

Okay, and you plotted increases and decrease of autism and speech disorders reported to VAERS, and the VAERS graph and the California Department of Developmental Services graphs roughly paralleled each other insofar as when cases increased and when cases decreased for each of autism and speech disorders?

David Geier: Yes.

You figured out confounding factors and you've found that the increases and decreases correlated with increasing and decreasing amounts of Thimerosal administered via the vaccine schedule?

David Geier: Yes.

Department of Education figures also bore this out and so you feel that your findings support a real effect and not a chance observation?

David Geier: Yes.

All right. Do other scientific studies from other researchers such as toxicology, molecular, biochemistry, clinical science, etc., implicate mercury as a possible factor in the autism epidemic?

David Geier: Absolutely. The best in some ways, or the most interesting one that I've come across, my father already mentioned and everybody always points to the Safe Minds *Medical Hypotheses* Study from 2001. The title of it I believe is "Autism: A Novel Form of Mercury Poisoning." Everybody always points to that as the study that implicates Thimerosal or mercury in autism. I like a study that I've come across from early 2000. One of the co-authors on the study was Thomas Burbacher who is the scientist who's done the research in monkeys showing Thimerosal goes into the brain and stays there for a very long time. But he, along with his colleagues, published in 2000 in the NIH's own journal of *Environmental Health Perspectives* that when you look at what mercury can do in tissue culture—meaning that it can kill neurons, it can cause neuro-degeneration, it can interfere in the signaling factors in neurons to prevent them from undergoing normal neuronal development—his comment was that it wouldn't be surprising if mercury could be causing autism.

So he put forward that hypothesis, or that review, of the literature in 2000, so that it was already apparent in 2000 before any of the modern evidence – biochemical, clinical, everything that we have – he already understood that mercury could be causing autism. So that this is something that's been known for a very, very long time in the literature; that mercury can cause the exact lesions that are seen in autism. This is nothing new even though they try to pretend now like this is some crazy parent in a basement somewhere that came up with the idea mercury could be causing autism. This is something supported by 40 or 50 or maybe even 60 years' worth of literature on the effects of mercury, and more specifically organic mercury on humans, animals, tissue cultures, all support our exact conclusion.

Mark Geier: Dr. Julie Gerberding has often said, "You know, why are you complaining now? They came out with Thimerosal in the '30's. Why didn't they complain then?" Why doesn't she go back and read the articles from the '30's and '40's 'cause we have. They complained and they complained vigorously. So vigorously that the American Medical Association actually recommended that it be removed way back around 1950. Those articles exist and you don't make them go away by simply not looking them up. We've spent hours in the library and those articles exist. As soon as Thimerosal came out, articles started coming out reporting massive problems with Thimerosal.

David Geier: We're talking within years and it's so bad – the history of Thimerosal – Eli Lilly in their own patent of Thimerosal said Thimerosal was toxic, they knew that ethylmercury came out of the Thimerosal, and that it was the ethylmercury that was mediating the adverse reactions in people. They even knew Thimerosal was ineffective at killing bacteria. This is completely obscene that they themselves said that in their own patent, tried to fix the problem but were unable to in the patent as they described, and it's just gone on every single decade, every single year. Practically since the introduction of Thimerosal, people have seen damage in animals, in people, in tissue culture. Any way you look at this, backwards, forwards, and upside down, there is no place for Thimerosal in medicine.

I'll leave you with one sort of parting thought about the history of Thimerosal. In 1956, a guy named Dr. Engley, who founded the University of Missouri's Microbiology Deparment that published an article where he specifically evaluated Thimerosal and showed that if you take Thimerosal and you introduce it into a vaccine at the level that it's present as a preservative, it's extremely ineffective at killing bacteria. He went out and collected over 1,000 bottles of vaccine that were in use in clinics and showed over 5% of those bottles he was able to find bacterial contamination in there, showing that the Thimerosal was completely ineffective. He then took human cells in tissue culture, grew them up and exposed them to Thimerosal and all kinds of other mercury compounds. He showed Thimerosal was the most toxic of all the mercurials he tested – the most toxic. When you extrapolate out to the minimum level of Thimerosal, he was able to show significant damage to the tissue culture cells. It was at five parts per billion of mercury. This is in 1956 he showed that.

Thomas Burbacher and the current monkey/primate study where he injected them mimicking the childhood vaccine schedule, showed that there was about 50 parts per billion of total mercury in the brain when he got done dosing. That means he found a level ten times higher than in 1956 researchers showed you could kill human cells in tissue culture. That's how much mercury went into not even "susceptible" monkeys; it's routine monkeys. If you look at the inorganic part – which was about half of that – that persists in the brain, he was unable to show any half-life. That was five times higher than Engley showed you could kill human cells in tissue culture. The levels we gave to these children, it's amazing we didn't kill them all.

Gentlemen, thank you for further illuminating this issue, for bringing up so many thought-provoking points, so many important points, and for speaking with us today.

Mark Geier: Thank you for having us.

Appendix VIII. A Summary of Scientific Literature Supporting the Exogenous Boosting Hypothesis

The Nature of Herpes Zoster: A long-term study and a new hypothesis.
(Proc R Soc Med. 1965 Jan;58:9-20.)
Hope Simpson RE.
The peculiar age distribution of zoster may in part reflect the frequency with which the different age groups encounter cases of varicella and, because of the ensuing boost to their antibody production have their attacks of zoster postponed.
PMID: 14267505

Immunologic evidence of reinfection with varicella-zoster virus.
(J Infect Dis. 1983 Aug;148(2):200-5.)
Arvin AM, Koropchak CM, Wittek AE.
Resistance to reinfection with varicella-zoster virus (VZV) was evaluated in immune adults who had household exposure to varicella. ***Sixty-four percent of 25 adults exposed to varicella had a fourfold or greater rise in IgG antibody to VZV or had a high initial IgG antibody titer to VZV that declined by fourfold.*** IgM antibody was detected in only 12% of 25 VZV-immune subjects. Seventy percent of 23 subjects exposed to varicella had IgA antibody to VZV compared with 13% of 23 subjects with antibody to VZV who had no recent exposure (P less than 0.001, chi 2 test). Enhanced cellular immunity was documented by an increase in lymphocyte transformation to VZV antigen from a mean +/- SE index of 7.8 +/- 1.30 to 15.3 +/- 2.56 (P = 0.01, paired t-test). ***The increase in immunity to VZV in many immune subjects exposed to VZV suggests the occurrence of subclinical reinfection.***
PMID: 6310001

The epidemiology of varicella-zoster virus infections: the influence of varicella on the prevalence of herpes zoster.
(Epidemiol Infect, 1992 Jun; 108(3):513-28)
Garnett GP, Grenfell BT.
Department of Animal and Plant Sciences, Sheffield University.
This paper uses mathematical models and data analysis to examine the epidemiological implications of possible immunologically mediated links between patterns of varicella and herpes-zoster incidence in human communities. A review of previously published reports does not clarify whether or not there is a relationship between the incidence of varicella and the incidence of zoster. However, new analysis of data collected by the Royal College of General Practitioners provides indirect evidence for the hypothesis that a high intensity of varicella transmission suppresses viral reactivation. The significance of this finding for proposed varicella vaccination campaigns is explored by a review of published data on the use of the vaccine. No significant difference is shown to exist between the risk of zoster caused by the vaccine and the wild virus. A mathematical model is then developed to take into consideration the influence of the prevalence of varicella on viral reactivation and the impact of vaccination with attenuated virus, which may be able to recrudesce. ***Under some conditions, mass application of such vaccines may have the impact of increasing zoster incidence. The results presented here indicate that, before starting any vaccination programme against varicella, its consequences need to be assessed in much more depth.***
PMID: 1318219

Cell-mediated immunity to varicella-zoster virus.
(J Infect Dis. 1992 Aug;166 Suppl 1:S35-41.)
Arvin AM.
Department of Pediatrics, Stanford University School of Medicine, California.
Natural varicella-zoster virus (VZV) infection and immunization with live attenuated varicella vaccine elicits T lymphocytes that recognize VZV glycoproteins, gpl-V, and the immediate early/tegument protein, the product of gene 62 (IE62). Proliferation or cytotoxicity assays, done under limiting dilution conditions to estimate responder cell frequencies, indicate no preferential recognition of VZV proteins by human T cells. Analysis of the primary cytotoxic T lymphocyte (CTL) response after vaccination demonstrates that both gpl and IE62 are targets of the early response. CD4(+)- and CD8(+)-mediated CTL recognition of these viral proteins can be detected with natural and vaccine-induced immunity. Responder cell frequencies for protein-specific T cell proliferation and CTL function are generally comparable in subjects with natural and vaccine-acquired immunity to VZV. ***Exogenous reexposure to VZV results in enhanced T cell proliferation and may be an important mechanism for maintaining virus-specific cellular immunity.*** Providing exogenous reexposure by giving varicella vaccine to individuals who have preexisting natural

immunity markedly increases the responder cell frequencies of T cells that proliferate in response to VZV antigen and the numbers of circulating CTL that recognize VZV proteins.
PMID: 1320649

[Incidence of herpes zoster in pediatricians and history of reexposure to varicella-zoster virus in patients with herpes zoster]
(Kansenshogaku Zasshi. 1995 Aug;69(8):908-12.)
[Article in Japanese]
Terada K, Hiraga Y, Kawano S, Kataoka N.
Department of Pediatrics, Kawasaki Medical School.
We found that pediatricians have enhanced specific cellular immunity to varicella-zoster virus (VZV) compared with the general population, which may be due to reexposure to VZV from children with chickenpox. There have been some reported that the varicella vaccine enhance the specific cellular immunity. To estimate the efficacy of varicella vaccine for protection against herpes zoster in the elderly, we investigated the incidence of herpes zoster in 500 pediatricians and family practitioners with their fifties and sixties, and history of reexposure to VZV in 61 patients with herpes zoster by questionnaires retrospectively. Thirty four of 352 pediatricians had a past history of herpes zoster. ***The incidence per 100,000 person-years of herpes zoster was 65.2 in those in their fifties and 158.2 in those in their sixties, which are 1/2 to 1/8 of other reports regarding the general population.*** Among 61 immunocompetent patients with herpes zoster, only 4 patients (6.6%) had the chance for reexpose to VZV before their herpes zoster. Only 7 (17.5%) of the 40 patients older than 50 years of age lived with their children less than 14 years of age. Twenty-three (57.5%) of them lived without their children and grandchildren. They are thought to be less chance to reexpose to VZV through children. We may think that the booster effect by reexposure to VZV plays an important role to prevent herpes zoster. Therefore, we can speculate that the varicella vaccine may protect against herpes zoster in the elderly by the enhanced specific cellular immunity due to the booster effect.
PMID: 7594784

The protective effect of immunologic boosting against zoster: an analysis in leukemic children who were vaccinated against chickenpox.
(J Infect Dis. 1996 Feb;173(2):450-3.)
Gershon AA, LaRussa P, Steinberg S, Mervish N, Lo SH, Meier P.
Department of Pediatrics, Columbia University College of Physicians and Surgeons, New York, New York 10032, USA.
Whether reexposure of varicella-immune persons to varicella-zoster virus would protect against or predispose to development of zoster was analyzed. The rate of zoster in 511 leukemic recipients of varicella vaccine who had 1 or > 1 dose of varicella vaccine and in those who did or did not have a household exposure to varicella was determined. A Kaplan-Meier life-table analysis revealed that the incidence of zoster was lower in those given > 1 dose of vaccine (P < .05). A Cox proportional hazards analysis showed that both household exposure to varicella and receipt of > 1 dose of vaccine were highly protective (P < .01) against zoster. ***Thus, the risk of zoster is decreased by reexposure to varicella-zoster virus, either by vaccination or by close exposure to varicella.***
PMID: 8568309

Varicella-zoster virus.
(Clin Microbiol Rev. 1996 Jul;9(3):361-81.)
Arvin AM.
Department of Pediatrics, Stanford University School of Medicine, California
94305-5119, USA.
Varicella-zoster virus (VZV) is a ubiquitous human alphaherpesvirus that causes varicella (chicken pox) and herpes zoster (shingles). Varicella is a common childhood illness, characterized by fever, viremia, and scattered vesicular lesions of the skin. As is characteristic of the alphaherpesviruses, VZV establishes latency in cells of the dorsal root ganglia. Herpes zoster, caused by VZV reactivation, is a localized, painful, vesicular rash involving one or adjacent dermatomes. The incidence of herpes zoster increases with age or immunosuppression. The VZV virion consists of a nucleocapsid surrounding a core that contains the linear, double-stranded DNA genome; a protein tegument separates the capsid from the lipid envelope, which incorporates the major viral glycoproteins. VZV is found in a worldwide geographic distribution but is more prevalent in temperate climates. Primary VZV infection elicits immunoglobulin G (IgG), IgM, and IgA antibodies, which bind to many classes of viral proteins. Virus-specific cellular immunity is critical for controlling viral replication in healthy and immunocompromised patients with primary or recurrent VZV infections. Rapid laboratory confirmation of the diagnosis of varicella or herpes zoster, which can be accomplished by detecting viral proteins or DNA, is important to determine the need for antiviral therapy. Acyclovir is licensed for

treatment of varicella and herpes zoster, and acyclovir, valacyclovir, and famciclovir are approved for herpes zoster. Passive antibody prophylaxis with varicella-zoster immune globulin is indicated for susceptible high risk patients exposed to varicella. A live attenuated varicella vaccine (Oka/Merck strain) is now recommended for routine childhood immunization. ***Memory T lymphocytes that recognize VZV antigens are maintained at frequencies of approximately 1 in 40,000 PBMC in immune adults. These responses may persist because of periodic reexposures of immune individuals to VZV during the annual varicella epidemics. This mechanism of exogenous reexposure is supported b y the observation that VZV is detected by PCR in oropharygeal secretions of close contacts of patients with varicella.***
PMID: 8809466

Universal vaccination against varicella [Correspondence].
(N Engl J Med, 1998 Mar 5; 338(10):683.)
Spingarn RW, Benjamin JA, Meissner HC.
To the Editor: Historically, chickenpox has been largely a benign disease affecting predominantly preschool and school-aged children. Times are changing: in Massachusetts, children enrolled in day-care programs will soon be required to be vaccinated against varicella (or have evidence of having had the disease). Although it is generally held that immunizing children is axiomatic for public health, vaccinating all children against chickenpox is a bad idea. ***It is unknown whether long-term immunity to varicella arises from an attack of the disease in childhood or from the virus's repeatedly (and naturally) boosting immunity because it is maintained in our communities. ... Yet policies of universal vaccination of children [against chickenpox] will serve, over time, to eradicate most, but not all, naturally occurring [chickenpox] and its immeasurable booster effect.***
PMID: 9490383

Lasting immunity to varicella in doctors study (L.I.V.I.D. study).
(J Am Acad Dermatol. 1998 May;38(5 Pt 1):763-5.)
Solomon BA, Kaporis AG, Glass AT, Simon SI, Baldwin HE.
Department of Dermatology, State University of New York Health Science Center at Brooklyn, USA.
Physicians, pediatricians (who have a greater incidence of exposure to VZV) were reported to have lower rates of HZ than psychiatrists (who had the lowest VZV exposure rates).
PMID: 9591824

Evidence for frequent reactivation of the Oka varicella vaccine strain in healthy vaccinees.
(Arch Virol Suppl. 2001;(17):7-15.)
Krause PR.
Laboratory of DNA Viruses, Division of Viral Products, Center for Biologics Evaluation and Research, Food and Drug Administration, Bethesda, Maryland 20892, USA. Serum antibody levels and infection rates were followed for 4 years in 4,631 children immunized with the recently licensed Oka strain varicella vaccine. Anti-VZV titers declined over time in high-responder subjects, but rose in vaccinees with low titers. Among subjects with low anti-VZV titers, the frequency of clinical sequelae and immunological boosting significantly exceeded the 13%/yr rate of exposure to wild type varicella. These findings indicate that the Oka strain of VZV persisted in vivo, and reactivated as serum antibody titers declined after vaccination. This mechanism may improve vaccine-associated long-term immunity. ***Pre-licensure clinical studies showed that mean serum anti-VZV levels among vaccinees continued to increase with time after vaccination. This was attributed to immunologic boosting caused by exposure to wild-type VZV in the community.***
PMID: 11339552

Contacts with varicella or with children and protection against herpes zoster in adults: a case-control study.
(Lancet. 2002 Aug 31;360(9334):678-82.)
Thomas SL, Wheeler JG, Hall AJ.
Infectious Disease Epidemiology Unit, London School of Hygiene and Tropical Medicine,
Keppel Street, London WC1E 7HT, UK.
BACKGROUND: Whether exogenous exposure to varicella-zoster-virus protects individuals with latent varicella-zoster virus infection against herpes zoster by boosting immunity is not known. To test the hypothesis that contacts with children increase exposure to varicella zoster virus and protect latently infected adults against zoster, we did a case-control study in south London, UK. METHODS: From 22 general practices, we identified patients with recently diagnosed zoster, and control individuals with no history of zoster, matched to patients by age, sex, and practice. Participants were asked about contacts with people with varicella or zoster in the past 10 years, and social and occupational contacts with children as proxies for varicella contacts. Odds ratios were estimated with conditional logistic regression. FINDINGS: Data from 244 patients and 485 controls

were analysed. On multivariable analysis, protection associated with contacts with a few children in the household or via childcare seemed to be largely mediated by increased access to children outside the household. Social contacts with many children outside the household and occupational contacts with ill children were associated with graded protection against zoster, with less than a fifth the risk in the most heavily exposed groups compared with the least exposed. The strength of protection diminished after controlling for known varicella contacts; the latter remained significantly protective (odds ratio 0.29 [95% CI 0.10-0.84] for those with five contacts or more). INTERPRETATION: ***Re-exposure to varicella-zoster virus via contact with children seems to protect latently infected individuals against zoster. Reduction of childhood varicella by vaccination might lead to increased incidence of adult zoster. Vaccination of the elderly (if effective) should be considered in countries with childhood varicella vaccination programmes.***
PMID: 12241874

Exposure to varicella boosts immunity to herpes-zoster: implications for mass vaccination against chickenpox.
(Vaccine. 2002 Jun 7;20(19-20):2500-7)
Brisson M, Gay NJ, Edmunds WJ, Andrews NJ.
Immunisation Division, PHLS Communicable Disease Surveillance Centre, London, UK.
We present data to confirm that exposure to varicella boosts immunity to herpes-zoster. We show that exposure to varicella is greater in adults living with children and that this exposure is highly protective against zoster (Incidence ratio=0.75, 95% CI, 0.63-0.89). The data is used to parameterise a mathematical model of varicella zoster virus (VZV) transmission that captures differences in exposure to varicella in adults living with and without children. Under the 'best-fit' model, exposure to varicella is estimated to boost cell-mediated immunity for an average of 20 years (95% CI, 7-41years). ***Mass varicella vaccination is expected to cause a major epidemic of herpes-zoster, affecting more than 50% of those aged 10- 44 years at the introduction of vaccination.***
PMID: 12057605

Varicella vaccination in England and Wales: cost-utility analysis.
(Arch Dis Child. 2003 Oct;88(10):862-9.)
Brisson M, Edmunds WJ.
Immunisation Division, PHLS Communicable Disease Surveillance Centre, London NW9 5EQ, UK.
AIMS: To assess the cost-effectiveness of varicella vaccination, taking into account its impact on zoster. METHODS: An age structured transmission dynamic model was used to predict the future incidence of varicella and zoster. Data from national and sentinel surveillance systems were used to estimate age specific physician consultation, hospitalisation, and mortality rates. Unit costs, taken from standard sources, were applied to the predicted health outcomes. RESULTS: In England and Wales, the annual burden of VZV related disease is substantial, with an estimated 651,000 cases of varicella and 189,000 cases of zoster, resulting in approximately 18,000 QALYs lost. ***The model predicts that although the overall burden of varicella will significantly be reduced following mass infant vaccination, these benefits will be offset by a significant rise in zoster morbidity. Under base case assumptions, infant vaccination is estimated to produce an overall loss of 54,000 discounted QALYs over 80 years and to result in a net cost from the health provider (NHS) and the societal perspectives. These results rest heavily on the impact of vaccination on zoster....Conclusion: Routine infant varicella vaccination is unlikely to be cost-effective and may produce an increase in overall morbidity. Adolescent vaccination is the safest and most cost-effective strategy, but has the least overall impact on varicella.***
PMID: 14500303

What does epidemiology tell us about risk factors for herpes zoster?
(Lancet Infect Dis, 2004 Jan.; 4(1):26-33)
Thomas SL, Hall AJ.
Infectious Disease Epidemiology Unit, London School of Hygiene and Tropical Medicine,
Keppel Street, London, UK.
Reactivation of latent varicella zoster virus as herpes zoster is thought to result from waning of specific cell-mediated immunity, but little is known about its determinants in individuals with no underlying immunosuppression. We systematically reviewed studies of zoster epidemiology in adults and analysed data from a large morbidity study to identify factors that might be modulated to reduce the risk of zoster. Annual zoster incidence in population-based studies varied from 3.6-14.2/10(3) in the oldest individuals. Risk factors identified in analytical studies that could explain this variation included age, sex, ethnicity, genetic susceptibility, ***exogenous boosting of immunity from varicella contacts,*** underlying cell-mediated immune disorders, mechanical trauma, psychological stress, and immunotoxin exposure. Our review highlights the lack of information about risk

factors for zoster. We suggest areas of research that could lead to interventions to limit the incidence of zoster. Such research might also help to identify risk factors for agerelated immune decline.
PMID: 14720565

What does epidemiology tell us about risk factors for herpes zoster?
(Lancet Infect Dis, 2004 Jan.; 4(1):26-33)
Thomas SL, Hall AJ.
Infectious Disease Epidemiology Unit, London School of Hygiene and Tropical Medicine, Keppel Street, London, UK.
Reactivation of latent varicella zoster virus as herpes zoster is thought to result from waning of specific cell-mediated immunity, but little is known about its determinants in individuals with no underlying immunosuppression. We systematically reviewed studies of zoster epidemiology in adults and analysed data from a large morbidity study to identify factors that might be modulated to reduce the risk of zoster. Annual zoster incidence in population-based studies varied from 3.6-14.2/10(3) in the oldest individuals. Risk factors identified in analytical studies that could explain this variation included age, sex, ethnicity, genetic susceptibility, ***exogenous boosting of immunity from varicella contacts,*** underlying cell-mediated immune disorders, mechanical trauma, psychological stress, and immunotoxin exposure. Our review highlights the lack of information about risk factors for zoster. We suggest areas of research that could lead to interventions to limit the incidence of zoster. Such research might also help to identify risk factors for age-related immune decline.
PMID: 14720565

Outbreak of varicella among vaccinated children--Michigan, 2003.
(MMWR Morb Mortal Wkly Rep. 2004 May 14;53(18):389-92)
Centers for Disease Control and Prevention (CDC).
On November 18, 2003, the Oakland County Health Division alerted the Michigan Department of Community Health (MDCH) to a varicella (chicken pox) outbreak in a kindergarten-third grade elementary school. On December 11, MDCH and Oakland County public health epidemiologists, with the technical assistance of CDC, conducted a retrospective cohort study to describe the outbreak, determine varicella vaccine effectiveness (VE), and examine risk factors for breakthrough disease (i.e., varicella occurring >42 days after vaccination). ***This report summarizes the results of that study, which indicated that 1) transmission of varicella was sustained at the school for nearly 1 month despite high vaccination coverage, 2) vaccinated patients had substantially milder disease (<50 lesions), and 3) a period of > or =4 years since vaccination was a risk factor for breakthrough disease.***

The incidence of varicella and herpes zoster in Massachusetts as measured by the Behavioral Risk Factor Surveillance System (BRFSS) during a period of increasing varicella vaccine coverage, 1998-2003.
(BMC Public Health. 2005 Jun 16;5(1):68 [Epub ahead of print])
W. Katherine Yih[1], Daniel R. Brooks[2], Susan M. Lett[3], Aisha O. Jumaan[4], Zi Zhang[5], Karen M. Clements[6], Jane F. Seward.[7]
[1]Department of Ambulatory Care and Prevention, Harvard Medical School and Harvard Pilgrim Health Care, Boston, USA;
[2]Department of Epidemiology, Boston University School of Public Health, Boston, USA;
[3]Division of Epidemiology and Immunization, Bureau of Communicable Disease Control, Massachusetts Department of Public Health, Boston, USA;
[4]Health Investigation Branch, Division of Health Studies, Agency for Toxic Substance and Disease Registry, Centers for Disease Control and Prevention, Atlanta, USA;
[5]Health Survey Program; Center for Health Information, Statistics, Research and Evaluation; Massachusetts Department of Public Health; Boston, USA;
[6]Applied Statistics, Evaluation and Technical Services; Bureau of Family and Community Health; Massachusetts Department of Public Health; Boston, USA;
[7]Viral Vaccine-Preventable Disease Branch, Epidemiology and Surveillance Division, National Immunization Program, Centers for Disease Control and Prevention, Atlanta, USA.
BACKGROUND: The authors sought to monitor the impact of widespread varicella vaccination on the epidemiology of varicella and herpes zoster. While varicella incidence would be expected to decrease, mathematical models predict an initial increase in herpes zoster incidence if re-exposure to varicella protects against reactivation of the varicella zoster virus. METHODS: In 1998-2003, as varicella vaccine uptake increased, incidence of varicella and herpes zoster in Massachusetts was monitored using the random-digit-dial Behavioral Risk Factor Surveillance System. RESULTS: Between 1998 and 2003, varicella incidence declined from 16.5/1,000 to 3.5/1,000 (79%) overall with >65% decreases for all age groups except adults (27% decrease). ***Age-***

standardized estimates of overall herpes zoster occurrence increased from 2.77/1,000 to 5.25/1,000 (90%) in the period 1999-2003, and the trend in both crude and adjusted rates was highly significant (p<0.001). Annual age-specific rates were somewhat unstable, but all increased, and the trend was significant for the 25-44 year and 65+ year age groups. CONCLUSIONS: ***As varicella vaccine coverage in children increased, the incidence of varicella decreased and the occurrence of herpes zoster increased.*** If the observed increase in herpes zoster incidence is real, widespread vaccination of children is only one of several possible explanations. Further studies are needed to understand secular trends in herpes zoster before and after use of varicella vaccine in the United States and other countries.
PMID: 15960856

Recurrence of herpes zoster in an immunocompetent adult male.
(J Ayub Med Coll Abbottabad. 2005 Jul-Sep;17(3):80-81)
Combined Military Hospital, Abbottabad
Raza N, Iqbal P, Anwer J.
Repeated and disseminated eruptions of herpes zoster are frequently detected in immunocompromised patients, but are rare in immunocompetent individuals. We report a case of recurrent herpes zoster in a young healthy male, who redeveloped herpes zoster in a different dermatome after one year. The authors write in their DISCUSSION, ***"Cellular immunity is more important than humoral immunity, both for limiting the extent of primary infection with Varicella Zoster Virus as well as for preventing reactivation of the latent virus."*** They also write, ***"Blocking of cell mediated defenses by rising levels of specific antibodies after exposure to exogenous Varicella Zoster virus or by some other mechanism may be a possibility."***
PMID: 16320806

Editorial: varicella immunization and herpes zoster
(Herpes: the journal of the IHMF, 2005 Dec; 12(3):59)
Department of Public Health, University of Rome, "Tor Vergata", Rome, Italy
Volpi A.
"Boosting VZV immunity can protect against zoster: re-exposure to VZV via contact with children protects latently infected individuals. Memory CD4 and CD8 cells that recognize VZV proteins are readily detectable in younger adults, in whom zoster is relatively rare, although the capacity of peripheral-blood T-cells in those who are latently infected with VZV appears to diminish with age.... [Cellular immunity] ... appears more likely to be a consequence of periodic boosting on exposure to VZV or zoster...

The decreasing incidence of VZV following universal childhood vaccination is of concern, because a reduced circulation of wild-type VZV could lead to more cases of zoster in older people, whose immunity is no longer being boosted by exposure to children with primary infection.
PMID: 16393520

Chickenpox, chickenpox vaccination and shingles
(Postgrad Med J. 2006 May;82(967):351-352)
Welsby PD.
Infectious Diseases Unit, Western General Hospital
"We know that exposure to chickenpox can significantly prevent or delay shingles (by exogenous boosting of immunity)... Having a child in the household reduced the risk of shingles for about 20 years..."
PMID: 16679476

Appendix IX. *Medical Veritas®:* The Journal of Medical Truth

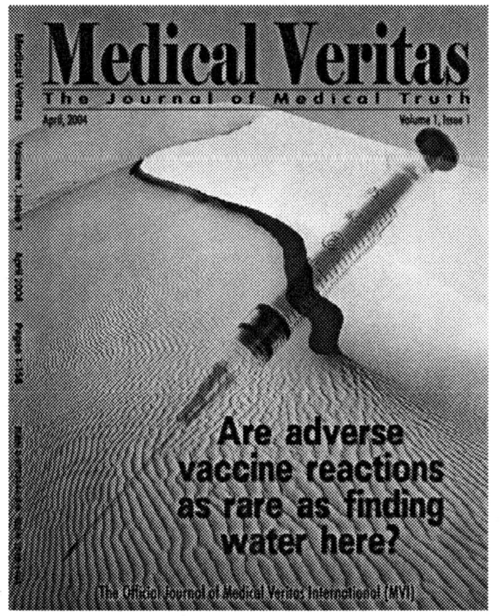

Concerned patients and even some healthcare providers are becoming aware of major deficiencies in medicine and are abandoning ship, disavowing current medical practice and turning increasingly toward alternative care. We, the editorial staff of *Medical Veritas®,* are dedicated to restoring objectivity and accuracy of reporting in medical science. Our peer-reviewed medical journal will aspire towards discovering and disclosing medical truth or "veritas"--whether about vaccines, medicines, disease mechanisms, or other medical/health concerns. Specifically, you will read honest opinions even when such opinions go contrary to vested interests and regimented medical practices. We are committed to uncovering medical truth by

- looking beyond the biased, self-serving, selective presentations of data;
- researching for forgotten or suppressed concepts and data;
- setting a model for other publications;
- encouraging others with inside information to come forward;
- providing a sounding board for presentations of views that may be in conflict with mainstream medicine or science.

Some physicians and researchers, even prominent ones, will be quick to argue that there is no such thing as medical or indeed scientific truth. We may appear to be somewhat arrogant in our choice of the word "Veritas" in our journal title in that even prominent scientists are wary of assuming they have all the answers. It is almost universally admitted that what we believe and consequently practice today is less than optimal and will be supplanted in the future by more accurate theories based upon improved understanding of disease mechanisms. Nevertheless, we can resist the current practice of "flavoring" data to meet financial and political objectives. Medical practice can be improved by full and honest disclosure of available data, research and analyses. We are committed to providing such disclosure and balanced information in *Medical Veritas* (Medical Truth). This journal will assist patients and conscientious healthcare providers in making informed medical decisions based on manuscripts of the highest integrity—presenting research that likely will not always harmonize with the interests of pharmaceutical companies and profit motives

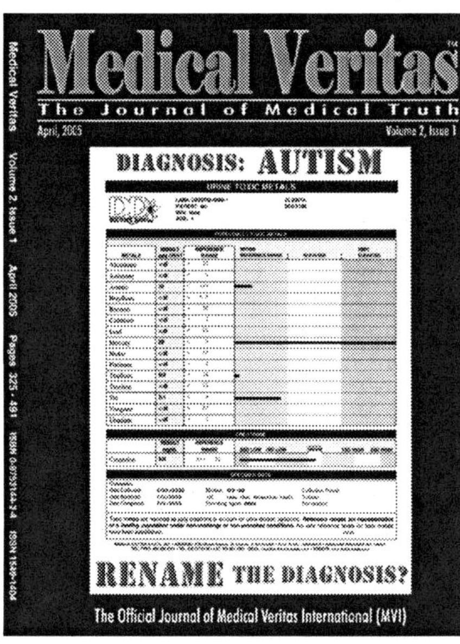

of present day health establishments. We will present evidence fundamental to deliberations of a court—reliable, authentic, accurate, and complete. We believe that a better-informed public will help to ensure better medical practice.

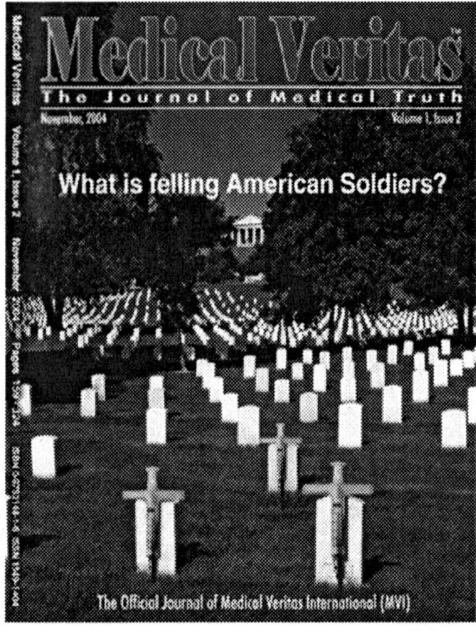

Adverse reactions to vaccines and other interventions invariably start as a small number of poorly described reports which are anecdotal and easily attributed to chance. As the numbers increase, those in authority in public health discern something might be wrong and closer scrutiny is needed. When the numbers reach the hundreds, decision makers have to persuade themselves that every adverse reaction is a false alarm—not a single one is a true association. When that happens, the numbers support a causal relationship except for the skeptics and those with conflicts of interest—who accept nothing but "scientific proof."

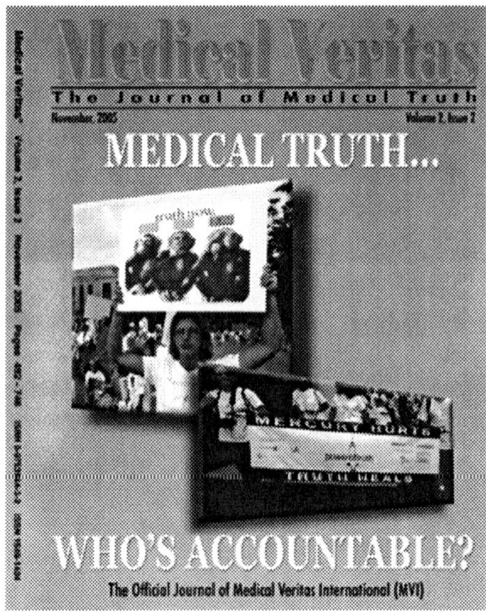

Public health officials and their respective medical establishments in the U.S. and U.K. often ignore important evidence, especially with regard to vaccines, stating "the weight of currently available scientific evidence does not support the hypothesis..." U.S. professor Donald W. Miller, Jr., MD and British lawyer Clifford G. Miller, Esq, explain, "Editors can subvert peer review by selecting only reviewers who will reject papers that run counter to—or praise papers that support—the interests of journal's advertisers or its owners. Lines of independent research contradicting conventional wisdom can systematically remain unpublished." They continue, "Such hard-to-publish research may prove that what the scientific community generally accepts as correct is, in fact, wrong. Research follows the funding, resulting in a wealth of publications favoring the funding interests. This can have a disproportionate effect on the 'weight' of evidence, especially for epidemiologic evidence in court." [On Evidence, Medical and Legal, Journal of American Physicians and Surgeons, Fall 2005;10(3):70–75].

Medical Veritas™ includes a special feature entitled *Forum* that provides real life accounts on specific topics, based on the personal perspective of parents and caretakers. These reports, combined with the more technical data, analyses, and results contained in other manuscripts throughout the journal will ultimately help all readers to see some underlying problems with the current medical system and encourage physicians and scientists to consider medical evidence instead of medical theories.

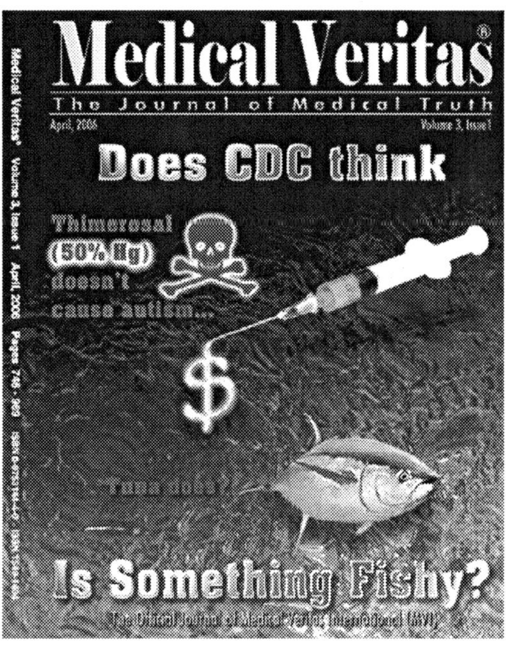

Some researchers and scientists carrying on clinical and epidemiological investigations and other research have found that virtually all favorable data and analyses generated are readily published in peer-reviewed medical journals, while negative or deleterious findings appear to be suppressed. Some researchers have found themselves resigning on ethical grounds in order to try to distance themselves from research fraud. Others have attempted to independently publish their data and analyses--only to receive directives from legal entities to "cease and desist publication in medical journals." We do not believe this to be an isolated occurrence, and we recognize other journals' tendencies toward positive bias. When individuals are subjected to censorship, experience intimidation, are not permitted to conduct research objectively, or when research data concerning a vaccine or other medication used in human populations is being suppressed or misrepresented, this is very disturbing and goes against all scientific norms--compromising professional ethics.

When full disclosure of both positive and deleterious effects of an intervention is lacking, this undermines stated aims of medical programs and can ultimately lead to recommendations for treatments that are ineffective and cause harm or death. Full disclosure is the characteristic aim of *Medical Veritas*, and we believe that this less-biased approach distinguishes it from other medical journals that may be prone to reporting only positive results of medical research.

Sincerely,

Gary S. Goldman, Ph.D.
Editor-in-Chief

Medical Veritas: The Journal of Medical Truth

April, 2004 ISSN 1549-1404 Volume 1, Issue 1

Table of Contents

Medical Veritas™: **The Journal of Medical Truth**
November, 2004 ISSN 1549-1404 Volume 1, Issue 2

Table of Contents

Medical Veritas™: The Journal of Medical Truth

April, 2005 ISSN 1549-1404 Volume 2, Issue 1

Table of Contents

Medical Veritas®: The Journal of Medical Truth

November, 2005 Volume 2, Issue 2

Table of Contents

Medical Veritas®: The Journal of Medical Truth

April, 2006 **Volume 3, Issue 1**

Table of Contents

Note:

Medical Veritas® journals can be ordered online at www.MedicalVeritas.com.

Alternativley, send payment payment of $40.00 plus $5.00 shipping/handling (please specify Volume Number and Issue desired, along with name, address, phone, and e-mail address) to:

Medical Veritas International Inc.
P.O. Box 847
Pearblossom, CA 93553

Medical Veritas International Inc. is a 501(c)(3) nonprofit organization. Its chief activity involves the publication of peer-reviewed findings, authored by scientists, healthcare providers, researchers and others, free of the influences of pharmaceutical companies and other vested interests. Unique in its field, MVI's journal, ***Medical Veritas***®, includes research and analyses by educated laypersons, as well as professionals.

By thoroughly investigating and reporting on the safety issues of medical interventions, free of the propaganda promoted by pseudo studies, ***Medical Veritas***® allows individuals to make truly informed decisions, resulting in major improvements to healthcare worldwide. As an example, ***Vol. 1, Issue 1***, has already been used successfully in court testimony. MVI accepts no advertising from entitities that could impact its ability to present truthful information. It relies solely on contributions from those who support this important mission. Your help is essential toward its success. *Any amount that you can give is deeply appreicated and is tax-deductable (under section 170 of the IRS Code) to the full extent permitted by law.*

Appendix X. Peer-review Manuscripts Concerning Safety, Adverse Reactions and Other Varicella Vaccine-Related Complications

[1] Braun MM, Mootrey GT, Seward JF, Rider LG, Krause PR. Postlicensure safety surveillance for varicella vaccine. JAMA 2000; 284:1271–9.

[2] Ravkina LI, Matsevich GR. Morphological changes in the central nervous system in post-vaccinal encephalomyelitis developing after chickenpox vaccination in children. Zh Nevropatol Psikhiatr Im S S Korsakova. 1970; 70(10):1465–71.

[3] Poser CM. Neurological Complications of Vaccinations. Mealey's Litigation Report, Thimerosal & Vaccines, 2003 Apr.;Volume 1, Issue #10.

[4] Sunaga Y, Hikima A, Ostuka T, Morikawa A. Acute cerebellar ataxia with abnormal MRI lesions after varicella vaccination. Pediatr Neurol. 1995 Nov; 13(4):340–2. [2 year old boy with staggering gait and difficulty speaking.]

[5] Singer S, Johnson CE, Mohr R, Holowecky C. Urticaria following varicella vaccine associated with gelatin allergy. Vaccine 1999 Jan 28; 17(4):327–9.

[6] Gerecitano J, Friedman-Kien A, Chazen GD. Allergic reaction to varicella vaccine. Ann Intern Med. 1997 May 15; 126(10):833–4.

[7] Sakaguchi M, Yamanaka T, Ikeda K, Sano Y, Fujita H, Miura T, Inouye S. IgE-mediated systemic reactions to gelatin included in the varicella vaccine. J Allergy Clin Immonol. 1997 Feb; 99(2):263–4.

[8] Naruse H, Miwata H, Ozaki T, Asano Y, Namazue J, Yamanishi K. Varicella infection complicated with meningitis after immunization. Acta Paediatr Jpn; 1993 Aug; 35(4):345–7.

[9] Lee SY, Komp DM, Andiman W. Thrombocytopenic Purpura following varicella-zoster vaccination. Am J Pediatr Hematol Oncol, 1986 Spring; 8(1):78–80.

[10] Matsubara K, Nigami H, Harigaya H, Baba K. Herpes zoster in a normal child after varicella vaccination. Acta Paediatr Jpn; 1995 Oct; 37(5):648–50.

[11] Hammerschlag MR, Gershon AA, Steinberg SP, Clarke L, Gelb LD. Herpes zoster in an adult recipient of live attenuated varicella vaccine. J Infect Dis, 1989 Sept; 160(3):535–7.

[12] Esmaeli-Gutstein B, Winkelman JZ. Uveitis associated with varicella virus vaccine. Am J Ophthalmol, 1999 Jun; 127(6):733–4.
A 16-year-old girl developed blurred vision in her left eye 7-days after receiving varicella vaccine.

[13] Wrensch M., Weinberg A, Wiencke J, Miike R., Barger G, Kelsey K. Prevalence of Antibodies to Four Herpesviruses among Adults with Glioma [Brain Tumor] and Controls. Am J of Epidem, 2001; 154(2):161–5.

[14] Uebe B, Sauerbrei A, Burdach S, Horneff G. Herpes zoster by reactivated vaccine varicella zoster virus in a healthy child. Eur J Pediatr, 2002 Aug; 161(8):442-444. Epub 2002 Jun 25.
A 27-month-old girl developed an impressive herpes zoster infection 16 months after varicella vaccination that was localized in three adjacent cervical

dermatome. VZV vaccine stain was identified by polymerase chain reaction.

[15] Naseri A, Good WV, Cunningham ET Jr. Herpes zoster virus sclerokeratitis and anterior uveitis in a child following varicella vaccination. Am J Ophthalmol. 2003 Mar; 135(3):415 7.

[16] Schwab J, Ryan M. Varicella zoster virus meningitis in a previously immunized child. Pediatrics, 2004 Aug;114(2):e273-e274.
A 5-year-old developed varicella-zoster meningitis and transient sensorineural hearing loss. Treatment with acyclovir resulted in full recovery.

[17] Wirrell E, Hill MD, Jadavji T, Kirton A, Barlow K. Stroke after varicella vaccination. J Pediatr, 2004 Dec; 146(6):845–7.
Two children presented with acute hemiparesis 5 days and 3 weeks, respectively, following varicella vaccination. Both showed unilateral infarction of the basal ganglia and internal capsule, a distribution consistent with varicella angiopathy. Both children had small patent foramen ovale (PFO), and one child also had severe iron-deficiency anemia, which may have predisposed the patient to this adverse effect. The authors state, "These two cases of stroke in temporal association with varicella vaccination may represent chance occurrence. However, the characteristic location of infarcts raises the possibility of varicella vasculopathy."

[18] Bronstein DE, Cotliar J, Votava-Smith JK, Powell MZ, Miller MJ, Cherry JD. Recurrent papular urticaria after varicella immunization in a 15-month-old girl. Pediatr Infect Dis J. 2005 Mar;24(3):269-270.
Varicella-like rash after immunization with the live attenuated varicella vaccine is relatively common. Such vaccine-associate rashes generally consist of fewer lesions than occur in chickenpox. We describe a 15-month-old girl who experienced the onset of recurring papular urticaria after varicella immunization. The rash was varicella-like and thought by us to be caused by vaccine virus.

[19] Binder NR, Holland GN, Hosea S, Silverberg ML. Herpes zoster ophthalmicus in an otherwise-healthy child. J AAPOS, 2005 Dec; 9(6):597-8.
A case of pediatric herpes zoster ophthalmicus in a child that had been vaccinated against varicella and otherwise had no known exposure to varicella-zoster virus and the initial presentation of HZO was a painful and diffuse subconjunctival hemorrhage that appeared before any of its classic signs were observed.

[20] Grossberg R, Harpaz R, Rubtcova E, Loparev V, Seward JF, Schmid DS. Secondary transmission of varicella vaccine virus in a chronic care facility for children. J. Pediatr. 2006 Jun.;148(6):842-4.
15-days after receiving varicella vaccine, a 16-year-old developed severe varicella. A 13-year-old and 39-year old were infected with 2 variant vaccine strains.

[21] Lohiya GS, Tan-Figueroa L, Reddy S, Marshall S. Chickenpox and pneumonia following varicella vaccine. Infect. Control Hosp. Epidemiol. 2004 July; 25(7):530.

[22] Levitsky J, Te HS, Faust TW, Cohen SM. Varicella infection following varicella vaccination in a liver transplant recipient. Am. J. Transplant. 2002 Oct;2(9):880-882.

[23] Huang W, Hussey M, Michel F. Transmission of varicella to a gravida via close contacts immunized with varicella-zoster vaccine. A case report. J. Reprod.

Med. 1999 Oct;44(10):905-907. Authors concluded, "It may not be as safe as previously thought for seronegative gravidas to be in close contact with people vaccinated with the varicella vaccine."

[24] Kohl S. Rapp J, La Russa P, Gershon AA, Steinberg SP. Natural varicella-zoster virus reactivation shortly after varicella immunization in a child. Pediatr. Infect. Dis J. 1999 Dec; 18(12):1112-1113.
Twelve days following varicella vaccination in his right arm, a 6-year-old male developed wild-type herpes zoster rash on his back and left arm.

[25] Salzman MB, Sharrar RG, Steinberg S, LaRussa P. Transmission of varicella-vaccine virus from a healthy 12-month-old child to his pregnant mother. J. Pediatr. 1997 Jul;131(1 Pt 1):151-154.
Author's write, "A 12-month-old healthy boy had approximately 30 vesicular skin lesions 24 days after receiving varicella vaccine. Sixteen days later his pregnant mother had 100 lesions. Varicella-vaccine virus was identified by polymerase chain reaction in the vesicular lesions of the mother. After an elective abortion, no virus was detected in the fetal tissue. This case documents transmission of varicella-vaccine virus from a healthy 12-month-old infant to his pregnant mother."

[26] Plotkin SA, Starr SE, Connor K, Morton D. Zoster in normal children after varicella vaccine. [Case Report; Letter] J Infect. Dis., 1989 May; 159(5):1000-1001.
Six months after varicella vaccination a 2-year-old male developed herpes zoster on the right side of his chest (T6 dermatome). A female was vaccinated at 1-year old. Two to three years after vaccination, she was exposed to wild-type varicella in school contacts and then one year later, at 4-years-old, developed herpes zoster over her right scapula. Author's state, "Our 2 cases demonstrate that zoster after receipt of Oka/Merck varicella vaccine can occur in normal children."

[27] Levin MJ, Dahl KM, Weinberg A, Giller R, Patel A, Krause PR. Development of resistance to acyclovir during chronic infection with the Oka vaccine strain of varicella-zoster virus, in an immunosuppressed child. J Infect Dis. 2003 Oct 1;188(7):954-959. Epub 2003 Sep 26.
A 1-year-old boy was vaccinated with the Oka strain of varicella just prior to the discovery of a tumor that required intensive antitumor therapy. Three months later he developed herpes zoster, which developed into chronic verrucous lesions that were refractory to treatment with acyclovir and which subsequently disseminated. DNA from a biopsy specimen of a chronic herpes-zoster lesion indicated that the Oka vaccine strain of the virus caused this severe complication. Analysis of this viral DNA demonstrated a mutation in the viral thymidine kinase gene. Plasmids containing this altered gene were unable to produce functional thymidine kinase in an in vitro translation system. The presence of this mutation would explain the clinical resistance to acyclovir. This is the first report of Oka-strain varicella virus causing severe disease after reactivation and of resistance to acyclovir during an infection caused by this virus.

Appendix XI. Adverse Reactions to Varicella Vaccination: 5 Example Cases

Case "A"

A 35-year old female, who had never had varicella, was exposed to infected children. Her physician recommended prompt vaccination. On May 18, 1998, she received a first dose of varicella vaccine. Approximately two hours following vaccination, a transient welt developed at the injection site with a 3-inch line of lymphangitis.

Eight days after vaccination, she developed a fever, sore throat, nausea, vomiting, malaise and dizziness. She noticed some bruises and had aching in her knees, hands and feet.

Seen by her physician because of an irregular heart rate, her ECG revealed supra ventricular extra systoles and left ventricular hypertrophy. Her CPK was elevated to 676. Her nausea and vomiting persisted for the next three months despite use of anti-nausea medication. She was admitted to a hospital for rehydration after losing 12 lbs – more than 10% of her previous healthy weight.

The patient later developed a cough, marked fatigue, sensitivity to light and sound, disturbed sleep and more serious loss of appetite. These symptoms along with dizziness persisted for weeks and she had difficulty going from her bed to the bathroom without assistance.

By the sixth month post-vaccination, she was seen by a neurologist and a physiatrist. Both thought that she could have Guillian-Barré syndrome. An EMG revealed involvement in an ulnar distribution.

Over time, the patient's nausea decreased and her fever subsided. Her joint pains became episodic but more intense during the attacks and she experienced some muscle weakness on and off. Gradually, she was able to work for a few hours at a time.

A VAERS report was finally, filed January 30, 2000 – about 1.5 years after the adverse reactions started.

Case "B"

A man who was vaccinated against varicella in 1995 developed encephalomyloneuritis and required hospitalization for months. He remains permanently disabled.

Case "C"

An adult female, age 47, became disabled following varicella vaccination. She worked as a research coordinator in the infectious disease unit of a Medical School. She and other immune employees were recruited as healthy controls for a *manufacturer-sponsored* vaccine study aimed at detecting the boosting effect of the vaccine. Her pre-study laboratory values were completely normal. She received a first dose of the vaccine in March and the second in May 2001. She developed diarrhea shortly after the second dose and by November 2001, she was quite ill and had serious intestinal difficulties.

She underwent a colonoscopy and was diagnosed with the rare and more serious collagenous colitis. While her lymphocytes decreased from 25 to 14%, her total white count, neutrophils and eosinophils increased. She was told that her collagenous colitis was autoimmune in nature.

She remains disabled and out of work. Her case was reported to VAERS.

Case "D"

A 17-month-old female toddler received the varicella vaccination on March 20, 1996. Her older brother reacted to all vaccinations and developed late-onset autism following his MMR. D's mother was initially fearful and refused the varicella vaccine for her daughter. Her physician reassured her by saying: "Do you think I would give the vaccination to my own children if I thought it wasn't safe?"

Her physician also informed her that state law mandates chickenpox vaccination but never told her that she could withhold her consent. The mother says that she felt "humiliated into allowing her daughter to receive the varicella vaccine."

Shortly afterwards, "D" began having joint pains, eczema and allergies. Her symptoms worsened at the age of 6. Her ANA became positive and she developed autoimmune thyroid disease with a high TSH. Her skin sensitivity also became more intense. Her physician was of the opinion that a virus probably triggered her autoimmune response.

Case "E"

This boy was born on June 30, 1998 and received the varicella vaccination on June 29, 2000.

Twenty-eight months following varicella vaccination (October 29, 2002), he developed break-through chickenpox with an estimated 30 to 40 lesions that were intensely itchy.

He was listless and had some rhinorhea but remained afebrile.

On June 12, 2003 (age 5), he had a unilateral shingles eruption on the back of his neck. He had moderate pain and the lesions were tender and sensitive to clothing. In spite of treatment with Acyclovir*, the rash lasted for 45 days.

Nine months later, on March 10, 2004, he had a recurrence of shingles affecting the left nipple and the left side of the back. This time, the pain was more severe. He was treated again with Acyclovir. The rash slowly subsided but left scars.

Two months later, on May 13, 2004, he had still another recurrence with moderate pain, in the same location as previously mentioned. He received a third course of Acyclovir and the rash resolved after a month.

Each of the three occurrences of the shingles rash was on his left side. He took Acyclovir Oral Suspension (200mg per 5ml): Two teaspoons 4 times a day for 5 days.

Appendix XII. Vaccination and Autoimmunity: Reassessing Evidence

Marc Girard, MSc, MD
1 bd de la République
78000-Versailles (France)
Phone: +33 01 39 67 01 10 Fax: +33 01 39 67 01 11
Email: agosgirard@free.fr

Abstract

The autoimmune risks of vaccines seem frequently overlooked. Whereas most available vaccinations are supposed to produce long-lasting immunity, the fact that they can also produce long-term detrimental immune effects seems to be ignored as evidenced by the short duration of safety studies during development. Likewise, whereas it seems natural to simply rely on surrogate markers, such as antibodies, to demonstrate vaccine efficacy, the levels of evidence required to acknowledge adverse effects is far higher. Reports to the Vaccine Adverse Event Reporting System (VAERS) are deemed more conclusive when reassuring than when suggesting significant toxicity. As a result of these blatant biases in clinical and/or epidemiological research, experts on autoimmunity and vaccine critics are limited to demonstrating theoretical mechanisms because evidence in practice is lacking.

Known as the bias of the selective assessment, this unbalance in the demonstration of the benefits as compared to the risks is the bête noire of evidence-based medicine. Therefore, when readjusted to the demonstrative level normally viewed as sufficient in clinical research in general and in vaccine science specifically, the corpus of data on the autoimmune hazards of vaccines appears certainly more impressive than generally recognized and calls for further research, for an overall reassessment of the benefit/risk ratio of vaccines including multiple vaccinations. Because vaccines are now aimed at preventing diseases which may be quite rare, the Hippocratic principle of prudence is more than ever a very topical issue.

Keywords: *benefit/risk ratio, bias, evidence-based medicine (EBM), Hippocratic principle, vaccination*

Competing interests: Dr Girard works as an independent consultant for pharmaceutical industry, including vaccine manufacturers and a number of their competitors. He received no funding for this paper.

1. Introduction

Although vaccine safety is obviously a major issue, its prime importance is often relegated to a secondary and unimportant role. A review of the medical literature reveals that more often than not, any legitimate question raised about the safety of any vaccine is likely to be ignored or interpreted as "myth", "fiction" or "misconceptions" [1-6].

A recent international conference held in Lausanne, Switzerland [6] may start to reverse this trend, help those scientists genuinely concerned with vaccines hazards regain their credibility, encourage others to come forth and put on the market genuinely safe vaccines, that will not need to be withdrawn following problematic post-marketing performances.

I will not speak in this debate as an immunologist, but as a specialist in drug research and as a medical expert witness with an extensive experience in criminal inquiries on drug scandals and data distortion. Thus, I would like to take the special issue of vaccines to illustrate the effects of quite general vices such as negligence, poor methodology, selective assessment, disregarding or rejection of data – and to suggest that, as a consequence, the autoimmune potential of vaccination could be greatly underestimated.

2. Negligence or carelessness

Several mechanisms can account for the autoimmune hazards of vaccines:

- An individual toxicity if a vaccine antigen mimics host antigens;
- A cumulative addition of the individual toxicities when several antigens are administered together;
- A potential interaction resulting when two vaccines administered together produce a reaction or a chain of reactions that neither would have induced independently.

Although theoretical, this multiple potential for autoimmune hazards should carry at its highest level the Hippocratic principle first not to harm. This should be all the more so since in developed countries most vaccines are administered to children and adults in perfect health, each of the exposed subjects has a tiny risk of developing a severe form of the infectious disease and the effectiveness of the vaccine is not assured.

Yet, strangely enough, caution is not always the rule with vaccination policy. In a country like France, and while epidemiological evidence is mainly lacking, up to 11 vaccinations (including one heptavalent pneumococcal vaccine) are recommended or mandated prior to the age of 1 year.

3. Data quality

The quality of the safety studies performed on vaccines is often questionable.

- They are usually of short duration in the range of days. Most safety studies during the development of Engerix B® (one product against hepatitis B) lasted 4 days as mentioned in the Physician Desk Reference (PDR). Yet, it is not easy to understand why products supposed to have beneficial effects in the long term could not also have detrimental effects within the same long term.

- Trials are usually carried out in developing countries, where reliable long term follow-up is most often not available.
- Even in developed countries, post-marketing surveillance depends mainly on systems such as the U.S. Vaccine Adverse Event Reporting System (VAERS) where almost every alert is discredited on the basis that spontaneous reporting does not permit reliable assessment [7,8].

Thus, when an immunologist addresses the issue of the autoimmune complications of vaccines, he starts with a long list of potential mechanisms but quite often is obliged to conclude that no trustworthy evidence is available. To be sure, lack of evidence is an expected result of such a poor surveillance system; but if reliable assessment of vaccines hazards is out of reach, it still remains to be re-assessed whether it is consistent with our Hippocratic principles to expose so many people in perfect health to such products.

Just as disturbing is the fact that the reliability of vaccine surveillance seems to fluctuate according to the trend of its results: very poor when suggesting a toxicity, quite satisfactory when no hazard is detected[78].

- After an analysis of the VAERS database suggested that cerebellar ataxia, autism, mental retardation and permanent brain damage were significantly increased following MMR vaccination [9], the UK Medicines and Healthcare Products Authority (MHRA) issued a statement dismissing the findings on the basis that "the authors failed to consider the limitations and biases inherent in VAERS data (...)"[79].
- About the same time, others published a re-assuring study on vaccines safety which therefore concluded that VAERS is not only important for detecting vaccine-associated adverse events, but it also serves to "reassure the general public concerning the safety of a new vaccine, as in the safety assessments of varicella vaccine and hepatitis A [10]." Interestingly this robust optimism on the reliability of the database did not attract any comment from the regulatory authorities about "the limitation and biases inherent..."

4. Selective assessment

In contrast with physics or chemistry data, drug research data is "soft" [11]: its significance often requires an interpretation. However, interpretation does not mean selective assessment of available evidence (as illustrated by the preceding examples). On the contrary, our main requirement to claim a minimum of scientific validity should be a strict, I should say an obsessive regularity in giving the same weight to data of the same reliability. For example, the concern should not be to assess whether severe toxicity is "certain" when the efficacy of vaccines is never certain.

When it comes to vaccines, where no assessment can be more than statistical, our only

---

[78] Exactly the converse of what should be expected on purely methodological grounds: reporting represent an alert for the least, whereas non-reporting leaves completely open the issue of an undetected toxicity (as illustrated by a number of examples in the history of pharmacy).

[79] Statement from the Medicines and Healthcare Products Regulatory Agency (MHRA): study on safety of MMR vaccine by Geier and Geier—conclusions are not justified. Internet-Document, page (2 pages), May 22, 2003.

concern should be to ascertain that the level of evidence for any toxic effect is the same, lower or higher than the level of evidence normally considered as "sufficient" to take medical or regulatory measures.

Let's consider one example. Tolcapone (Tasmar®) is a drug that was licensed for use in some severe forms of Parkinson's disease. In Sept 1998, further to a safety alert, all international reports of liver injury were reviewed by the European Agency for the Evaluation of Medicinal Products (EMEA). At the time, in an indication where severely disabled patients may have been willing to accept a high level of risk in the hope of even a modest benefit, a total of ten serious cases worldwide, generally of questionable causality and of which only 3 were published, was sufficient to justify drug withdrawal [12]: it would be interesting to compare this level of "significance" with that requested by governmental agencies to admit that there might be a problem with, for example, sudden infant death syndrome, for which hundreds or even thousands of cases have been reported following vaccination... [8,13].[80]

So, let us take as a unit of measure the level of evidence normally deemed as "sufficient" even for drugs aimed at curing even severe diseases. *My point is to show that with such a natural unit of measure, evidence of toxicity for some vaccines is already far higher than usually claimed by experts or agencies.*

Consider, amongst others, the case of hepatitis B vaccine (HBV). It has been repeated that no significant problem was ever reported outside France and that the French problem was an artefact due to media coverage.

This is not true.

Besides the overwhelming predominance of reports about adverse events following hepatitis B vaccination, it is clear (Table 1) that this predominance was evident and blatant as compared to other vaccines of far larger exposure—before any media coverage which began in 1996. When one compares the reaction of governmental agencies to the many HBV problems to those resulting from only three publications on tolcapone (above), the bias is immediately noticeable: by the end of 1994, when dozens of publications were already available and many problems had been publicised, the French Minister of Health launched a national universal campaign of hepatitis B vaccination. Ten years later, universal vaccination in other countries remains an issue [14,15].

The data of the French health system (Fig. 1) reveal a clear increase in neurological and autoimmune complications after the mass campaign (red arrow) was launched. As differences in the absolute frequencies render maintaining a vivid representation difficult, it may be useful to examine the evolution of multiple sclerosis (MS) as compared to the number of vaccine units sold (Fig. 2).[81]

---

[80] The exaggeration of the European authorities in precautionary measures in this instance was further confirmed by the fact that the withdrawal was lifted some years later (http://www.emea.eu.int/human docs/PDFs/EPAR/tasmar/034397en8a.pdf); in Autumn 2005, the drug was re-introduced on the market.

[81] One may note that even considered alone, this graph (which concern dozens of millions of vaccinated subjects) is an impressive denial of Sadovnick and Schefele's paper which concluded that the vaccine was safe as no change in the frequency of neurological complications was observed after a program of vaccination was implemented [19]: although this paper was only based upon a tiny population (less than 300 000 students) and

Table 1. Published case reports on various vaccine hazards in REACTIONS database

Vaccine	*Number of case reports*	
	prior to 1995	*1983-2004*
Hepatitis B (HBV)	42	102
Measles or MMR	20	40
Tetanus or DTP	13	27
Haemophilus influenzae type b (Hib)	4	7
Polio or DTP	3	3

But returning to the original graph (Fig. 1) reveals another interesting trend, namely the time lag of about 1 year between the increase in MS and the subsequent increase in unspecified "neuro-muscular disorders" which was not evident prior to 1996. In fact the first increase had an important impact on media coverage and from then on, because of the stubborn denials of health agencies as well as of experts, it became scientifically "incorrect" to make a formal diagnosis of MS in a person exposed to hepatitis B vaccine: this reluctance is clearly illustrated by the time lag and the subsequent dramatic increase. The addition of both curves (Fig. 3) gives a clearer picture of the effects of the mass campaign on the prevalence of severe neuro-muscular diseases. It should be pointed out that this dramatic evolution, affecting thousands of citizens who were in perfect health prior to their exposure, only represents the more severe cases.

The clear evidence graphically demonstrated in these exhibits were completely ignored by the regulatory agencies as well as by "experts" panels until I made them public starting in 2002. Those willing to go on ignoring the health catastrophe that was caused in France by hepatitis B vaccination have contended ever since then that the data – if not "myth" or "fiction" – simply corresponded to artefacts related to better diagnosis of multiple sclerosis and to the recent wider availability of therapy using interferon.

Obviously, evidence supporting these claims is weak:

- Due to the abovementioned climate of scientific correctness, enormous time and energy were spent to narrow the criteria for the diagnosis of MS. This resulted in a significant increase of unspecified "severe neuro-muscular disorders" (the second curve) which, as clinical experience confirmed, included genuine cases of multiple sclerosis MS which for one (generally lame) reason or another were not labeled as such. This general tendency was facilitated by the fact that often drug-induced diseases are generally *atypical* and a little different from the "classical" illness. In this particular case, it is striking that quite often, the lesions in the white substance as detected on MRI examination are unusually tiny and modest when compared to those normally seen in non-iatrogenic instances of MS. In

---

paid no attention to the real exposure (implementation of a program may not alter vaccinations practices), it is classically included amongst the hard arguments of every experts panel or "consensus" conference contending that there is no significant hazard with HBV.

addition, and for unexplained reasons, the size of these tiny lesions is often disproportionate to their clinical expression, which may be severe so that in most cases, this perplexing disproportion between small anatomical lesions and significant symptomatic expression, far from being interpreted as an interesting clue towards exogenous etiology, was on the contrary an easy pretext to evoke a non-neurological disorder such as hysteria or cardio-vascular disorders, etc. Although such a context of reluctance to make a diagnosis of MS should have automatically led to a *decrease* in observed MS cases, the opposite occurred and newly diagnosed cases of MS increased significantly as clearly demonstrated in the attached graphs: in other words, increase in neuromuscular disorders occurred in spite of repeated efforts to reduce the number of newly diagnosed post-vaccinal MS.

- It is also evident from the figures supplied by the manufacturers that significant increases in the sales of interferon did not begin prior to 1997, a full two years after the impressive increase shown in Figure 2.

5. Data rejection or dissimulation

The unprecedented potential of HBV to induce MS is also evident from a number of additional clues [16,17], such as the alarming epidemics of paediatric MS. The French regulatory authorities have kept unpublished the existence of a cohort of about 800 children who developed MS, some as young as of 2 years old. Similarly disturbing studies revealing a significant increase in lupus erythematosus (LE) and Graves' disease post hepatitis B vaccination are still unpublished [16] and it is likely that they will remain so.

There are other forms of data dissimulation. Figure 4 shows the corrected proof of a paper which was accepted and had already received a digital object identifier (DOI). After repeated requests about failure to access it in "author's gateway," I received a one sentence explanation from the editor of the journal:

Dear Dr. Girard,

On the basis of the advice I have received I have decided not to go ahead with your publication.
Signed, Emeritus Professor of Science and Engineering Ethics (...)

This should be a matter of concern for every scientist that an unidentified "advice" is sufficient to justify the rejection of a paper at this step of the publication process. This should be all the more so since, apparently, the editor responsible for this unusual shift in publication rules claims to be in charge of teaching scientific ethics...

6. Conclusion

Many other examples of poor methodology, selective assessment or dissimulation of data could be given. This suggests that research and development on vaccines are still **at the zero-level of evidence-based medicine** (EBM) [18].

As assessed with the same units of measure used with other drugs, some vaccines and specifically the hepatitis B vaccine have **an unacceptable benefit/risk ratio**, especially in countries where the diseases they claim to control are not endemic.

For obvious reasons of profit, the threats to the scientific and medical ethics of our job have reached a worrying level: it is **the personal responsibility of each** of us to resist – and to support those who are the most under pressure.

References

[1] Kimmel SR. Vaccine adverse events: Separating myth from reality. Am Fam Physician 2002 Dec 1; 66(11):2113–20.

[2] MacIntyre CR, Leask J. Immunization myths and realities: Responding to arguments against immunization. Journal of Paediatrics & Child Health 2003 Sep-2003 Oct 31;39(7):487–91.

[3] Bedford H, Elliman D. Misconceptions about the new combination vaccine. BMJ 2004 Aug 21; 329(7463):411–2.

[4] Begg N, Nicoll A. Myths in medicine. Immunisation. BMJ 1994 Oct 22;309(6961):1073–5.

[5] Girard M. Misconceptions about misconceptions. Br Med J 2005. Available online at :http://bmj.bmjjournals.com/cgi/eletters /329-7463/411#72515

[6] Vaccination, infection & autoimmunity: Myth and reality. Lausanne, Swiss, 26-28 Oct 2005

[7] Anonymous. Report of the working group on the possible relationship between hepatitis B vaccination and the chronic fatigue syndrome. CMAJ 1993 Aug 1;149(3):314–9.

[8] Silvers L, Ellenberg S, Wise R, et al. The epidemiology of fatalities reported to the vaccine event reporting system 1990-1997. Pharmacoepidemiol Drug Saf 2001;10:279–85.

[9] Geier M, Geier DA. Pediatric MMR vaccination safety. International Pediatrics 2003;18:108–13.

[10] Zhou W, Pool V, Iskander JK, English-Bullard R, Ball R, Wise RP, Haber P, Pless RP, Mootrey G, Ellenberg SS, et al. Surveillance for safety after immunization: Vaccine Adverse Event Reporting System (VAERS)—U.S., 1991-2001. MMWR Surveill Summ 2003 Jan 24;52(1):1–24.

[11] Feinstein A. Clinical biostatistics. II. Statistics versus science in the design of experiments. Clin Pharmacol Ther 1970;11:282–92.

[12] CSM. Withdrawal of tolcapone (Tasmar). Currents Problems 1999(25 Feb):1.

[13] Zinka B, Rauch E, Buettner A, Rueff F, Penning R. Unexplained cases of sudden infant death shortly after hexavalent vaccination. Vaccine 2005 May 18.

[14] Girard M. Hepatitis B: how to manipulate the media machine. Br Med J 2005. Available online at :http://bmj.bmjjournals.com/cgi/ eletters/329-7474/1059#87547.

[15] Beeching NJ. Hepatitis B infections. BMJ 2004 Nov 6; 329(7474):1059-60.

[16] Girard M. Autoimmune hazards of hepatitis B vaccine. Autoimmun Rev 2005 Feb;4(2):96–100.

[17] Comenge Y, Girard M. Multiple sclerosis and hepatitis B vaccination: Adding the credibility of molecular biology to an unusual level of clinical and epidemiological evidence. Med Hypotheses 2005 Sep 19.

[18] Girard M. Hepatitis B universal vaccination: learning from the French experience. Red Flags 2005. Available online at http://www.redflagsdaily .com /articles/2005_aug10.html.
[19] Sadovnick AD, Scheifele DW. School-based hepatitis B vaccination programme and adolescent multiple sclerosis [letter]. Lancet 2000 Feb 12;355(9203):549–50.

Figure 1. Data of Health Insurance System, France

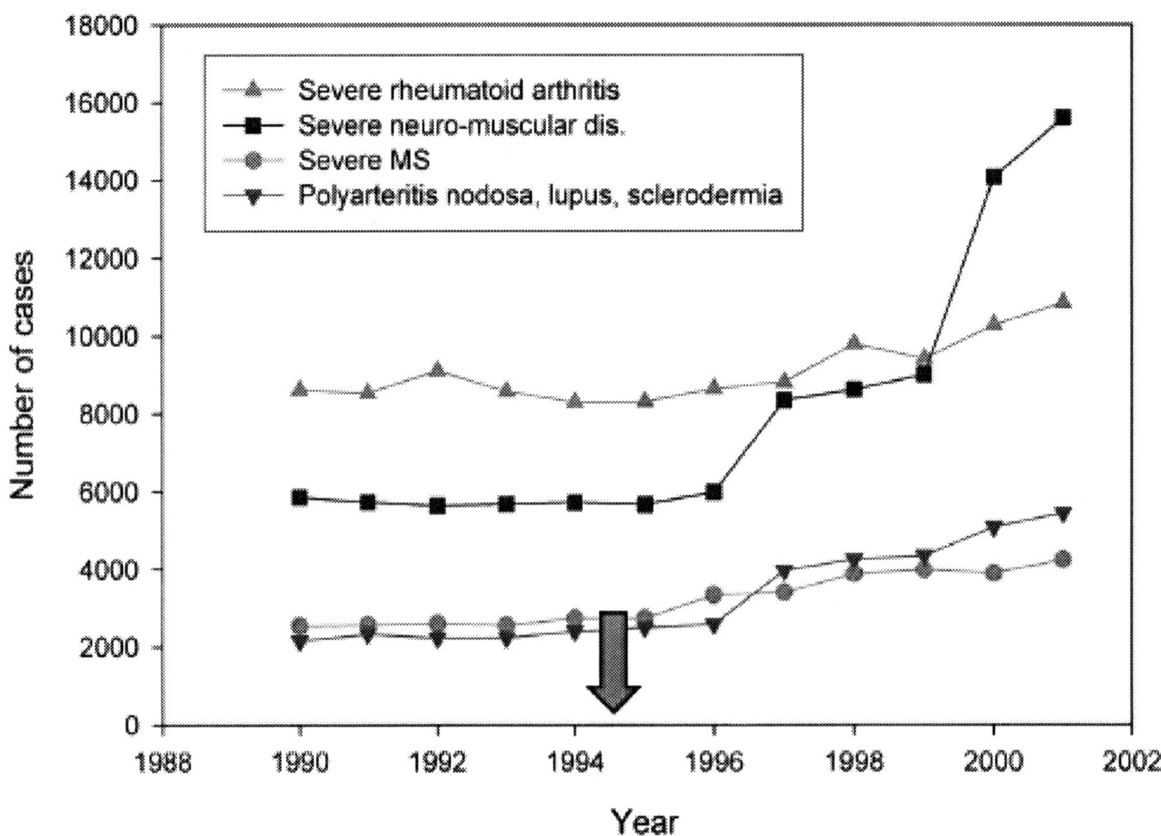

Figure 2. Multiple Sclerosis and Number of Vaccine Units Sold, 1982-2000, France

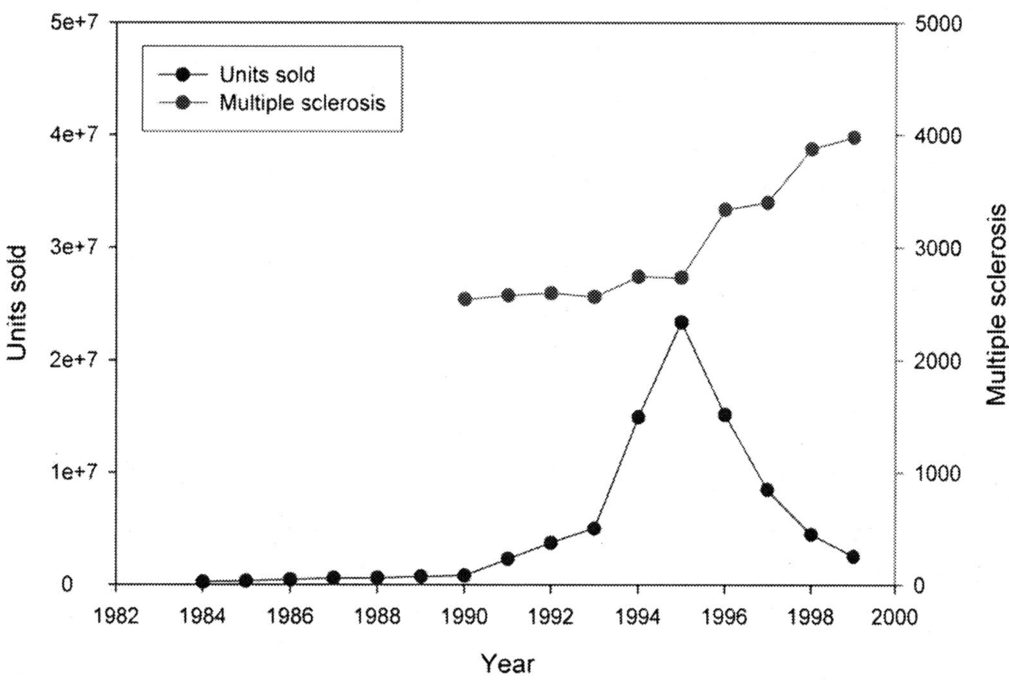

Figure 3. Data from Health Insurance System, France

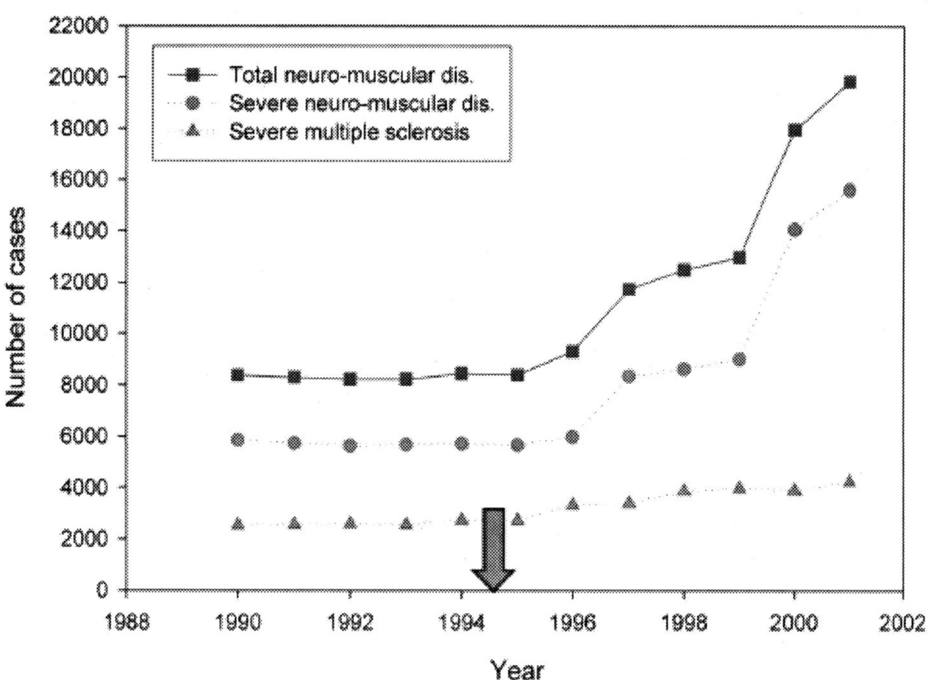

Figure 4.

Page 1 of corrected proof Letter to the editor of *Vaccine* available as "Article in Press" subsequently cancelled

Letter to the editor

Sir,

According to a recent editorial [1], the revelation of a potential conflict of interest for one of the researchers who claimed that there might be a link between MMR vaccination and autism [2] was "a dramatic twist".

In February 2000, in the context of the debate on hepatitis B vaccination, the French Agency sharply criticized an epidemiological study for its inconsistencies over time, and concluded that it should be "discarded": in spite of this, this investigation is now included in any expert review on this subject as a paper by Zipp et al. [3], without any methodological criticism or mention of any link with manufacturers. Likewise, when Scrip reported the conclusions the *Viral Hepatitis Prevention Board* as the WHO's voice, it seemed self-evident that in spite of being created and sponsored by industry, this board was "independent" [4]: it would have been sufficient to check on MEDLINE whether some of its members had any other qualification than being manufacturers employees for being included in the group of "experts", for not to speak about WHO's overestimation of hepatitis B risks in order to facilitate the inclusion of the vaccination in national programs [5].

While a study by Jick et al. showing no increase in autism after MMR vaccination was given media coverage (BMJ 2004;328:364), we are still awaiting the complete publication of a study co-authored by the same epidemiologist which suggests a sharp increase in neurological hazards of vaccination against hepatitis B [6], confirming an impressive body of surprisingly neglected evidence. Different authors sent me various noticeable contributions concerning this vaccination (e.g., on its benefit/risk ration in low endemic countries, or on an observed cross-relation between hepatitis B components and auto-antibodies produced by a patient suffering from a post-vaccinal neurolupus) the publication of which was systematically rejected in reference to the sacred requirements of "scientific rigour", whereas investigations showing no vaccine risk are regularly published in the greatest journals, in spite of their blatant biases [7] or gross methodological deficiencies [8]. Everybody knows that selective quotation or publication of favourable results by manufacturers is one of the most tricky means of distorting evidence; but if (perhaps subconsciously) editors develop the same kind of selective requirements to accept or reject manuscripts, the consequences will be even worse since one part of available evidence will be labeled "of poor quality" by neutral authorities: yet, my experience and that of an increasing number of colleagues suggest that for the time being and everything being otherwise equal, it is more difficult to publish results or reviews suggesting vaccine toxicity as compared to those refuting the hazards or exemplifying benefits.

When, based upon Vaccine Adverse Even Reporting System (VAERS) data, Geier and Geier published a paper showing significant hazards with MMR vaccination [9], their conclusions were discarded by A. Breckenridge on the basis of the allegedly well-known shortcomings of VAERS data [10], whereas Zhou et al. [11] are still undisputed for claiming that VAERS is a useful surveillance system when in confirms the overall safety of vaccines. The same holds true when VAERS is used to deny any risk of sudden infant death, whereas case/control studies of correct methodology are still lacking on this crucial topic.

When the promoters of a universal campaign of vaccination against hepatitis B organized an "international consensus conference" in Paris (10-11 September 2003), P. Van Damme—amongst most others—was presented to the public as a WHO's collaborator working in Antverp University, without any word of his links with the vaccine manufacturers as reflected by contemporary papers [12]. Co-author of an abovementioned biased study [7] favouring the vaccination and well-known promoter of hepatitis B vaccination, R. Chen was invited to discuss and criticize the (not yet fully published!) study from the Boston Group, whereas none of the researchers having documented either the toxicity of the vaccine or its problematic benefit in low-endemic countries was even informed of this "consensus" meeting.

Whereas the claimed purpose of vaccination is to produce beneficial immunity on the long run, it is scientifically correct to accept that most vaccines are devoid of long-term hazards (e.g., in terms of auto-immunity) since in most cases the mean…

Appendix XIII. About the Researcher

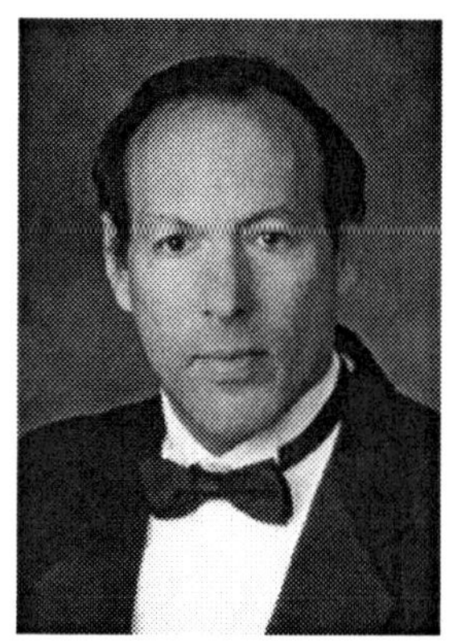

Gary S. Goldman holds a Ph.D. in Computer Science from Pacific Western University in Los Angeles and graduated with honors in 1977 from California State University, Fullerton (CSUF) with a double major: B.S. Engineering and B.S. Computer Science. He was elected member of the Phi-Kappa-Phi honor society and in 1976 received the Outstanding University Engineering Student Award, presented by the Orange County Engineering Education Council (OCEC). At graduation he received a special Merit Award in recognition of scholarly commitment and outstanding Academic Achievement in Computer Science, presented by CSUF.

Gary S. Goldman also received a special Merit Award in recognition of an attitude of enthusiasm and for outstanding service to the Division of Engineering at CSUF presented by Dr. Eugene Hunt, Chairman. At CSUF, Goldman was employed as a computer consultant assisting faculty/staff and students with computer applications. He later served as a part-time assistant professor for the Engineering and Quantitative Methods departments instructing both graduate and undergraduate courses in statistics, programming, digital simulation, and digital logic design and switching theory.

In 1980, as vice-president of Systems Development of Cascade Graphics Development, he developed the first microcomputer-based computer-aided drafting (CAD) system (prior to the well known *AutoCad* product). Dr. Gilbert McCann, then professor emeritus of CalTech, served on the board of directors of this company. Goldman engaged in computer consulting tours to South Africa, Germany, Holland, England and Canada. Goldman holds a U.S. patent (#4223255, granted September, 1980) for a micro-programmed, high-efficiency motor-in-a-wheel called "Power Wheel," for use in electric vehicular applications. This invention was featured on the front cover of the Fall, 1980 issue of *Science and Mechanics*.

After operating one year independently, Cascade Graphics Development was acquired by an international petrochemical company. In the early 1980's, Dr. Goldman assisted with the integration of the graphics system and voice input technology. This product, unique for its time, permitted disabled persons to be productive and generate high quality drawings. He recalls hiring a quadriplegic who accomplished fulfilling and productive work on this system. Dr. Goldman automated the design of vertical cylindrical heaters, including programs that first designed, then produced the configuration of convection coils as well as performing the necessary tube-wall thickness calculations for the piping. Dr. Goldman wrote a heuristic program that designed earth retaining walls with and without traffic loads and provided the complete materials list and drawing for the project. Goldman's program could produce a 100-foot long wall along any given terrain in five minutes—a task that previously took several engineers an entire week to accomplish. He also developed a specialized curve fitting routine, used by pilot Burt Rutan, suitable for aircraft wing design.

He co-developed the Goldman/Blake remediation program for children who suffer specific visual process deficits; this program was used in a pilot study at the Hope-Haven Hospital in Florida. In 1976, he served on a development team that produced the first Interactive Graphics Terminal, IGT-100, at

CalComp (California Computer Products, Anaheim, CA) writing software and systems level routines that permitted the editing of drawings prior to their being electronically plotted.

For 30 plus years, Goldman has served as a computer consultant responsible for the automation of a wide variety of businesses, improved production, and conversion of databases. He has authored and presented numerous manuscripts contributing to engineering and computer science disciplines and enjoys writing heuristic programs (developing algorithms based on ones knowledge and intuition concerning a problem).

Dr. Goldman served for eight years (from January, 1995 until his resignation in October of 2002) as Research Analyst for the Varicella Active Surveillance Project in Antelope Valley, in a cooperative project with the Centers for Disease Control and Prevention (CDC, Atlanta, GA).

Presently, Dr. Goldman serves as a consulting computer scientist and is on the board of directors of *Pearblossom Private School, Inc.* which provides distance education to over 5,000 independent study students each year in grades K through 12 throughout the United States (see www.PearblossomSchool .com)

Since 2004 he has served as Editor-in-Chief of the peer-reviewed journal, *Medical Veritas: The Journal of Medical Truth* (see www.MedicalVeritas.com). Through this endeavor Dr. Goldman has had the privilege of interfacing with world-renowned scientists, researchers, and physicians, some of which include Dr. Bonnie S. Dunbar, cell-biologist; Dr. Yash Paul, consulting physician; Dr. M. A. Al-Bayati, toxicologist; Dr. Paul G. King, chemist; Dr. Boyd E. Haley, chemist; Dr. Mark R. Geier, geneticist; Dr. Andrew J. Wakefield, gastroenterologist, etc. Dr. Goldman has studied adverse reactions caused by the Hepatitis B vaccine, MMR vaccine, anthrax vaccine, deleterious effects of instant or early cord clamping (ICC/ECC) and various birthing positions, vaccine induced autoimmune problems, shaken baby syndrome (SBS), hyperbaric oxygen therapy (HBOT), Thimerosal-containing vaccines, autism, and other medical topics.

His biography is included in Marquis' 8th Edition 2005-2006 Who's Who in Science and Engineering and 23rd Edition (2006) of Who's Who in the World. Dr. Goldman has also created a medical research search facility at www.Pubmednci.com.

In 2006, Dr. Goldman was interviewed as a guest speaker on *Radio Liberty* by host Dr. Stanley Monteith regarding varicella vaccination. He has also addressed the Zostavax® vaccination on *AutismOne Radio.* Articles regarding his research have appeared in *Mothering Magazine* ("Trading Chickenpox for Shingles?" in Nov./Dec. 2005 issue, page 33), and in *Nexus: Colorado's Holistic Journal* (Sept./Oct. issue Letter to the Editor).

Recent Publications, Abstracts, etc.

[1] The impact of vaccination on varicella incidence, conditional on school attendance and temperature, in Antelope Valley, CA. Goldman GS, Glasser JW, Maupin TJ, Peterson CL, Mascola L, Chen RT, and Seward, JF. Presentation by J.W. Glasser at 16th International Conference on Pharmacoepidemiology (ICPE); Barcelona, Spain; August 22, 2000; Pharmacoepidemiology and Drug Safety; 9(Suppl 1):S67.

[2] Varicella active surveillance: use of capture-recapture methods to assess completion of surveillance data. Peterson CL, Maupin T, Goldman G, Mascola L. 37th Interscience Conference on Antimicrobial Agents and Chemotherapy. September 28 - October 1, 1997, Toronto, Canada; Abstract H-111, page 233.

[3] Decline in varicella incidence and hospitalizations in sentinel surveillance areas in the United States, 1995-2000. Seward J,

Watson B, Peterson C, Mascola L, Pelosi J, Zhang J, Jumaan A, Maupin T, Goldman G, Perella D, Waites C, Tabony L, Wharton M. The 4th International Conference on VZV, March 3-5, 2001, Oral Presentation, La Jolla, California. VZV Research Foundation in partnership with Columbia University College of Physicians and Surgeons.

[4] Breakthrough varicella cases since vaccine licensure in the Varicella Active Surveillance Project. April 2001 Supplement of Pediatric Research, Presented April 28-May 1, 2001 Pediatric Academic Societies Meeting, Baltimore, Maryland. Galil K[1], Watson B[2], Peterson C[3], Mascola L[3], Pelosi J[4], Seward J[1], Zhang J[5], Maupin T[3], Goldman G[3], Perella D[2], Waites C[4], Tabony L[4], Wharton M[1]. Centers for Disease Control and Prevention, Atlanta[1], GA; Philadelphia Department of Public Health, Philadelphia, PA[2]; Los Angeles County Department of Health, Los Angeles, CA[3]; Texas Department of Health, Austin, TX[4]; Dyntel Corporation, Atlanta, GA[5]. Publication no. 843.

[5] Knowledge, attitudes, and practices of healthcare providers regarding varicella vaccination in sentinel surveillance area, 1996, 1997, and 1999. Maupin T, Goldman G, Peterson C, Mascola L, Seward J. Poster Session, April 28-May 1 2001, Pediatric Academic Society Annual Meeting, Baltimore, Maryland.

[6] Varicella Eepidemiology: six years of active surveillance data following implementation of the varicella vaccination program. Peterson C, Mascola L, Maupin T, Goldman G, Seward J, Presented at the 39th Annual Meeting of the Infectious Diseases Society of America (IDSA), Abstract 943, October 25-28, 2001; San Francisco, California.

[7] Varicella disease after introduction of varicella vaccine in the United States, 1995-2000. Seward JF, Watson BM, Peterson CL, Mascola L, Pelosi JW, Xhang JX, Maupin TJ, Goldman GS, Tabony LJ, Brodovicz KG, Jumaan AO, Wharton M. JAMA 2002; 287(5):606-611.

[8] Second varicella infections: are they more common than previously thought? Hall S, Maupin T, Seward J, Jumaan AO, Peterson C, Goldman G, Mascola L, Wharton M. Pediatrics. 2002 Jun;109(6):1068-73.

[9] Varicella susceptibility among adolescents in an active surveillance site. Maupin T, Goldman G, Peterson C, Mascola L, Seward J, Jumaan A, 36th National Immunization Conference of the CDC, May 1, 2002, Denver, Colorado.

[10] Varicella susceptibility and incidence of herpes-zoster among children and adolescents in a community under active surveillance. Goldman G. *Vaccine,* 2003 Oct. 1; 21(27-30):4238-42.

[11] Incidence of herpes-zoster among children and adolescents in a community with moderate varicella vaccination coverage. Goldman G. *Vaccine,* 2003 Oct. 1; 21(27-30):4243-49.

[12] Using capture-recapture methods to assess varicella incidence in a community under active surveillance. Goldman G. *Vaccine*, 2003 Oct 1; 21(27-30):4250–55.

[13] Cost-benefit analysis of universal varicella vaccination in the U.S. taking into account the closely related herpes-zoster epidemiology. Goldman G. *Vaccine*, 2005 May; 23(25):3349–55.

[14] An investigation of the association between MMR vaccination and autism in Denmark. Goldman G, Yazbak EF, *Journal of Association of American Physicians and Surgeons*, Fall 2004; 9(3):70–5.

[15] Response to Letter to Editor by Jumaan: Goldman's role in the Varicella Active Surveillance Project. Goldman GS. *Vaccine*, 2004 Sep 3; 22(25-26):3232–6.

[16] Annual Summary, 1995, 1996, 1997, 1998, 1999, 2000, 2001, Antelope Valley Varicella Active Surveillance Project, Los Angeles County Department of Health Services (LACDHS); Centers for Disease Control and Prevention (CDC) Cooperative Agreement No. U66/CCU911165-10; Maupin T, Goldman G, Peterson C, Mascola L.

[17] Universal varicella vaccination: Efficacy trends and effect on herpes-zoster. Goldman GS. *International Journal of Toxicology*, 2005 July-Aug.;24(4):205–13.

[18] The Case against Universal Varicella Vaccination. [Commentary] Goldman GS. *International Journal of Toxicology*, 2006 Sept.-Oct.; 25(5):313–17.

Appendix XIV. Reporting to the Vaccine Adverse Event Reporting System (VAERS)

If you or your child experiences an adverse vaccine reaction, it should be reported to the Vaccine Adverse Event Reporting System (VAERS), whose website is located at www.vaers.org

The Vaccine Adverse Event Reporting System is a national vaccine safety surveillance program co-sponsored by the Centers for Disease Control and Prevention (CDC) and the Food and Drug Administration (FDA). While only a small proportion of adverse reactions are generally reported to VAERS, this nevertheless helps to identify safety concerns associated with vaccines.

In particular, if you or your child experiences an adverse vaccine reaction to the *varicella vaccine*, especially a reactivation of shingles or other condition, Dr. Gary S. Goldman would appreciate hearing from you via e-mail: pearblossominc@aol.com

A physician should file the VAERS report, however anyone is permitted to file one. Vaccine recipients or their parents or guardians are encouraged to seek the help of their health care professionals and, where appropriate, legal counsel in filling out the VAERS form.

....Adverse Event reports should also be filed when you or your child receives the wrong vaccine, is administered vaccines that are not meant to be administered at the same time, is administered when you or your child is ill, or is administered without obtaining your written informed consent.

Reporting an adverse event to VAERS is not the same as filing an injury compensation claim; this kind of claim is discussed next.

Appendix XV. Filing for Vaccine Injury Compensation

If you or your child has experienced an injury that you believe may have been caused by a vaccine, please contact Dr. Gary Goldman via e-mail, at pearblossominc@aol.com and start a claim for compensation by filing a petition with the Vaccine Injury Compensation Program (VICP). The website for VICP is www.hrsa.gov/osp /vicp

Vaccines currently covered under the VICP are: diphtheria, tetanus, pertussis, (DTP, DTaP, DT, TT, or Td), measles, mumps, rubella (MMR or any components), polio (OPV or IPV), hepatitis B, Haemophilus influenzae type b, varicella (chicken pox), rotavirus and pneumococcal conjugate, whether administered individually or in combination.

Vaccine-Related Injury Compensation

- Reasonable compensation for past and future non-reimbursable medical, custodial care, and rehabilitation costs.
- $250,000 cap for actual and projected pain and suffering, emotional distress.
- Lost earnings.
- Reasonable attorneys' fees and costs.
- Deadline for filing: Within 36 months after appearance of first symptoms.

Compensation for Vaccine-Related Death

- $250,000 for the estate of the deceased.
- Reasonable attorneys' fees and costs.
- Deadline for filing: Within 24 months of death and within 48 months after the onset of the vaccine-related injury from which the death occurred.

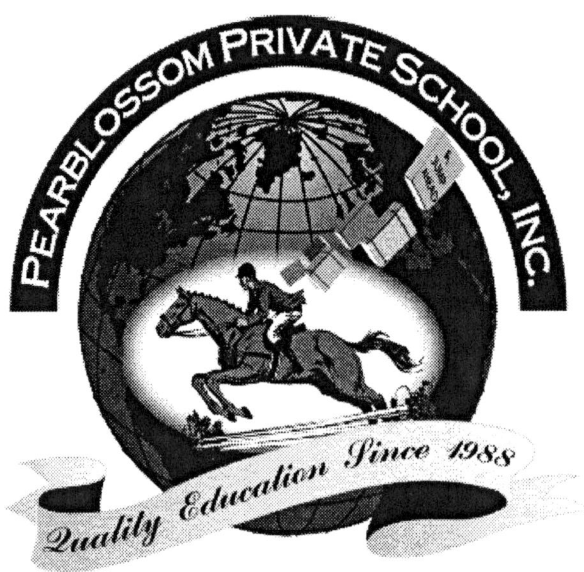

Pearblossom Private School, Inc. has provided quality educational programs to thousands of students throughout the United States since 1989. Its state-of-the-art "Same-Day E-Mail Grading," developed and implemented by the director in 1998, continues to provide fast turnaround times and accurate grading of student tests. We have automated our shipping department, reduced the time to prepare official transcripts and report cards, developed student identification cards, and instituted many other changes and innovations in an effort to provide fast and efficient service.

Teacher of the year candidate answers questions from toll-free hotline ...

Through word of mouth referrals, Pearblossom Private School, Inc. currently processes some 4,500 student enrollments each year, from virtually every state. Since we operate year round, enrollments are accepted on a continuous basis throughout the year. The helpful staff and quality curriculum further distinguish Pearblossom Private School, Inc. from other would-be competitors. Additionally parents and/or students can call our toll-free hotline to receive concise, easy-to-follow strategies for solving occasional questions that may arise during the course of studying materials or taking tests. Finally our informative newsletters add to a most satisfying educational experience.

User-friendly software allows the student to send answers to completed tests via E-mail.

High School Program (Grades 9 through 12)

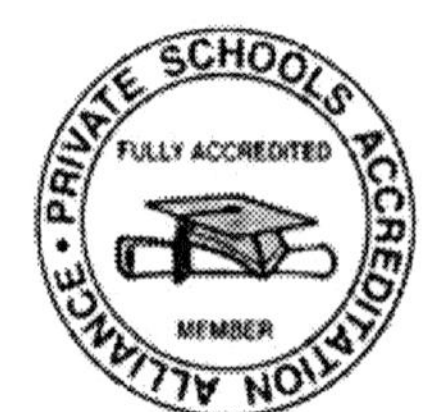

Our high school students are provided with the most comprehensive textbooks available. A high school diploma is issued to those students who satisfactorily complete the requirements. Students who have computers are provided with Windows software that has master end-of-chapter tests for both core subjects and electives. User friendly software allows the student to send the answers to completed tests via e-mail. These tests are graded and returned the same day they are received by *Pearblossom Private School, Inc.* Grading includes a list of the missed questions and the percentage correct on each submitted chapter test as well as a progress report that details the scores for each test taken to date in the given subject.

Students may improve their test scores by correcting any missed questions, but may only resubmit a test one time after the initial grading. Those students who do not possess home computers can take the hard copy version of the standardized tests and simply send their answers to us for manual grading.

Middle School Program (Grades 7 & 8)

This program consists of six outstanding textbooks in the following subject areas: (1) grammar and composition, (2) literature, (3) history, (4) science, (5) health and (6) mathematics.

The middle school program is combined into a single combination 7th/8th grade, since 8th grade is practically a complete review of material previously presented in 6th and 7th grades. Tests for each subject are graded by Pearblossom Private School, Inc. and are available in standard hard copy format or computer format for Same-Day Grading. A consumable Grammar Workbook is also included in the program and serves as a mini-course in grammar, usage, and mechanics. Earth or Life Science can be specified to adapt the program to the student's interests. General mathematics or Pre-algebra are options available depending on the student's math skills.

Elementary Program (Grades K through 6)

Each student is provided with the following consumable work-books: (1) spelling book, (2) mathematics book, (3) phonics, (4) writing, (5) language arts, (6) reading, (7) Super Workbook.

Please note, however, that both the subjects of the individual elementary books and the quantity of consumable workbooks provided in addition to the Super Workbook are subject to change and availability.

Depending on the grade level, the 600-800-page Super Workbook contains a well-planned course of study organized to teach the basic academic curriculum. The Kindergarten program is appropriate for preschool children aged 3 1/2 years and older and includes a book that teaches children to read in "100 easy lessons." No flash cards, lesson plans, additional books, or machines are necessary. The parent who completes this program will know more about teaching reading than most public school teachers, because the parent will have carefully observed and participated in the step by step development of his/her child's reading skills. Our elementary school students are issued grades based on their performance on lessons in a Super Workbook. Those parents that have computers are provided easy-to-use software that maintains student grades and computes overall averages in all subjects.

The "Hot Line" Advantage Examples of topics that have been explained to students include balancing chemical or nuclear reaction equations, computing probabilities, trigonometry and its application to real life, solving simultaneous equations in two or more unknowns, graphing inequalities, matrix operations, and many more.

Informative Newsletter

Our bimonthly newsletter contains interesting material for parents and students alike, including discussions of various home schooling topics, lessons in mathematics, pre algebra, or algebra, thinking challenges, information on newly available electives, highlights concerning student projects and achievements, and much more.

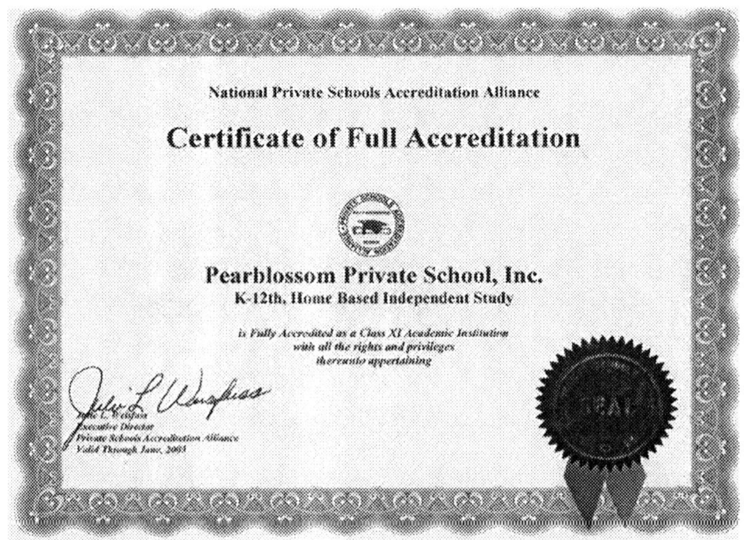

National Private Schools Accreditation Alliance

Certificate of Full Accreditation

Pearblossom Private School, Inc.
K-12th, Home Based Independent Study

is Fully Accredited as a Class XI Academic Institution
with all the rights and privileges
thereunto appertaining

Executive Director
Private Schools Accreditation Alliance
Valid Through June, 2003

We are members of the Better Business Bureau, no. 9-13011559, and our program is fully and nationally accredited by the National Private School Association Group (toll-free telephone number, 1-800-840-0939). Pearblossom Private School, Inc. is listed in the California Private School Directory, identification no. 19-64246-7069792. (Accreditation granted by any group does not guarantee credit transferability. Please check specific policies of acceptance at the receiving organization or institution. Also check the home schooling requirements of your local school district superintendent prior to enrolling.)

Toll-Fee Phone: 1-800-309-3569 between 9:00 am and 3:00 pm Pacific Standard Time
Outside the United States: Phone: 1-661-944-0914
For more information and to enroll online see www.PearblossomSchool.com

Printed in the United States
69858LV00005B/68

9 780978 838300